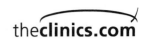

EMERGENCY MEDICINE CLINICS OF NORTH AMERICA

Ophthalmologic Emergencies

GUEST EDITORS
Joseph H. Kahn, MD and
Brendan Magauran, MD

CONSULTING EDITOR
Amal Mattu, MD

February 2008 • Volume 26 • Number 1

SAUNDERS

An Imprint of Elsevier, Inc.
PHILADELPHIA   LONDON   TORONTO   MONTREAL   SYDNEY   TOKYO

W.B. SAUNDERS COMPANY
A Division of Elsevier Inc.

1600 John F. Kennedy Boulevard, Suite 1800 • Philadelphia, Pennsylvania 19103-2899

http://www.theclinics.com

EMERGENCY MEDICINE CLINICS　　　　　　　　　**Volume 26, Number 1**
OF NORTH AMERICA　　　　　　　　　　　　　　　**ISSN 0733-8627**
February 2008　　　　　　　　　　　　**ISBN-13: 978-1-4160-5852-6**
Editor: Patrick Manley　　　　　　　　　　　**ISBN-10: 1-4160-5852-4**

The ideas and opinions expressed in *Emergency Medicine Clinics of North America* do not necessarily reflect those of the Publisher. The Publisher does not assume any responsibility for any injury and/or damage to persons or property arising out of or related to any use of the material contained in this periodical. The reader is advised to check the appropriate medical literature and the product information currently provided by the manufacturer of each drug to be administered to verify the dosage, the method and duration of administration, or contraindications. It is the responsibility of the treating physician or other health care professional, relying on independent experience and knowledge of the patient, to determine drug dosages and the best treatment for the patient. Mention of any product in this issue should not be construed as endorsement by the contributors, editors, or the Publisher of the product or manufacturers' claims.

Emergency Medicine Clinics of North America (ISSN 0733-8627) is published quarterly by Elsevier Inc., 360 Park Avenue South, New York, NY, 10010-1710. Months of issue are February, May, August, and November. Business and Editorial Offices: 1600 John F. Kennedy Boulevard, Suite 1800, Philadelphia, PA 19103-2899. Customer Service Office: 6277 Sea Harbor Drive, Orlando, FL 32887-4800. Periodicals postage paid at New York, NY, and additional mailing offices. Subscription prices are $109.00 per year (US students), $212.00 per year (US individuals), $339.00 per year (US institutions), $145.00 per year (international students), $285.00 per year (international individuals), $400.00 per year (international institutions), $145.00 per year (Canadian students), $261.00 per year (Canadian individuals), and $400.00 per year (Canadian institutions). International air speed delivery is included in all *Clinics'* subscription prices. All prices are subject to change without notice. POSTMASTER: Send address changes to *Emergency Medicine Clinics of North America*, Elsevier Periodicals Customer Service, 6277 Sea Harbor Drive, Orlando, FL 32887-4800. Customer Service: 1-800-654-2452 (US). From outside the United States, call 1-407-563-6020. Fax: 1-407-363-9661. E-mail: JournalsCustomerService-usa@elsevier.com.

Emergency Medicine Clinics of North America is covered in *Index Medicus, Current Contents/Clinical Medicine, EMBASE/Excerpta Medica, BIOSIS, SciSearch, CINAHL, ISI/BIOMED,* and *Research Alert.*

Printed in the United States of America.

CONSULTING EDITOR

AMAL MATTU, MD, Program Director, Emergency Medicine Residency; and Associate Professor, Department of Emergency Medicine, University of Maryland School of Medicine, Baltimore, Maryland

GUEST EDITORS

JOSEPH H. KAHN, MD, FACEP, Associate Professor of Emergency Medicine, Boston University School of Medicine; Director of Medical Student Education, Department of Emergency Medicine, Boston Medical Center, Boston, Massachusetts

BRENDAN MAGAURAN, MD, MBA, Assistant Professor of Emergency Medicine, Boston University School of Medicine;, Medical Director, Department of Emergency Medicine, Boston Medical Center, Boston, Massachusetts

CONTRIBUTORS

MATTHEW R. BABINEAU, MD, Department of Emergency Medicine, Beth Israel Deaconess Medical Center, Boston, Massachusetts

SHARON P. BORD, MD, Resident, Department of Emergency Medicine, Boston University Medical Center, Boston, Massachusetts

JAMES M. DARGIN, MD, Chief Resident, Department of Emergency Medicine, Boston University School of Medicine, Boston Medical Center, Boston, Massachusetts

DAVID H. DORFMAN, MD, Associate Professor of Pediatrics, Boston University School of Medicine; and Director of Fellowship Pediatric Emergency Medicine, Boston Medical Center, Boston, Massachusetts

DAVID K. DUONG, MD, MS, Emergency Medicine Residency, Boston Medical Center, Boston, Massachusetts

WILLIAM G. FERNANDEZ, MD, MPH, Boston Medical Center, Department of Emergency Medicine, Boston University School of Medicine, Boston, Massachusetts

JOSEPH H. KAHN, MD, FACEP, Associate Professor of Emergency Medicine, Boston University School of Medicine; Director of Medical Student Education, Department of Emergency Medicine, Boston Medical Center, Boston, Massachusetts

JEAN E. KLIG, MD, FAAP, Assistant Professor, Division of Pediatric Emergency Medicine, Boston University School of Medicine, Boston Medical Center, Boston, Massachusetts

MEGAN M. LEO, MD, Emergency Medicine Residency, Boston Medical Center, Boston, Massachusetts

JUDITH LINDEN, MD, Associate Residency Director, Department of Emergency Medicine, Boston University Medical Center, Boston, Massachusetts

ROBERT A. LOWENSTEIN, MD, Associate Director, Department of Emergency Medicine, Quincy Medical Center, Quincy; Assistant Professor, Department of Emergency Medicine, Boston University School of Medicine, Boston Medical Center, Boston, Massachusetts

BRENDAN MAGAURAN, MD, MBA, Assistant Professor of Emergency Medicine, Boston University School of Medicine; Medical Director, Department of Emergency Medicine, Boston Medical Center, Boston, Massachusetts

AHMED R. MAHMOOD, MD, Resident Physician, Department of Emergency Medicine, Boston Medical Center, Boston, Massachusetts

CHRISTOPHER M. McSTAY, MD, Assistant Professor of Emergency Medicine, Department of Emergency Medicine, New York University/Bellevue Hospital Center, New York, New York

ELIZABETH L. MITCHELL, MD, Assistant Professor of Emergency Medicine, Department of Emergency Medicine, Boston University School of Medicine, Boston Medical Center, Boston, Massachusetts

JORMA B. MUELLER, MD, Emergency Medicine Residency, New York University/ Bellevue Hospital Center, New York, New York

ANEESH T. NARANG, MD, Clinical Instructor, Department of Emergency Medicine, Boston Medical Center, Boston, Massachusetts

KIMBALL A. PRENTISS, MD, Clinical Instructor in Pediatrics, Boston University School of Medicine; and Fellow in Pediatric Emergency Medicine, Boston Medical Center, Boston, Massachusetts

DEREK A. ROBINETT, MD, Instructor of Emergency Medicine, Boston University School of Medicine; Attending Physician, Department of Emergency Medicine, Boston Medical Center, Boston, Massachusetts

LEON D. SANCHEZ, MD, MPH, Department of Emergency Medicine, Beth Israel Deaconess Medical Center, Boston, Massachusetts

JEFFREY I. SCHNEIDER, MD, Assistant Professor, Boston University School of Medicine; and Department of Emergency Medicine, Boston Medical Center, Boston, Massachusetts

JORDAN SPECTOR, MD, Boston Medical Center, Department of Emergency Medicine, Boston University School of Medicine, Boston, Massachusetts; Department of Emergency Medicine, Albert Einstein Medical Center, Philadelphia, Pennsylvania

MICHAEL VORTMANN, MD, Resident Physician, Department of Emergency Medicine, Boston University School of Medicine, Boston Medical Center, Boston, Massachusetts

CONTENTS

This article is a review of the anatomy of the eye and its surrounding tissues. A working knowledge of the functional anatomy of the eye will aid the emergency physician in performing a thorough yet efficient physical examination of the eye. A goal-directed physical examination of the eye will allow the emergency physician to attempt to identify (or exclude) visionthreatening disease processes and facilitate communication with the ophthalmologist.

Ophthalmologic emergencies account for up to 3% of visits to emergency departments in the United States. Although isolated ocular complaints are rarely life-threatening, they can lead to significant short- and long-term morbidity, including permanent visual loss. The role of the emergency physician in management of ocular emergencies is similar to that for other chief complaints: to recognize and diagnose emergency conditions, to provide appropriate initial therapy, and to ensure correct disposition. This article reviews several of the essential ophthalmologic procedures that are within the scope of emergency medical practice. Slit lamp examination, foreign body removal, use of ultrasound, tonometry, and other emergency ophthalmologic procedures are discussed.

The red eye is one of the most frequent presenting complaints in the emergency department setting. A wide spectrum of disease processes may present as a red eye, ranging from benign self-limiting etiologies to serious vision-threatening ones. The emergency physician must be adept at recognizing "red flags" from the history and physical examination that necessitate immediate treatment and referral. In addition, it is imperative for the emergency physician to recognize the need for immediate versus elective ophthalmologist consultation for the various conditions. This article includes a discussion of the key historical features, clinical presentations, physical examination findings, and management of the more common causes of the red eye.

Managing the inflamed or infected eye in the emergency setting presents a diagnostic and therapeutic challenge to the emergency physician; the causes and prognoses range from benign, self-limited illness to organ-threatening pathology. A careful history, with attention to comorbid illnesses and time course, is paramount, as is knowledge of the complete ophthalmologic examination. Much of the organ morbidity is ameliorated with prompt therapy in the emergency department and by initiating ophthalmologic consultation. In this article, the authors discuss the diagnosis and treatment of several types of eye infection, including conjunctivitis, episcleritis, keratitis, uveitis, hordeolum and chalazion, dacryocystitis, and cellulitis.

Acute monocular visual loss is an alarming symptom for the patient and the emergency physician. This article focuses on the presentation, diagnosis, and management of several causes of acute monocular visual loss with suggestions for when to emergently involve an ophthalmologist. Topics discussed include temporal arteritis, optic neuritis, retinal artery occlusion, retinal vein occlusion, retinal detachment, and retinal vasculitis.

Trauma to the eye represents approximately 3% of all emergency department visits in the United States. Rapid assessment and examination following trauma to the eye is crucial. A thorough knowledge of potential injuries is imperative to ensure rapid diagnosis, to prevent further damage to the eye, and to preserve visual capacity. This article describes the aspects of the eye examination that merit special attention in the case of trauma. It then discusses the eye injuries most likely to be seen in the emergency department and their appropriate treatment.

Chemical or radiant energy injuries to the eyes are considered ocular burns. The majority of these injuries are occupation-related. Chemical burns are by far more common and represent a true emergency. Thermal and UV injuries are associated with severe pain, but often result in less long-term sequelae than chemical injuries do. The term "biologic exposure" refers to an exposure to human blood or other body fluid. This article describes patterns of these injuries and exposures, with particular emphasis on emergent management and including acute diagnostic and treatment considerations.

Neuro-ophthalmologic disorders arise from all areas of the neuro-ophthalmologic tract. They may be expressed simply as loss of vision or double vision, or as complex syndromes or systemic illnesses, depending on the location and type of lesion. Problems may occur anywhere along the visual pathway, including the brainstem, cavernous sinus, subarachnoid space, and orbital apex, and may affect adjacent structures also. A firm understanding of the neuroanatomy and neurophysiology of the eye is essential to correct diagnosis.

Examining the young child who presents to the emergency department with a visual or ocular complaint can be a challenge. This article discusses basic concepts of visual and behavioral development and methods for an accurate ocular examination in young children. Topics reviewed include conjunctivitis, orbital and periorbital cellulitis, lacrimal system infections, congenital issues, misalignment, and oncology.

FORTHCOMING ISSUES

RECENT ISSUES

ELSEVIER
SAUNDERS

Emerg Med Clin N Am
26 (2008) xi

EMERGENCY
MEDICINE
CLINICS OF
NORTH AMERICA

Erratum

An Emergency Medicine Approach to Neonatal Hyperbilirubinemia

James E. Colletti, MD, FAAEM, FAAP[a],
Samip Kothori, MD[b], Danielle M. Jackson, MD[c],
Kevin P. Kilgore, MD[c], Kelly Barringer, MD[c]

[a]Department of Emergency Medicine, Mayo Clinic College of Medicine,
200 First St. SW, Rochester, MN 55905, USA
[b]Department of Pediatrics, University of Arizona, 150 N. Campbell Avenue,
Tucson, AZ 85724, USA
[c]Department of Emergency Medicine, Regions Hospital, 640 Jackson Street,
Mail Stop 11102F, St. Paul, MN 55101, USA

The above article, which appeared in the November 2007 issue ("Pediatric Emergencies in the First Year of Life"), contained a misspelling of the second author's name. The correct spelling is Samip Kothari, MD.

0733-8627/08/$ - see front matter © 2008 Elsevier Inc. All rights reserved.
doi:10.1016/j.emc.2007.12.001   *emed.theclinics.com*

ELSEVIER
SAUNDERS

Emerg Med Clin N Am
26 (2008) xiii–xiv

EMERGENCY
MEDICINE
CLINICS OF
NORTH AMERICA

Foreword

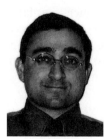

Amal Mattu, MD
Consulting Editor

Noted English writer Max Beerbohm was quoted as saying "...the eyes are the window of the soul." Beerbohm may have been discussing human nature, but the eyes are no less important in medicine. The eyes provide important information regarding a patient's neurologic status, including the cranial nerves, cortical and brainstem function, toxic and metabolic disorders, atherosclerotic disease, diabetes, connective tissue disease, thyroid disease, and a myriad of other systemic ailments in addition to intrinsic ophthalmologic disorders. Though the eyes may be important to the physician, they are even more important to the patient; none of the other four major senses (touch, taste, hearing, smell) are as important as vision. The ability for a person to function well in our society is influenced tremendously by the ability to see. Vision is so important of a sensation, in fact, that an entire specialty is devoted to the maintenance of this sensation.

Therefore, it is vital for emergency physicians to have an excellent understanding of ophthalmologic emergencies. Emergency physicians must have a sound knowledge of the anatomy and physiology of the eye, be well-versed in proper examination techniques, and be able to recognize intrinsic and extra-ocular manifestations of disease. Emergency physicians also should have proficiency in proper management of these conditions to ensure preservation of vision in high-risk conditions. Acute visual complaints often receive less attention than other perilous conditions, such as chest pain in a busy emergency department (ED), but the consequences of misdiagnosis are equally disastrous for the patient and in terms of medicolegal risk.

0733-8627/08/$ - see front matter © 2008 Elsevier Inc. All rights reserved.
doi:10.1016/j.emc.2007.12.003   *emed.theclinics.com*

In this issue of *Emergency Medicine Clinics of North America*, guest editors Drs. Kahn and Magauran have assembled an outstanding group of authors to educate us on this vital aspect of our specialty. Important articles are devoted to proper examination techniques and procedures, and subsequent articles are devoted to the myriad of ophthalmologic conditions—medical, toxic, and traumatic—that are encountered in ED patients. The articles are organized primarily in a complaint-based format, rather than a disease-based format, which simulates the real-world experience of patient presentations in the ED. Articles also are devoted to ophthalmologic manifestations of systemic disease, neuro-ophthalmologic conditions, and pediatric issues. This issue also includes an immensely practical article that focuses on conditions that require emergency ophthalmologic consultation, an article that is worth posting in every ED and urgent care center.

I congratulate the editors and authors on producing an outstanding addition to the *Clinics* series. This issue should be considered required reading not only for practicing emergency physicians, but also for emergency medicine trainees and for any other health care providers who manage patients who have acute ophthalmologic complaints in their daily practice. This issue certainly provides us all with a "window" into better patient care and decreased medicolegal risk.

Amal Mattu, MD
Program Director
Emergency Medicine Residency
and
Associate Professor
Department of Emergency Medicine
University of Maryland School of Medicine
110 S. Paca Street, 6th Floor, Suite 200
Baltimore, MD 21201, USA

E-mail address: amattu@smail.umaryland.edu

ELSEVIER
SAUNDERS

Emerg Med Clin N Am
26 (2008) xv–xvi

EMERGENCY
MEDICINE
CLINICS OF
NORTH AMERICA

Preface

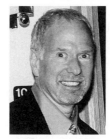 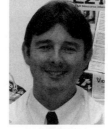

Joseph H. Kahn, MD, FACEP   Brendan Magauran, MD, MBA
Guest Editors

With more than 2 million visits annually to United States emergency departments, patients who have complaints involving the eye and its surrounding tissues are encountered frequently by the emergency physician. Eye complaints represent the full range of disease, from trivial (uncomplicated subconjunctival hemorrhage) to life-threatening (intracranial aneurysm). This issue attempts to provide a framework to approach patients who have eye complaints.

The issue begins with "Physical Exam of the Eye," which reviews the anatomy of the eye, including its innervation and blood supply and suggests how to perform a rapid, yet thorough, physical exam of the eye. There is an article entitled "Ophthalmologic Procedures" that reviews commonly performed ophthalmologic procedures, such as measurement of visual acuity, tonometry, and slit lamp evaluation, and infrequently used procedures, such as paracentesis and lateral canthotomy, with a discussion of ocular ultrasound. The subsequent articles approach the patient who has eye complaints in one of two ways: a system-based approach and a problem-based approach.

The system-based articles include "Ocular Infection and Inflammation," which discusses topics from conjunctivitis to scleritis and orbital cellulitis. The next system-based article is entitled "Trauma to the Globe and Orbit," and is a comprehensive article that covers topics ranging from corneal abrasion to hyphema, ruptured globe, and retro-orbital hemorrhage. Another system-based article is "Neuro-Ophthalmology," which presents a detailed discussion of the unique ocular findings seen in neurologic

doi:10.1016/j.emc.2007.12.002   *emed.theclinics.com*

diseases, including afferent papillary defect, Argyll Robertson pupil, and Adie's tonic pupil. The final system-based article is "Ophthalmologic Complications of Systemic Disease," which covers topics ranging from diabetes to acquired immunodeficiency syndrome.

The first of the problem-based articles is "The Red Eye," and it discusses the differential diagnosis and treatment of this very common emergency department presentation, which ranges from conjunctivitis to acute angle closure glaucoma. Another problem-based article is "Acute Visual Loss," and it discusses central retinal artery occlusion, retinal detachment, and other causes of this condition that can be alarming for the physician and the patient. The next problem-based article is "Eye Exposures," which attempts to guide the emergency physician in the management of conditions ranging from alkali exposures to biologic exposures to health care workers. The final problem-based article is entitled "The Painful Eye," which discusses topics including uveitis and optic neuritis. There is a separate article entitled "Pediatric Ophthalmology in the Emergency Department" that provides guidelines for the evaluation and management of ocular complaints in children of various age groups. The final article, entitled "Conditions Requiring Emergency Ophthalmologic Consultation," cuts through the myriad of ophthalmologic complaints that patients present with and presents those diagnoses, such as endophthalmitis and corneal ulceration, that require immediate attention by an ophthalmologist.

We thank all of the authors who so carefully researched and wrote the articles in this edition of *Emergency Medicine Clinics of North America.* We also thank our families for their support as we revised and assembled this issue. We thank Patrick Manley and the staff at Elsevier for their guidance and patience. We especially thank those of you who read this edition; we sincerely hope that you find it worthwhile.

Joseph H. Kahn, MD, FACEP
Brendan Magauran, MD, MBA
Department of Emergency Medicine
Boston Medical Center
1 Boston Medical Center Place
Boston, MA 02118, USA

E-mail addresses: jkahn@bu.edu; brendan.magauran@bmc.org

EMERGENCY
MEDICINE
CLINICS OF
NORTH AMERICA

ELSEVIER
SAUNDERS

Emerg Med Clin N Am
26 (2008) 1–16

The Physical Examination of the Eye

Derek A. Robinett, MD[a,b],
Joseph H. Kahn, MD, FACEP[a,b],*

[a]*Boston University School of Medicine, 80 East Concord Street, Boston, MA 02118, USA*
[b]*Department of Emergency Medicine, Boston Medical Center,
1 Boston Medical Center Place, Boston, MA 02118, USA*

There are more than 2 million visits annually to United States emergency departments for complaints involving the eye and its surrounding tissues [1]. Approximately one half of these visits are related to trauma to the eye and its adnexal tissues, 3% of which require admission to the hospital [1,2]. Six percent of eye injuries presenting to emergency departments annually are related to the use of drugs and/or alcohol [1]. Most of these patients are treated initially by emergency physicians, with or without ophthalmology consultation. Performing a complete, accurate, and efficient physical examination of the eye allows the emergency physician to treat most eye complaints and to communicate effectively with the ophthalmologist on call. The physical examination of the eye requires a Snelling Chart (or substitute), a light source, ophthalmoscope, slit lamp, a method for determining intraocular pressure, proparicaine ophthalmic solution, and fluorescein stain [3].

Knowledge of the anatomy of the eye is essential in emergency medicine. To properly diagnose ocular problems, one should have full knowledge of the eye, orbit, cranial nerves, musculature for the control of eye movements, and blood supply of the eye.

The orbit

The orbit is composed of four walls. The roof of the orbit is comprised of the frontal bone and the lesser wing of the sphenoid bone. The lateral wall is made of the zygomatic bone and the greater wing of the sphenoid bone. The lateral wall and roof are separated by the superior orbital fissure. The floor of the orbit is composed primarily of the maxilla. However, portions of the zygomatic and palatine bones contribute to the floor. The medial wall is formed by portions of multiple bones including the ethmoid, lacrimal,

* Corresponding author.
 E-mail address: jkahn@bu.edu (J.H. Kahn).

0733-8627/08/$ - see front matter © 2008 Elsevier Inc. All rights reserved.
doi:10.1016/j.emc.2007.11.007   *emed.theclinics.com*

sphenoid, frontal, and maxilla. The anterior portion of the orbit is narrower than the area behind the rim, which adds protection [4–7].

The orbit lies in close proximity to the paranasal sinuses (Fig. 1), allowing sinus infections to spread to the periorbital tissues (preseptal cellulitis) and into the orbit itself (orbital cellulitis) [8]. These conditions will be discussed in detail in an article by Mueller and McStay elsewhere in this issue.

The external eye

The external anatomy of the eye is made up of the eyebrows, the eyelids, and the lacrimal apparatus. The eyebrows consist of thick skin and hair with muscle fibers underneath. The eyelids function to protect the eyeball by closing. They are made of thin skin covering the orbicularis oculi muscle. This muscle closes the lids. Beneath the muscle is areolar tissue followed by a fibrous connective tissue layer called the "tarsal plate." The lids are covered on their posterior surface by mucosa called the "palpebral conjunctiva." Between the orbit and tarsal plate lies fascia that makes up the orbital septum.

The lacrimal apparatus is composed of the lacrimal gland, lacrimal sac, canaliculi, and the nasolacrimal duct. Many accessory lacrimal glands also exist. The lacrimal gland produces tears that coat the anterior portion of the eye. The tears are drained through the canaliculi to the lacrimal sac. The lacrimal sac drains into the nasal cavity via the nasolacrimal duct [5,6].

During examination of the external structures surrounding the eye, many diseases and injuries should be looked for specific to the structures being examined. Examination of the lids may reveal chalazion, hordeolum, or lid cellulitis, all of which will be discussed by Mueller and McStay in an article found elsewhere in this issue. Abnormalities of the orbicularis oculi muscle may be seen in seventh cranial nerve palsies. Lid lag (ptosis) may be seen in third cranial nerve palsies and in Horner's syndrome. These entities will be discussed by Duong, Leo, and Mitchell in an article found elsewhere in this issue. Conjunctivitis

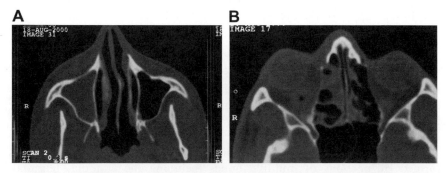

Fig. 1. (*A*) Axial cross sections of the maxillary sinus and orbit. The sinus is completely occluded with, in this case, pus. (*B*) Dorsally, of the eyeball, an expansile process with visible gas inclusions is visible. Gas-producing microorganisms are the likely source of this hypodense area. (*From* Blake FAS, Siegert J, Wedl J, et al. The acute orbit: etiology, diagnosis, and therapy. J Oral Maxillofacial Surg 2006;64:91; with permission.)

may involve the inner lining of the eyelids (palpebral conjunctiva). The palpebral conjunctiva lining the upper lid is a common site for occult ocular foreign bodies. All elements of the tear-producing and collecting system are subject to infection (dacrocystitis) or obstruction and require special attention in the setting of trauma, because lacerations to these structures may require repair by an ophthalmologist. These injuries will be discussed in an article by Bord and Linden elsewhere in this issue.

The eyeball

A review of daytime presentations to an ophthalmologic emergency department in Sydney, Australia found the following five most common diagnoses: conjunctivitis, keratitis, cataract, corneal abrasion, and iridocyclitis [9].

The conjunctiva

A thin mucous membrane covers the posterior lids and anterior sclera. This is the conjunctiva. It is continuous with the skin at the margin of the lid. In the United States, more than 500,000 patients present to the emergency department annually for inflammation of the conjunctiva [1]. Conjunctivitis will be discussed in detail in the article "Ocular Infection and Inflammation" by Mueller and McStay and "The Red Eye" by Mahmood and Narang elsewhere in this issue.

Tenon's capsule

Tenon's Capsule (also called the fascia Bulbi) is a fibrous globe that envelops the eyeball from the optic nerve to the limbus. Tubular reflections of the capsule enclose each extraocular muscle at its site of attachment and fuse with the fascia of these muscles and attach to adjacent orbital structures. These reflections limit the movement of these muscles [5,6].

The sclera and episclera

The fibrous coating of the eye is the sclera. This protective coating is made almost entirely of collagen. It is white in color and very dense. Anteriorly, it is continuous with the cornea. The episclera is a thin layer of elastic tissue that covers the anterior sclera [4,6].

Inflammation of these layers may be associated with connective tissue disorders. Scleritis is usually painful, whereas episcleritis is not. The redness associated with episcleritis blanches with instillation of phenylephrine drops, whereas the redness associated with scleritis does not. See the article by Mueller and McStay for a detailed discussion of these diseases.

The cornea

The transparent structure covering the anterior of the eye is the cornea. It is composed of five separate layers: the epithelium, Bowman's layer, the stroma, Descemet's layer, and the endothelium. The epithelium is highly prone to damage [6].

Corneal abrasions and foreign bodies comprise the majority of corneal abnormalities presenting to emergency departments. Other entities include keratitis, corneal ulcers, corneal perforation, and corneal exposures. Proparicaine to make the patient comfortable and fluorescein instillation to visualize corneal defects, in conjunction with slit lamp evaluation, are essential to evaluate the cornea. Corneal abnormalities are discussed in the articles "The Painful Eye" by Dargin and Lowenstein and "Ocular Infection and Inflammation" by Mueller and McStay in this issue.

The anterior chamber

Between the cornea and iris is the anterior chamber. The anterior chamber is filled with aqueous humor. The aqueous is formed by the ciliary body. It is drained from the anterior chamber by the trabecular meshwork. The trabecular meshwork is a series of collagen and elastic tissue with trabecular cells that form a filter. The ciliary muscle can contract and increase the size of the filter pores. This enhances the drainage of the aqueous. The aqueous is absorbed at a venous channel (the canal of Schlemm) where the iris and cornea join. This is the angle of the anterior chamber [4–7].

People with a narrow anterior chamber angle are at risk for acute angle closure glaucoma (Figs. 2 and 3). This vision-threatening, sometimes elusive diagnosis will be discussed in the article by Mahmood and Narang in this issue.

The uvea

The uvea consists of the iris and the ciliary body (anterior uvea) and the choroid (posterior uvea) [6].

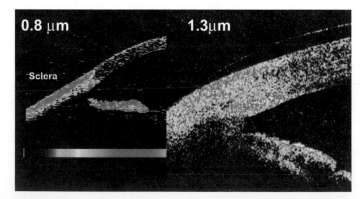

Fig. 2. Anterior-segment optical coherence tomography using 1.3-μm wavelength light provides better detail of anterior chamber angle anatomy. (*From* Radhakrishnan S, Huang D, Smith SD. Optical coherence tomography testing. Ophthalmol Clin North Am 2005;18:376; with permission.)

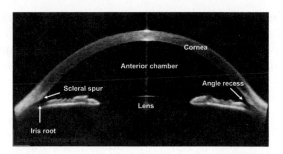

Fig. 3. Anterior segment optical coherence tomography image shows anterior chamber angle anatomy. (*From* Radhakrishnan S, Huang D, Smith SD. Optical coherence tomography testing. Ophthalmol Clin North Am 2005;18:376; with permission.)

The iris

The amount of light entering the eye is controlled by the iris. It is an extension of the ciliary body. It is a flat surface with a central, round opening (the pupil). The posterior surface of the iris is heavily pigmented. The stroma of the iris contains the sphincter and dilator muscles. The size of the pupil is controlled by parasympathetic innervation (contraction) and sympathetic innervation (dilation) [4–7].

The iris is the site of abnormalities of both traumatic and atraumatic etiologies. Iritis (anterior uveitis) may be infectious, rheumatologic, or idiopathic. Trauma may cause traumatic iritis, traumatic midriasis, or tears of the iris. Anterior uveitis will be discussed in the articles entitled "The Red Eye" by Mahmood and Narang and "The Painful Eye" by Dargin and Lowenstein in this issue.

The ciliary body

The ciliary body is composed of a series of veins and capillaries. The epithelium covering this body produces the aqueous. The ciliary muscle is made up of a series of muscle fibers arranged in a longitudinal, circular, and radial direction. These fibers can contract to change the shape of the lens and provide for different focal lengths [6].

The choroid

The choroid lies between the retina and sclera. It is comprised of a series of blood vessels that provide flow to the outer portion of the retina. There are three layers of these blood vessels [6].

Posterior uveitis, or choroiditis, is a vision-threatening emergency requiring urgent treatment. It is discussed in detail in the article by Mueller and McStay elsewher in this issue.

The lens

The lens is approximately 4 mm thick and 9 mm in length. It is convex, colorless, and transparent. It is held behind the iris by the zonule. The zonule connects to the ciliary body. As one ages, the lens becomes larger and less flexible. The lens contains no nerves or blood vessels [6].

The lens may be dislocated in the setting of trauma. Also, trauma may cause cataract formation. See the article by Bord and Linden elsewhere in this issue.

The retina

The specialized neural tissue lining the posterior, inner part of the globe is the retina. It is semitransparent and multilayered. It is composed of ten layers containing nervous tissue, pigmented epithelial cells, and photoreceptors. The retina is easily detached from its epithelium, except at the optic disk [4–6].

Retinal detachment, a vision-threatening ophthalmologic surgical emergency, can be recognized by historical features (visual loss, floaters, flashing lights) and on physical examination (elevated portion of retina on fundoscopic examination). This will be discussed in detail in the by Vortmann and Schneider found elsewhere in this issue.

The vitreous

Making up two thirds of the volume and weight of the eye, the vitreous fills the space between the lens and retina. It is clear and gelatinous. It is composed of collagen and hyaluronic acid but is 99% water [4–6].

Vitreous floaters are defined as dots or spots floating in the field of vision that change position when the patient shifts his or her gaze to a different direction [10]. They may be from blood or debris in the vitreous fluid. They may be caused by retinal detachment or hemorrhage.

The extraocular muscles

The extraocular muscles control the movements of the eye. There are six extraocular muscles.

The rectus muscles

The eye has four rectus muscles that are named by their insertion: medial, lateral, superior, and inferior. They originate from a common site, a ring shaped tendon called the annulus of Zinn. These muscles adduct, abduct, elevate, and depress the eye [4–6].

The oblique muscles

There are two oblique muscles of the eye. They provide some upward and downward movement of the eye but primarily provide rotational movement. These muscles are the superior oblique and the inferior oblique [4–6].

Disorders of upward gaze in a traumatized eye may be caused by orbital floor fracture with inferior rectus entrapment. This will be discussed in detail in the article by Bord and Linden elsewhere in this issue. Inability to move the eye, associated with proptosis, may be caused by orbital cellulitis or orbital hemorrhage.

Innervation of the eye

The eye is innervated by the cranial nerves listed below.

The optic nerve (II)

The optic nerve is composed mainly of visual fibers. It arises from the retina and consists of approximately one million axons. After leaving the globe, the nerve becomes myelinated. Each nerve is then enwrapped in a sheath of fibrous tissue that is contiguous with the meninges. It passes through the orbit and joins the nerve from the other eye at the optic chiasm. At the chiasm, nasal fibers from each optic nerve cross to the opposite tract. These axons then course to the lateral geniculate nucleus. After a synapse at the lateral geniculate nucleus, the nerves end in the primary visual cortex of the occipital lobes [4–6].

The oculomotor nerve (III)

The oculomotor nerve originates from the brainstem. It passes through the cavernous sinus and splits into inferior and superior branches. The superior branch innervates the superior rectus muscle. The inferior branch innervates the inferior and medial rectus muscles and the inferior oblique muscle. The inferior branch also provides parasympathetic innervation to the ciliary body [4–6].

The trochlear nerve (IV)

The trochlear nerve begins on the dorsal surface of the brain stem. It travels along the lateral wall of the cavernous sinus. It innervates the superior oblique muscle [4–6].

The trigeminal nerve (V)

The trigeminal nerve begins in the pons and forms the trigeminal ganglion. It then splits into three divisions. The first division is the ophthalmic division (V_1). The ophthalmic division passes through the cavernous sinus and divides to provide sensation to the brow, forehead, cornea, iris, and ciliary body. It also provides sensation to the conjunctiva, eyelids, and the tip of the nose. The second division is the maxillary division (V_2). It passes through the infraorbital canal and forms the infraorbital nerve. This provides sensation to the lower lid and cheek. The third division is the mandibular division (V_3). It provides sensation over the lower portion of the face and mouth. It also provides innervation to eight of the muscles of the face and jaw [4–6].

The abducens nerve (VI)

Originating between the medulla and pons, the abducens nerve passes within the cavernous sinus. It innervates the lateral rectus muscle [4–6].

Multiple disorders involve the innervation of the eyes. Optic neuritis may herald the onset of multiple sclerosis. It causes decreased visual acuity, an afferent papillary defect, and pain on eye movement. Fundoscopic examination may be normal (if the inflammation is retrobulbar) or may reveal edema of the optic disc (if the inflammation is anterior) [11].

Unilateral or bilateral abducens nerve palsy (inability to abduct one or both eyes) may be an early sign of increased intracranial pressure [12]. A posterior communicating artery aneurysm may compress the ophthalmic nerve, causing lid lag and ophthalmoplegia [12]. These entities will be discussed in detail in the article by Duong, Leo, and Mitchell found elsewehere in this issue. Furthermore, trauma can cause an orbital hemorrhage, which may lead to increased orbital pressure and ischemia of the optic nerve.

The blood supply of the eye

The first branch of the intracranial section of the internal carotid artery is the ophthalmic artery. The ophthalmic artery and its subsequent branches supply the main blood source to the eye and its structures. After the ophthalmic artery enters the orbit, the first branch is the central retinal artery. As the artery continues to course within the orbit, multiple other branches supply the structures of the eye until the most superficial branches reach the eyelids. Here they form arcades that anastomose with the external carotid artery.

The main venous drainage of the eye occurs via the superior and inferior ophthalmic veins. These two veins receive the drainage from the eye including the central retinal vein. They then empty into the cavernous sinus. The venous supply of the periorbital skin is contiguous with the deeper venous structures. Superficial skin infections can therefore spread via the venous system into the cavernous sinus and deeper structures [4–6].

The blood supply to the eye can be threatened in several ways. Embolization of plaque or clot to the central retinal artery can cause central retinal artery occlusion and acute painless monocular visual loss. Central retinal vein occlusion also causes visual loss over a longer time period than central retinal artery occlusion. Inflammation of the ophthalmic artery can result from temporal arteritis, causing painless visual loss, which may be unilateral or bilateral [11]. These disorders will be discussed in the article by Vortmann and Schneider in this issue. Also, trauma can disrupt the blood supply to the eye.

Physical examination of the eye

In performing the physical examination of the eye, one should be able to evaluate both anatomy and function of each eye. The evaluation of the anatomy should focus on whether the problem arises from the globe, the orbit, or the external structures. The evaluation of the function of the eye should include vision, alignment, and movements. Generally, the physical examination of the eye should begin with a measurement of visual acuity (an exception to this is when ocular exposure to toxic substances requires irrigation before visual acuity measurement [13]—in this case, a quick measurement of ocular pH can precede irrigation if it can be achieved in a few seconds and does not delay irrigation), then the examiner should start peripherally with the periorbital area and work centrally to examine the orbits, lids, the extraocular muscles, the conjunctiva, sclera and episclera, the uvea, the intraocular pressure, the cornea, the pupils, the anterior chamber, and the fundus.

Vision

The standard way to test vision is by reading a Snellen chart at 20 feet (Fig. 4). Each eye should be tested separately. The vision is then assigned a two-digit score (for example, 20/50) for each eye. The first number represents the distance from the chart, and the second digit represents the smallest line readable by the patient. Recording the vision separately for each eye, even if the vision is the same in each eye, is essential (for example, visual acuity: right eye 20/50, left eye 20/50). If a patient can read three letters on the next line, this can be recorded as, for example, 20/50 +3. If a patient gets 2 letters wrong on the last line, this can be recorded as, for example, 20/50 −2

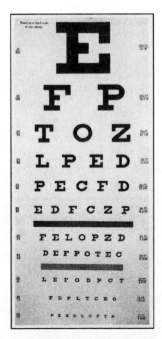

Fig. 4. Standard Snellen chart. (*From* Knicstcdt C, Stamper RL. Visual acuity and its measurement. Ophthalmol Clin North Am 2003;16:159; with permission.)

[12]. Patients who cannot read English can generally be tested with a tumbling E chart, in which the patient identifies the orientation of the letter E (facing to right, left, up, down) [14]. Testing vision in children will be discussed in detail in the article by Prentiss and Dorfman in this issue.

If the subject wears glasses and they are unavailable, vision can be tested through a pinhole. By reading the Snellen chart through multiple pinholes, the image is transmitted centrally through the lens onto the retina, excluding peripheral light. This allows for a clearer image to be formed and substitutes for eyeglasses [6].

If the patient cannot read the chart, he or she should be moved closer to the chart until he or she is 5 feet away. If he or she is still unable to read the chart, the examiner should test vision by having the patient count fingers at 2 feet. If the patient cannot count fingers accurately, the next step is to test whether he or she can detect hand motion. If the patient is unable to detect hand motion, the next step is to determine if he or she has light perception. The eye not being tested must be completely covered to test for light perception. If the patient can perceive light, the examiner can check to see if the patient can determine which direction the light is coming from (light perception with projection) or not (light perception without projection) [12]. If the patient is unable to detect light in an eye, that eye is considered totally blind (no light perception) [6].

Near vision may be tested at the bedside with a near-vision card, held 14 inches from the patient's face [12,15]. Poor performance on near-vision testing can be caused by acute visual impairment but may also be caused by presbyopia [16], which is age-related chronic impairment of near vision [12].

External examination

To begin the physical examination of the eye, one should start with the external structures. The eyelids and surrounding areas should be examined for swelling, erythema, warmth, skin growths, and tenderness. Trauma or infection (periorbital cellulites or zoster) may become apparent on evaluation of the peri-orbital region.

Proptosis can easily be identified with gross inspection of the orbits. Unilateral proptosis may be caused by orbital cellulitis, orbital hemorrhage, cavernous sinus thrombosis, or tumors. Bilateral exophthalmos is most commonly caused by hyperthyroidism [12]. Proptosis can be quantified by the ophthalmologist using an exophthalmometer [14]. Enophthalmos may be caused by an orbital blow-out fracture. The bony structures should be palpated to ascertain tenderness [6].

Lid evaluation may find ptosis, which may be congenital or acquired. Newly acquired ptosis may represent Horner's syndrome, third nerve palsy, botulism, or myasthenia gravis [10]. Inability to close the lids may result from weakness of the orbicularis oculi muscle, as in seventh cranial nerve palsy. It is important to flip the upper lid if you are searching for a foreign body. Careful evaluation of the lids may reveal infections of the lid (lid cellulitis) or dacrocystitis, which is an infection of the tear collection system (puncta, canaliculi, nasolacrimal duct). Other lid findings include hordeolum and chalazion. A hordeolum is an acute inflammation of a meibomian gland, and a chalazion is a chronic obstruction and inflammation of a meibomian gland [10,11].

Extraocular movements

When testing extraocular movement, special note should be made of the range, symmetry, smoothness, and speed of the eye movements. Nystagmus can also be observed. To test these movements, the patient is asked to fixate on a target with both eyes. The examiner then moves the target in four directions [6]. Disorders of ocular motility may be caused by cranial nerve dysfunction, extraocular muscle entrapment, or increased pressure within the orbit (orbital cellulitis or hemorrhage).

Examination of the conjunctiva

It is important to evaluate the conjunctiva lining the lids (palpebral conjunctiva) and the conjunctiva on the surface of the eye (bulbar conjunctiva). Conjunctival injection (prominence of vessels) may be diffuse or perilimbal (radiating outward from the limbus, which is where the cornea meets the sclera). Diffuse conjunctival injection usually results from inflammation or infection within the conjunctiva itself (conjunctivitis), whereas perilimbal injection may be the result of inflammation or infection within the uvea or anterior chamber. Chemosis refers to edema of the conjunctiva [11]. Conjunctivitis will be discussed in detail in the article by Mahmood and Narang found elsewhere in this issue.

Examination of the conjunctiva may also reveal a subconjunctival hemorrhage, which may be spontaneous or traumatic. Although these usually are benign and self-limited, severe subconjunctival hemorrhages (360° of bulbar conjunctiva) may be secondary to ruptured globe or coagulopathy [10].

Examination of the sclera and episclera

Inflammation of the episclera and sclera may be difficult to distinguish from conjunctivitis. Episcleritis is usually painless and causes injection of a sector of episcleral vessels. These vessels will blanche with application of phenylephrine. Vision usually is preserved. It is self-limited and may be associated with collagen vascular diseases [11].

Scleritis causes injection of scleral vessels with a characteristic violaceous color. It is painful and often causes decreased vision. The injection will not clear with topical phenylephrine. It is associated with collagen vascular diseases and certain infections (zoster, tuberculosis, syphilis). Treatment depends on severity but often includes systemic steroids [11]. See the article by Mahmood and Narang in this issue for detailed discussion of scleritis and episcleritis.

Examination of the uvea

Inflammation of the anterior uvea (anterior uveitis, iritis, iridocyclitis) can be detected by the associated photophobia and unilateral constricted pupil that results from ciliary spasm as well as cells and flare in the anterior chamber. Causes include trauma, viral, Reiter's Syndrome, sarcoidosis, juvenile rheumatoid arthritis, and retinoblastoma, and it often is idiopathic [11]. The iris should also be examined for traumatic tears at the papillary margin and for iridodialysis (separation of the iris from the ciliary body) [11].

Inflammation of the posterior uvea can be seen as exudates around retinal vessels and hazy vitreous humor. It can be caused by cytomegalovirus, toxoplasmosis, sarcoidosis, syphilis, herpes, and other causes [10]. Anterior and posterior uveitis will be discussed in the article by Mahmood and Narang in this issue.

Intraocular pressure

The intraocular pressure (IOP) should be measured if glaucoma is suspected. There is a detailed description of various tonometers in the article by Babineau and Sanchez elsewhere in this issue. High pressures may result from acute angle–closure glaucoma, open-angle glaucoma, hyphema, carotid-cavernous fistula, retro-bulbar hemorrhage, and other causes [10]. Low IOP may be seen in ruptured globe, retinal detachment, ocular ischemia, glaucoma medications, and other conditions.

Examination of the cornea

Corneal evaluation is accomplished with the aid of proparicaine, fluorescein, and the slit lamp. Defects in the corneal surface will appear bright yellow-green under the cobalt blue light on the slit lamp when stained with fluorescein [17]. It is an essential part of the emergency eye examination to carefully evaluate the cornea with the slit lamp for foreign bodies, abrasions, and ulcerations [17]. Many causes of infection and inflammation of the cornea (keratitis) have specific patterns of fluorescein uptake on slit lamp examination (herpes simplex, herpes zoster, adenovirus, ultraviolet keratitis) [11]. Corneal edema, seen in acute angle closure glaucoma, will appear to the examiner as a "steamy" cornea, and the patient will see "halos" around lights. Keratitis will be discussed in detail in the article by Dargin and Lowenstein in this issue.

Examination of the pupils

On gross examination, the pupils are symmetric and circular. As many as 20% of normal individuals may have anisocoria (unequal pupils) of less than 1 mm [18,19]. Anisocoria also may be caused by uveitis, trauma, uncal herniation, oculomotor nerve palsy, or Horner's Syndrome and iatrogenically by dilating or constricting drops or nebulized ipratropium [20]. The examiner should test the pupils' response to direct light. As the pupil reacts to direct light, a consensual response (constriction of the opposite pupil) will also occur. After the examiner notes the degree and speed of response of both the direct and consensual response in each eye, one should swing the light between the two eyes (swinging flashlight test) [15]. Each pupil should constrict with both direct and consensual light. If the pupil dilates as the light is swung to it from the opposite pupil, this means that the pupil constricts more vigorously to consensual light than direct light, the hallmark of an afferent papillary defect. This is referred to as a "Marcus Gunn pupil" (Fig. 5) [4–6]. The Marcus Gunn pupil is also discussed in the article by Duong, Leo, and Mitchell in this issue.

Examination of the anterior chamber

Hyphema (blood in the anterior chamber) and hypopyon (layer of white blood cells [WBCs] in the anterior chamber) often can be seen without magnification, but a slit lamp evaluation is essential to adequately evaluate the anterior chamber. With a slit lamp, inflammation of the anterior chamber will be seen as cells (WBCs floating in the aqueous) and flare (increased protein causing the aqueous to appear cloudy) [10]. Cells and flare in the anterior chamber can be seen in uveitis, scleritis, and trauma [11]. The use of the slit lamp is discussed in detail in the article by Babineau and Sanchez in this issue (Fig. 6).

The depth of the anterior chamber can be approximated using a penlight. The penlight is shone tangentially across the cornea from the temporal side. If the entire cornea is illuminated, this implies a deep anterior chamber with

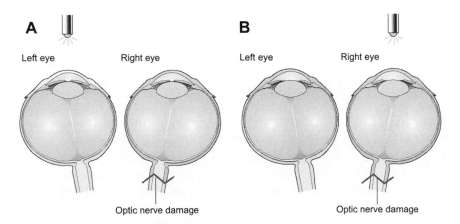

Fig. 5. Testing for relative afferent papillary difference. (*A*) The right optic nerve is damaged. The light is shone in the left eye; both pupils constrict (the direct and consensual light reflex). (*B*) The light is moved to the right eye, and there is no afferent limb to the reflex, thus both pupils dilate. (*From* James B, Benjamin L. Ophthalmology: investigation and examination techniques. China: Butterworth Heinemann (an imprint of Elsevier); 2007; with permission.)

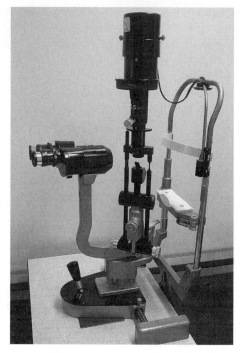

Fig. 6. An overall view of the slit lamp. (*From* James B, Benjamin L. Ophthalmology: investigation and examination techniques. China: Butterworth Heinemann (an imprint of Elsevier); 2007; with permission.)

a wide open angle. If the nasal portion of the cornea is in shadow, this implies a shallow anterior chamber with a narrow angle [21].

Ophthalmoscopy

The use of a hand-held ophthalmoscope enables the examiner to visualize the fundus. In a darkened room, the patient fixes his vision across the room, and the examiner then brings the ophthalmoscope as close as possible to examine each eye. The dial on the ophthalmoscope can then be adjusted to focus the image. This allows for examination of the structures in the retina. The examiner notes the optic disk, the vasculature, and the macula (Fig. 7). Dilation of the pupil can assist in the visualization of the retina. Examination of the periphery of the retina requires the use of an indirect ophthalmoscope and usually is performed by an ophthalmologist [4–6].

Summary

This article has provided a review of the anatomy of the eye and its surrounding tissues. A working knowledge of the functional anatomy of the eye will aid the emergency physician in performing a thorough yet efficient

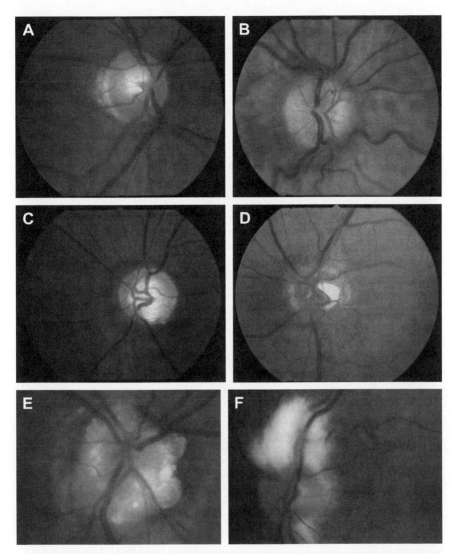

Fig. 7. Examples of optic disc abnormalities. (*A*) Normal disc: Note the distribution of the neuroretinal rim around the disc. (*B*) A swollen disc: The margin is not clearly demarcated; the patient had papilloedema. (*C*) The cup is enlarged, the neuroretinal rim thinned, and the inferior-superior-nasal-temporal pattern lost. The patient has glaucoma. (*D*) New vessels are growing at the disc: this patient had diabetes. (*E*) The disc has an irregular lumpy appearance and optic disc drusen. (*F*) Myelinated nerve fibers at the disc margin. (*From* James B, Benjamin L. Ophthalmology: investigation and examination techniques. China: Butterworth Heinemann (an imprint of Elsevier); 2007; with permission.)

physical examination of the eye. A goal-directed physical examination of the eye will allow the emergency physician to attempt to identify (or exclude) vision-threatening disease processes and facilitate communication with the ophthalmologist.

References

[1] Nash EA, Margo CE. Patterns of emergency department visits for disorders of the eye and ocular adnexa. Arch Ophthalmol 1998;116:1222–6.

[2] Nawar EW, Niska RW, Xu J. National hospital ambulatory medical care survey: 2005 emergency department summary. Advance Data from Vital and Health Statistics 2007;386:1–32.

[3] Khaw PT, Shaw P, Elkington AR. Injury to the eye. BMJ 2004;328:36–8.

[4] Lang G. Ophthalmology: a pocket textbook atlas. 2nd edition. New York: Thieme Medical Publishers; 2007.

[5] Goodman R. Ophto notes: the essential guide. 1st edition. New York: Thieme Medical Publishers; 2003.

[6] Riordan-Eva P, Whitcher J. Vaughan & Ashbury's general ophthalmology. 16th edition. New York: The McGraw-Hill Companies; 2004.

[7] Schlote T, Rohrbach J, Grueb M, et al. Pocket atlas of ophthalmology. 1st edition. New York: Thieme Medical Publishers; 2007.

[8] Blake FAS, Siegert J, Wedl J, et al. The acute orbit: etiology, diagnosis, and therapy. J Oral Maxillofac Surgery 2006;64:87–93.

[9] Kumar NL, Black D, McClellan K. Daytime presentations to a metropolitan ophthalmic emergency department. Clin Experiment Ophthalmol 2005;33:586–92.

[10] Kunimoto DY, Kanitkar KD, Makar MS, editors. The Wills eye manual: office and emergency room diagnosis and treatment of eye disease. 4th edition. New York: Lippincott Williams & Wilkins; 2004.

[11] Kaiser PK, Friedman NJ, Pineda R II. The Massachusetts eye and ear infirmary illustrated manual of ophthalmology. 2nd edition. China: Saunders; 2004.

[12] Leitman MW. Manual for eye examination and diagnosis. 7th edition. Massachusetts: Blackwell; 2007.

[13] Knoop K, Trott A. Ophthalmologic procedures in the emergency department—Part I: immediate sight-saving procedures. Acad Emerg Med 1994;1:408–12.

[14] James B, Benjamin L. Ophthalmology: investigation and examination techniques. China: Butterworth Heinemann; 2007.

[15] Chern KC. Emergency ophthalmology: a rapid treatment guide. Singapore: McGraw-Hill; 2002.

[16] Knoop K, Trott A. Ophthalmologic procedures in the emergency department—Part II: routine evaluation procedures. Acad Emerg Med 1995;2:144–50.

[17] Knoop K, Trott A. Ophthalmologic procedures in the emergency department—Part III: slit lamp use and foreign bodies. Acad Emerg Med 1995;2:224–30.

[18] Adams RD, Victor M, Ropper AH. Adams and Victor's Principles of Neurology. 7th edition. New York: McGraw-Hill; 2001.

[19] Trobe J. Anisocoria. The eyes have it. Available at: http://www.kellogg.umich.edu/theeyeshaveit/symptoms/anisocoria.html. Accessed October 8, 2007.

[20] Iosson N. Nebulizer-associated anisocoria. N Engl J Med 2006;354:e8.

[21] Sparks BI. Tangential penlight angle estimation. J Am Optom Assoc 1997;68:432–4.

ELSEVIER
SAUNDERS

Emerg Med Clin N Am
26 (2008) 17–34

EMERGENCY
MEDICINE
CLINICS OF
NORTH AMERICA

Ophthalmologic Procedures in the Emergency Department

Matthew R. Babineau, MD*,
Leon D. Sanchez, MD, MPH

Department of Emergency Medicine, Beth Israel Deaconess Medical Center, One Deaconess Road, West Campus Clinical Center, 2nd Floor, Boston, MA 02215, USA

Ophthalmologic emergencies account for up to 3% of visits to emergency departments in the United States [1]. Although isolated ocular complaints are rarely life-threatening, they can lead to significant short- and long-term morbidity, including permanent visual loss. The role of the emergency physician in management of ocular emergencies is similar to that for other chief complaints: (1) recognize and diagnose emergency conditions, (2) provide appropriate initial therapy, and (3) ensure correct disposition. This article reviews several of the essential ophthalmologic procedures that are within the scope of emergency medical practice.

Visual acuity testing

A simple but vital part of the ophthalmologic examination is a test of visual acuity. This is essential for all patients who have ocular or visual complaints. The affected and non-affected eyes should be tested individually, and then together, using a Snellen chart or equivalent. If the patient wears corrective lenses during the examination (or is not wearing lenses that are usually used), this should be noted. A critical part of the visual acuity examination is that decreased visual acuity should be rechecked using a pinhole card. A pinhole corrects for most refractive errors, by ensuring that only light striking the lens perpendicularly reaches the retina. Initially abnormal visual acuity that corrects with a pinhole indicates a problem with the lens, and is less concerning to an emergency physician. If this does not correct the visual problems, it indicates pathology that is more likely located within the retina or central nervous system.

---

* Corresponding author.
E-mail address: mbabinea@bidmc.harvard.edu (M.R. Babineau).

0733-8627/08/$ - see front matter © 2008 Elsevier Inc. All rights reserved.
doi:10.1016/j.emc.2007.11.003
emed.theclinics.com

Slit lamp examination

Along with visual acuity, pupillary movements, extra-ocular muscle movements, and fundoscopy (all reviewed elsewhere in this issue), the slit lamp examination is an essential aspect of a complete ophthalmologic examination [2]. The slit lamp is an illuminated biomicroscope that allows a magnified, stereoscopic view of the eye and surrounding structures [2]. It is especially useful for evaluation of the anterior segment of the eye, and should be a standard part of the examination in all ophthalmologic complaints [3].

Despite some manufacturer-specific differences in slit lamps, some general principles apply to the use of this device. Each unit has an illumination system and an observation system. The illumination system is a light source that projects through the slit aperture and onto the patient's eyes. This part should be mobile to allow different angles of light projection. Most systems have a rheostat mechanism that allows the examiner to change the shape and size of the slit beam, as well as a means to change the filter on the beam (neutral, cobalt blue, and red-free) [4]. The observation system is a binocular microscope, which typically allows magnification from 6X to 40X. The observation system is mounted on a chassis, which can be moved horizontally with a joystick device. Often the handle of the joystick can be rotated to allow for vertical movement of the observation system.

To perform the examination, the patient is asked to place his chin on the chin rest, with the forehead resting on the forehead bar. Efforts should be maintained to ensure that the patient is in a comfortable position, because this will lead to a more efficient examination [5]. The chin rest is adjusted so that the patient's eyes rest at the level of the black marker on the vertical pole next to the patients face [3]. The height of the slit lamp is adjusted so that the slit beam is centered on the patient's eyes. The patient should be asked to fix his gaze on a specific location (such as the examiner's ear) [5].

Initially, the examiner should adjust the diopter rings on the ocular piece to account for his or her individual refractive error and accommodation [6]. This will also account for any misalignment in the instrument [6]. This is done by using the focusing rod on the instrument [7]. The slit beam should be set on a low-voltage, wide beam, and should be at 45° from the patient-clinician axis [4]. The microscope should be set at its lowest magnification, and the joystick is used to move the device on the chassis until the eye is in focus. Once the eye is in focus, the clinician begins a systematic examination of individual structures. Although any system may work, the authors recommend using the mnemonic L-L-L-L-L-C-C-C (Table 1). If any abnormality is detected, the beam should be narrowed to help assess the depth, extent, and level of the abnormality. At this time, the magnification can also be increased for further evaluation.

Assessment of the anterior chamber (the region between the cornea and iris) is perhaps the most difficult part of the examination. The purpose of the

Table 1
Mnemonic for systematically assessing all portions of the eye, eyelid and adnexae during routine slit lamp examination

	Stands for	Example of pathology
L	Lids (eyelids)	Lacerations, edema, meibomian cyst
L	Lashes (eyelashes)	Discharge, inverted eye lash
L	Lacrima	Discharge, plugging, cannalicular lacerations
L	Lens (and iris)	Opacification/cataract, dislodgement, pupil shape and function, synechiae, iridodialysis, blood vessels
L	Limbus	Injection
C	Conjunctiva (and sclera)	Hyperemia, follicles, chemosis, foreign body
C	Cornea (and iris)	Edema, foreign body, abrasions, ulcers, opacification, keratitic precipitates
C	Chamber (anterior)	Cells/flare, hyphema/hypopion, shallow chamber

anterior chamber examination is mainly to assess the depth of the chamber (narrow in acute closed angle glaucoma), and to assess for the presence of "cells and flare" (present in inflammatory conditions such as uveitis).

To assess anterior chamber angle depth, use low magnification and a narrow slit beam at 60° from the patient-clinician axis [8]. The beam is centered as close to the limbus as possible, and normal to the cornea [4]. The depth is assessed by comparing the width of the cornea as seen by the light beam with the depth of the aqueous, which is represented by the darker section between the iris and the posterior aspect of the cornea [4]. An aqueous-to-cornea ratio of smaller than 1:4 (eg, a thin dark section compared with the corneal thickness) indicates a dangerously narrow angle, whereas a ratio of greater than 1:2 indicates an open angle [4]. To assess for cells and flare, the slit beam should be between 45° and 60°, and focused onto the front of the cornea. The examiner should assess the space between the focused beam of light (on the cornea), and the more diffuse light (on the lens), using the pupil as a dark background. In normal patients, this area should be completely clear. "Flare" appears as scattered light, and is caused by the presence of inflammatory proteins in the aqueous humor; cells appear as small, floating particulate matter within the aqueous (Fig. 1) [3].

Flourescein examination

The flourescein examination is another important aspect of a complete ophthalmologic examination. It is used to detect defects in the corneal epithelium [3,9]. It should be done in all evaluations of ocular trauma, foreign body, or suspected infection (including conjunctivitis, because symptoms of herpetic keratitis can occasionally mimic conjunctivitis) [10]. The only absolute contraindication to the procedure is a flourescein allergy.

Sodium flourescein is a water-soluble dye that flouresces in an alkaline environment (such as that encountered below the corneal epithileum), and

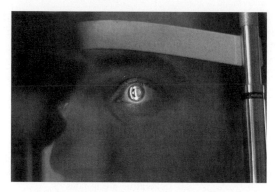

Fig. 1. Positioning for examination of the anterior chamber. Note the following: forehead is resting on the forehead bar; the patient's eyes rest at the level of the black marker on the vertical pole next to the patients face; two strips of light are visible, one at the cornea, the second at the iris with a clear anterior chamber.

not in the acidic environment (such as the tear film) [10]. Therefore, when instilled into the eye, defects in the corneal epithelium will show up as bright green when viewed under a blue light (on the slit lamp, or with a Wood's lamp). Deep corneal defects may allow penetration of flourescein into the anterior chamber. Although this is not a contraindication to the examination (the substance is nontoxic), it may cause a "flare" appearance on examination of the anterior chamber [10].

To perform the flourescein examination, a blue light source is first passed over the eye. Certain infectious organisms (eg, some species of *Pseudomonas* bacteria) may fluoresce under a blue light even without flourescein. Then an individually wrapped flouroscein paper is moistened with sterile water or the patient's own tear film. Many practitioners use topical anesthetic to wet the strip. This is not recommended by some authors, because the anesthetic solution may cause some patients to develop a superficial punctate keratitis, thereby confounding the examination [10]; however, in patients who have significant pain or blepharospasm and are refusing to open the eye, the use of topical anesthetic is advised [10]. The strip is then touched to the tear well, and removed. The patient is asked to blink several times to distribute the dye in a thin film over the entire surface of the eye. Too much dye can impair the examination by causing the eye to become flooded with flourescein. The eye is then inspected with a blue light source, and areas of green fluorescence, indicating corneal disruption, are noted [9].

A variation of this standard flourescein examination, the Seidel test, is used to test for a globe injury or full-thickness corneal disruption. To perform the test, a large amount of flourescein is instilled into the eye (preferably over the area of suspected perforation), which makes the eye appear orange. The globe is then examined for a dark stream interrupting the flourescein, indicating leakage of aqueous humor, and suggesting the diagnosis of globe rupture [10,11].

Note that in the past, bottles containing flourescein dye were used directly to instill the solution into the eye, but this practice is now discouraged because of the possibility of these solutions becoming contaminated with bacterial flora, particularly *Pseudomonas* [9,10].

Tonometry

Tonometry is the determination of intraocular pressure (IOP). Elevated intraocular pressures are associated with vision loss. The main indications of the procedure are to confirm a clinical diagnosis of acute angle closure glaucoma and to determine a baseline IOP after a blunt eye injury [10]. It can also be used to determine baseline IOPs in patients who have conditions such as iritis, or risk factors for open angle glaucoma [10].

With any method of tonometry, an intraocular pressure of 12 to 20 mmHg is considered normal. With an intraocular pressure of greater than 30 mmHg, especially in the context of abnormal optic disks or with visual field defects, therapy for glaucoma should be promptly initiated, and ophthalmologic consultation is warranted. IOPs between 20 and 30 mmHg require urgent follow-up with ophthalmology [9].

Tonometry should be avoided in suspected penetrating eye injuries, because it can worsen the defect and lead to extrusion of intraocular contents. Other relative contraindications to tonometry include eye infection (unless using a sterile cover), patients who have corneal defects, or patients who cannot remain relaxed and may induce corneal injury with sudden, rapid movements [9,10]. Corneal abrasions are rarely caused by tonometry [9].

There are several distinct methods of tonometry. The simplest is direct palpation of the globe. In this method, patients are instructed to look downward, but keep the eyes open. The clinician's index finger is used to gently palpate the globe through the eyelid, with just enough pressure applied to indent the globe slightly. This procedure is repeated on the unaffected eye as well, and the examiner qualitatively compares the amount of pressure required to indent each eye [10]. One study, comparing digital palpation with Goldmann tonometry, found digital palpation to be insensitive, accurately identifying only five of seven eyes that had an IOP greater than 30 mmHg [12]. In clinical practice, it may be more useful as a quick screening tool to test for asymmetric intraocular pressures between the two eyes.

Impression tonometry is the most common method used in most emergency departments. Impression tonometry measures intraocular pressure by measuring the amount of corneal indentation produced by a certain amount of force [13]. The two types of impression tonometry typically used by emergency physicians are Schiotz tonometry and a portable handheld instrument that provides readings that correlate closely with Goldmann tonometry.

With Schiotz tonometry, the first step is to ensure that the tonometer is functioning properly. Most Schiotz tonometers come with a metal test button in the kit. The tonometer can be lowered onto the test button to verify that the plunger is freely mobile with various amounts of pressure. If not, it can lead to falsely low readings, and should be cleaned with an alcohol solution [9]. To begin, the patient is placed in a supine position and asked to gaze straight ahead at a distant object. Topical anesthetic is instilled into the eyes. The clinician then separates the eyelids, taking care to avoid exerting manual pressure on the globe while doing so (this could lead to a falsely elevated reading). The tonometer is held in the patient's line of sight, and the patient is instructed that the procedure will not be painful (anxiety can cause tension in extra-ocular muscles and elevate the IOP) [10]. The tonometer foot is lowered onto the cornea, held loosely between the examiner's index finger and thumb. With the tonometer vertical, the clinician reads the number from the scale on the top of the tonometer. If the reading is low (<4 or <5), additional weight should be added to the scale and the above procedure repeated [9]. The reading is compared with a conversion table (based on the scale weight), thus yielding an intraocular pressure reading. This is compared between both eyes.

The other type of impression tonometry frequently used in the emergency department is the handheld digital device, which is used is used in a similar fashion to the Schiotz tonometer. Although somewhat less accurate, especially at high IOPs, its measurements have good interexaminer reliability, and it can be used with the patient in any position [10]. The pen must be calibrated at least once per day (see package insert for instructions on calibration). To use the device, the eye is instilled with topical anesthetic, and the patient is asked to relax and maintain his gaze fixed on a distant object. A fresh latex cover is placed over the end of the pen. The device is held in the same manner as a pen, and touched lightly four times to the cornea at a perpendicular angle. With each touch, the probe records an IOP. After the fourth touch, a final beep sounds and the liquid crystal display (LCD) screen displays the average IOP measurement in mmHg, along with a series of dashes. The dashes correspond to the statistical variance of the four measurements (with more dashes indicated a higher variance between the individual measurements). A single dash indicates that all measurements were within 20% of each other. If four dashes appear, it indicates that too few valid readings were obtained, and the process should be repeated [10]. The probe may need to be recalibrated if this problem continues.

Applanation tonometry is a very accurate method of tonometry that is less frequently used in the emergency department setting. This device is typically found attached to the slit lamp, and is performed as a part of the slit lamp examination. The patient is arranged in the slit lamp apparatus as described previously, and topical anesthesia and flourescein dye are instilled. The cobalt blue filter is selected and the aperture set so the beam is fully open (as would be done for an evaluation of corneal abrasion) [10]. The illumination apparatus is angled at 45° to 60°, and directed such that it shines through the applanation prism. The pressure knob of the tonometer is turned to its lowest setting (10 mmHg), so that when corneal contact is placed, there will be only light pressure. The instrument is brought toward the patient's eye with the joystick control. Once contact is made with the cornea, a diffuse bluish glow will be visible throughout the limbus. When the operator looks through the ocular pieces, he will see two blue semicircles bordered by an arc of green light [10]. The semicircles may pulse in synchrony with the patient's heartbeat. The pressure knob is adjusted such that the ends of the semicircles are in contact and aligned. If they overlap it indicates the tonometer pressure is too high. If they are not in contact, it indicates that the pressure is too low (Fig. 2) [10].

There are several sources of error with applanation tonometry. Accommodation, Valsalva maneuver, and vertical gaze can cause large errors in readings [14]. Furthermore, repeated measurements can cause a false underestimation of intraocular pressure. Other sources of error are similar to those in the above-described methods, with the important exception that ocular rigidity does not affect the measurements [10].

Other methods of tonometry, such as the McKay-Marg method and pneumatic tonometry, are less frequently used, and discussion of these methods can be found elsewhere in this issue.

Lid eversion

Lid eversion is a simple but essential task for the emergency practitioner to be familiar with. It is useful primarily for inspecting the tarsal conjunctiva and fornices, as well as to localize a foreign body located in one of these areas.

To evert the upper lid, the patient is instructed to look downwards. The clinician grasps the eyelids at the lid margin with the thumb and index finger. The upper lid is gently pulled downward and outward, and a cotton-tipped applicator is used to press on the superior aspect of the tarsal plate, over the lid. The examiner then turns this lid rapidly outward and upward over the cotton swab. The lashes can be held against the superior orbital rim to keep the lid everted while the adnexal structures are inspected [10]. To return the lid to normal position, the examiner releases his grip on the lid margin, and the patient is simply instructed to look upward [9].

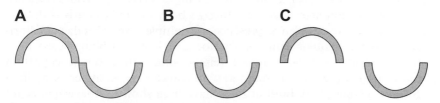

Fig. 2. Schematic representation of visualized semicircles while using applanation tonometer. (*A*) Alignment indicating correct pressure reading. (*B*) Pressure reading is too high. (*C*) Pressure reading is too low.

The lower eyelid is smaller, and lacks a tarsal plate, and therefore is not suitable to eversion; however, full inspection of the fornices and deep adnexae can be readily accomplished via directly pulling at the base of the eyelid.

Foreign body removal

Ocular foreign bodies represent a high-risk chief complaint because they can be vision-threatening in both the short and long term. The two tasks that face the emergency clinician in this situation are: (1) to determine if the foreign body is superficial or intraocular, and (2) to remove superficial foreign bodies.

Intraocular foreign bodies (IOFBs) are diagnosed through a variety of modalities. First, gross inspection is performed, looking for features that suggest perforation, such as prolapse of intraocular contents, changes in pupillary anatomy, or conjunctival edema [15]. Lid eversion is performed to assess for forniceal foreign bodies. The slit lamp examination may reveal a foreign body in the anterior chamber (~15% of IOFBs) [15], and the entire surface of the eye should be inspected, with and without flourescein [10]. Posterior foreign bodies are more difficult for the emergency physician to assess by direct visualization; however, this may be the only opportunity to do so before the foreign body is obscured by vitreal hemorrhage or cataract formation [15]. The practice of pupillary dilation is currently controversial; although it is helpful in determining location of IOFBs, it may compound problems (ie, if it pulls out iris that is plugging a corneal laceration) [15].

If an IOFB is suspected based on the examination, ophthalmology should be consulted immediately. The priority of the emergency provider is then to prevent further globe injury. The patient should be kept quiet, with the head of the bed elevated, and a shield should be placed over the eye (taking care to make sure pressure points are directed onto the orbits, and not the globe). Tonometry or other procedures that place pressure on the eye should be avoided [10]. In these patients, systemic antibiotics should be given, as should antiemetics (to prevent increased intraocular pressures from vomiting) [15].

When the initial ophthalmologic examination is complete, further imaging is often necessary. It is important that the emergency provider does not stop the evaluation after a corneal foreign body or single IOFB is discovered, or he may overlook the presence of multiple foreign bodies. Historically, plain radiographs (anteroposterior and lateral orbital views) have been used to look for radiopaque foreign bodies, with precise localization performed by using various radiographic markers (ie, Comberg's method or Sweet's method) [15]. Both of these have been shown to have significant inaccuracy, and to miss radiolucent or small foreign bodies. Ultrasonography (US) is an increasingly popular modality, because of its immediate availability for emergency physicians familiar with the practice (see below for a complete discussion of this topic). At present, CT scans are considered the gold standard, and have the highest accuracy in diagnosis and localization [16]. The physician should request 3 mm sections through the orbit, unless a foreign body was seen on plain radiography, in which case 6 mm sections are acceptable [17]. MRI is not considered a first-line diagnostic modality, because it is contraindicated in the case of known or suspected metallic IOFB (70%–90% of cases) [15], and is typically more difficult to obtain than the other studies mentioned above.

If a foreign body has been found to penetrate the globe through using any of these modalities, emergent ophthalmologic consultation is indicated. The emergency physician should take care to note visual acuity, lens damage, presence of vitreal hemorrhage, type of IOFB, and entry site, because these are shown to be the most important indicators of final visual outcome [18].

If an uncomplicated (ie, not intraocular, multiple, or deeply embedded) ocular foreign body is discovered, the emergency physician should attempt to remove it. The exception is when the patient is uncooperative, in which case ophthalmology should be consulted to remove it [10].

To remove the foreign body, the eye is anesthetized with topical anesthetic, and a slit lamp examination is performed. The patient is asked to move the eye to a position such that the foreign body is rotated to the highest point of the cornea [9]. Successful removal can often be achieved by gentle jet stream irrigation [10], which may be especially useful if there is more than one foreign body [11]. Another method is to use a cotton-tipped applicator that has been moistened with topical anesthetic [15]. This can be rolled over the foreign body to gently lift the object off of the ocular surface. If these less invasive methods are unsuccessful, needle removal is often required. A 25-gauge needle is placed on a tuberculin syringe. The foreign body is approached tangentially to the globe (viewed through the slit lamp), and the beveled edge is used to gently scrape it off of the cornea [15]. Although this procedure may inspire some degree of anxiety in both the clinician and the patient, the corneal epithelium is resilient and should not be perforated with careful manipulation. Many practitioners now recommend avoidance of the "spud" device, because there may be a risk of increased corneal scarring [9,15].

Multiple corneal foreign bodies can be removed with the same methods, though may be more amenable to jet stream irrigation [11]. If there are diffusely located foreign bodies (ie, from an explosion), however, the patient should be referred to ophthalmology, where most of the corneal epithelium will be removed to decrease the scarring. Another special situation involves rust rings. These can often be removed with a needle (as described above) or with a pressure sensitive drill, but are not a true emergency [10]. Many will wash out spontaneously, and the others can be referred nonemergently to ophthalmology for removal [15]. During the next 24 to 48 hours after formation, the iron will often necrose the surrounding epithelial cells and allow the ring to then be removed intact [10]. Delayed removal may be especially indicated in the case of a rust ring that is deep or located in the center of the visual field, because this may allow time for the rust to migrate to the corneal surface, thus facilitating extraction [11].

Once the foreign body has been removed, the eye should be irrigated profusely. Studies have shown a lack of consensus among providers regarding further management of these injuries [19]. Topical nonsteroidal anti-inflammatory drugs (NSAIDs) have been shown to provide effective analgesia in several randomized clinical trials [20,21], and should be prescribed, with or without systemic analgesics (NSAID or opioid). Some authors recommend using a cycloplegic for pain caused by ciliary spasm, although this practice is not routine [11,15,19,22]. Artificial tears may help with superficial irritation [11]. Topical antibiotics and a tetanus booster may be given, although both of these practices are controversial with superficial injuries [9,10,23]. One prospective study where removed corneal foreign bodies were cultured showed that 32.7% grew positive cultures, mostly staphylococcal and streptococcal species [24]. *Pseudomonas* species are more common in patients who wear contact lenses [25], therefore mandating treatment with a quinolone antibiotic. Patching is not generally recommended, because studies have shown no significant improvement in patient comfort or healing rate [26,27]. Topical steroids should be avoided, because they may promote fungal ulceration. Topical anesthetics should also be avoided, because these agents may hide pain associated with retained foreign body or corneal ulceration [28].

Patients who have only superficial injuries do not need ophthalmology follow-up unless symptoms persist [10]. Patients who have large or central defects, purulent discharge, or anterior chamber reactions, but without globe penetration, can be discharged with 24-hour follow-up with ophthalmology for repeat examination and evaluation of infection [9,11].

Contact lens removal

The removal of contact lenses is a simple procedure that emergency physicians should be comfortable with. The patient should be asked whether he wears "soft" or "hard" lenses, because this may affect the method of removal. The first task is to localize the contact lens. Often the patient may not be able to sense the lens if it is in a conjunctival fornix. The patient is examined in the standard fashion. The upper lid is everted. If the patient has significant pain or blepharospasm, the eye should be topically anesthetized. Note that flourescein dye can be used to help localize the lens, although it will permanently stain a soft lens.

When the lens is encountered, gentle pressure should be applied with a cotton-tipped applicator or a gloved finger [29]. If it is loose, it may be slid over the cornea, and the patient can remove it as usual [29]. A soft lens can be safely removed from any part of the eye. If the lens is somewhat adherent, gentle irrigation with a plastic catheter may moisten it and allow it to be moved to a position where it can be easily removed from the eye [30]. If it continues to be adherent, the practitioner should attempt to remove the lens directly by gently compressing it between a gloved thumb and forefinger to break the suction with the globe, then remove it.

If these steps fail, there are devices available that can help in removal. For soft lenses, rubber-tipped forceps can be used to squeeze the lens and allow removal [29]. For hard lenses, suction-cup removers can be used. The suction cup should be moistened with saline, and then applied gently directly to the front of the lens [30]. Once a seal is formed, the lens should be pulled off perpendicularly to the globe.

After removal, a flourescein examination should be performed to evaluate for the presence of corneal abrasions. These should be treated as any other corneal abrasion, with the caveat that if topical antibiotics are prescribed, it should be a quinolone (rather than a macrolide) to cover *Pseudomonas* and other organisms more common in contact-lens wearers [25,30]. The patient should be instructed not to wear the lens for at least 24 hours, or until free of any symptoms [29].

Eye irrigation

The foundation of emergency treatment for chemical burns is immediate and copious irrigation, because this has been shown to have the greatest effect on visual prognosis [31].

There are two broad types of chemical burn: acid and alkali. Acid burns produce a coagulative necrosis, and therefore, after the initial injury, the deeper structures may be somewhat protected from further injury (with the notable exception of hydrofluoric acid burns). Alkali burns produce a liquefactive necrosis and penetrate more rapidly into the anterior chamber (within minutes) [32].

Despite these differences, the treatment of ocular chemical burns is the same. When a patient presents with an ocular burn, irrigation should begin immediately, even in triage [33], especially because in practice, immediate, on-site irrigation occurs only in 40% to 50% of patients [34]. Physical examination should initially be limited to, at most, a very rapid visual acuity measurement and the determination of pH [3].

Measurement of ocular surface pH is a simple task. One simply touches the end of a piece of pH litmus paper to the tear well and compares the resulting color to the color scale located on the side of the container that holds the strips. The shelf life of the strips is roughly 5 years according to the manufacturer. There are several methods of irrigating the eye. Eye showers are available at many workplaces, but the actual amount of irrigant they deliver to the corneal surface and conjunctival fornices may be limited by blepharospasm caused by pain. In the emergency department, the ideal device to use is a Morgan lens. The Morgan lens is a molded lens that is applied directly to the eye surface, and can be directly attached to a length of intravenous (IV) tubing to allow continuous irrigation of the eye. To insert the lens, the patient should be instructed to look down, as the upper lid is grasped and the superior end of the lens is placed under the lid. This procedure is repeated with the lower lid. At this point, the lens is connected to the tubing from the irrigant, and the solution is allowed to bathe the eye. If the Morgan lens is not available, the eye can be directly irrigated with the cut end of IV tubing. This often requires an assistant to manually retract the eyelids throughout the procedure, however; otherwise, blepharospasm is likely to limit the amount of irrigant that reaches the corneal surface [15].

The irrigant is instilled until the pH of the eye returns to normal (pH 6.8–7.4) [9]. After irrigation, the practitioner should wait for 5 minutes before checking the pH, because earlier measurements may give a falsely reassuring pH by measuring the pH of the irrigant solution [11]. After achieving a normal pH, the eye should be continually irrigated for at least 30 more minutes [34]. Some authors recommend episodic irrigation for up to the following 24 hours [34].

There may be controversy regarding the specific type of irrigant to be used. Whereas different features make some solutions preferable to others, the most important factor is rapid institution of therapy, and it is essential to not delay irrigation while setting up the equipment or finding the best buffer solution [9]. Irrigation works by mechanical and chemical means. Mechanically, a volume of liquid coursing over the eye serves to remove any excess particles or drops of the offending agent. In this way, even tap water or other nonsterile fluid is a suitable irrigant if used immediately [11,34].

The preferred buffer solutions are amphoteric (universal) buffers that may help to limit further damage to the eye caused by exothermic chemical reactions between the irrigant and the offending agent [9]. Ethylenediaminetetraacetic acid (EDTA) used to be the primary amphoteric buffer, but has now been largely replaced by diphoterine [34,35]. Notably, acidic solutions should not be used to neutralize an alkaline burn, and alkaline solutions should not be used to neutralize an acidic burn [11]. Another consideration in use of buffers is the osmolarity. Because the cornea has a higher osmolarity (420 mOsm/L) than other areas in the human body, use of a hypotonic solution can lead to increased corneal water uptake, and therefore, exacerbate corneal edema from a burn [34,36]. This will also allow deeper corneal penetration of corrosive materials [34]. Therefore, osmotic solutions—normal saline (NS), lactated Ringer's solution (LR), or balanced salt solution (BSS)—are often preferred to nonosmotic solutions such as tap water. The pH of the solution is also a factor in the choice of irrigant. Normal saline has a pH of 4.5 to 7.0, lactated Ringer's is 6.2 to 7.5, and balanced salt solution is 7.1 to 7.4 [37]. For all of these reasons, many authors prefer BSS or LR as an irrigant, although isotonic NS is considered to be an appropriate substitute if others are unavailable [32], and even tap water irrigation has been shown to decrease the severity of ocular burns [36,38]. Each of these solutions has been shown to have equal tolerability to patients

[39], although warmed solutions have been shown to be better tolerated than room temperature [40].

Following adequate irrigation, it is important to do a complete ophthalmologic examination to rule out any retained foreign bodies, corneal injuries, or other injuries that need attention [9,11]. Some authors recommend sweeping the fornices with a moistened cotton-tipped applicator to remove any remaining particles of caustic material or necrotic conjunctiva. All patients, even those who have minor burns, should receive a tetanus shot, topical antibiotics, and oral analgesics, and be instructed to follow up with ophthalmology within 24 hours. Cycloplegics and pressure patches are controversial. For more severe burns, and especially those caused from alkali exposure, hospitalization may be warranted for intravenous antibiotics and further ophthalmologic care. In these cases, ophthalmologic consultation is required before institution of therapy such as cycloplegics, topical steroids, and further therapy. Prognosis depends on the depth of the injury, with opacification of the cornea and greater than 50% area of conjunctival ischemia being predictive of a poor outcome (Table 2).

Paracentesis

Anterior chamber paracentesis is a rare procedure in the emergency department; however, it is one that emergency providers should feel comfortable performing. The primary indication in the emergency setting is in the treatment of central retinal artery occlusion. In this disease, there is acute embolization to the central retinal artery, which is manifested by a painless loss of vision in the affected eye, and appears as a pale optic disc or a cherry red spot on fundoscopy. Immediate treatment is indicated if the patient presents within 24 to 48 hours of symptom onset, because once the retina has infarcted, vision loss is permanent [13]. Even with appropriate treatment, successful return of full visual acuity is rare [13].

Initial treatment is directed at improving retinal blood flow and trying to dislodge the clot into a more distal branch of the retinal artery. Common maneuvers include supine positioning (which improves retinal blood flow),

Table 2
Classification and prognosis of chemical ocular burns

Grade	Corneal findings	Conjunctival ischemia	Prognosis
I	Only epithelial loss.	None	Very good
II	Some edema and haze.	<1/3 of limbus	Some permanent scarring may occur.
III	Significant haziness	<1/2 limbus	Variable, usually some visual impairment
IV	Opaque	>1/2 limbus	Poor

Data from Cheh AI, Reensta-Buras WR. Ocular. http://www.emedicine.com/emerg/topic736.htm. Accessed August 3, 2007.

digital orbital massage (to diminish intraocular pressure and possibly dislodge the clot), and intravenous acetozolamide or topical B-blockers to further decrease intraocular pressure [41]. Carbogen therapy involves inhalation of a 5% CO2/95% O2 mixture of gas. The carbon dioxide may dilate retinal arterioles, thereby enhancing the delivery of oxygen-rich blood to the ischemic retina [42]. This should be done for 10 minutes every 2 hours, and continued for 48 hours. Hyperbaric oxygen therapy may provide similar benefits, but must be initiated soon after symptom onset (within 12 hours, and preferably within 2 hours) [42]. If these techniques fail to restore vision or are unavailable, however, anterior chamber paracentesis should be attempted.

To perform the procedure, the eye is topically anesthetized. The provider prepares a 30-gauge needle on a tuberculin syringe. The patient is positioned in the slit lamp apparatus as described above. The anterior chamber is carefully entered at the limbus, with the bevel facing the examiner. The clinician then removes 0.1 to 0.2 cc of aqueous, until the chamber becomes slightly shallower. The needle is withdrawn and the patient should then be given a topical antibiotic [41].

Lateral canthotomy

Lateral canthotomy is another rarely indicated but potentially vision-sparing procedure that emergency practitioners must be familiar with. The purpose of the procedure is to emergently relieve retro-orbital pressure after trauma. With significant retrobulbar hemorrhage, the optic nerve can become ischemic, leading to permanent visual loss within 90 to 120 minutes of ischemic time [43]. Although retrobulbar hemorrhage is now often diagnosed based on CT scan findings in the trauma victim, signs of retrobulbar hemorrhage include acute loss of visual acuity, elevated IOP (>40 mm Hg), and proptosis [43]. There are other more subtle findings suggestive of the diagnosis, including afferent pupillary defect, optic nerve pallor, and severe eye pain [43], but these findings alone should not merit canthotomy without confirmatory findings.

To perform the procedure, the patient is placed in the supine position, and 1 to 2 cc of 1% lidocaine with epinephrine is injected into the lateral canthus. The eye is then irrigated with normal saline to ensure a clean, noncontaminated working surface. A straight Kelly clamp is used to crimp the skin at the lateral canthus, then promptly removed. This serves two functions: it helps with hemostasis, and it marks the location for the canthotomy. At this point, an assistant may be useful to laterally retract the lid, thereby reducing the risk of inadvertent globe injury. Small scissors are used to make a 1 to 2 cm lateral incision along the line formed by the crimped Kelly clamp. The lower eyelid is then retracted to exposure the lateral canthus tendon, which can then be cut with the scissors. A small amount of blood should be expressed at this time. The intraocular pressure should be less than 40 mm Hg if the procedure is successful, and the patient should have improved visual acuity. If the pressure continues to remain elevated, the superior canthus can be cut in the same way [43].

Ocular ultrasonography

Bedside US, performed by emergency physicians, is a procedure that is gaining popularity in the emergency department. It can be a rapid, safe, and noninvasive method to make several diagnoses, and may be especially useful in the trauma patient where periorbital swelling limits direct visualization of the eye and surrounding structures [1]. It is also useful in nontraumatic eye complaints, because patients who have new-onset visual loss can be rapidly evaluated for retinal detachment or central retinal artery or vein occlusion (Table 3) [1].

To perform ocular US, a linear 10-mHz transducer (also known as a "vascular" probe) is used. The power output and gain settings should be minimized, because this decreases artifact from eyelid echoes and allows better visualization of ocular structures [44]. The patient is asked to close his eyes, and ultrasound gel is applied to the closed eye. The clinician should take care to avoid putting excessive pressure on the globe while performing the scan, and if there is a possibility of globe rupture, the scan should be performed without the transducer touching the eyelid (instead using a larger amount of ultrasound gel) [44]. The scan is done in both sagittal and transverse planes, as well as with two-dimensional Doppler imagining if there is suspicion of central retinal artery or vein occlusion [1,44]. The imaging can typically done by an experienced sonographer within 60 to 90 seconds [1].

There are few prospective studies regarding the role of ocular US in the emergency department. In one study by Blaivas and colleagues [1], 61 consecutive patients who had ocular complaints were enrolled, all of whom had bedside ocular US followed by a "confirmatory" study (either CT of orbits or formal ophthalmologic examination). The scans were done by experienced attending physicians or residents who had undergone a 1-hour lecture

Table 3
Ocular pathology visible with ultrasonography, and sonographic findings

Pathology	Ultrasonographic appearance
Retinal detachment	Band of echogenic material within vitreous body
Vitreous detachment	Collection of echogenic material between vitreous body and retina
Vitreous hemorrhage	Echogenic material within vitreous body
Retrobulbar hemorrhage	Hypoechoic lucency deep to retina
Lens dislocation	Lens in abnormal position within globe
Globe rupture	Difference in globe size between eyes; scleral folds
Intraocular foreign body	Echogenic foreign body visualized within globe
Central retinal artery/vein occlusion	Absence of Doppler flow at posterior retina

Data from Legome E, Pancu D. Future applications for emergency ultrasound. Emerg Med Clin N Am 2004;22:817–27.

and a 1-hour hands-on teaching experience. Of these 61 patients, the correct diagnosis was made by bedside US in 60, yielding test characteristics of: sensitivity 100% (95% CI 94–100), specificity 97% (95% CI 88–99), positive predictive value (PPV) 96% (95% CI 88–99), negative predictive value (NPV) 100% (95% CI 94–100) [1]. There have been no studies that look at how bedside ocular US changes decision-making regarding treatment, further diagnostic studies, or disposition [1,44].

Another novel use of bedside ocular US is in the evaluation of the optic nerve sheath diameter (ONSD) in a patient who has possible increased intracranial pressure (ICP). The scan is performed as above, and the ONSD is measured in each eye at a distance of 3 mm behind the globe. The ONSD measurement is then an average of both eyes [45]. An increased ONSD (>5.0 mm in adults, >4.5 mm in children age 1–15years, or >4.0 mm in children less than 1 year old) is considered abnormal and indicative of elevated intracranial pressure [45–47]. One study [46] has shown abnormal ONSD to have a 100% sensitivity (95% CI 68–100) for CT findings consistent with increased ICP, and a specificity of 63% (95% CI 50–76). Furthermore, this had a sensitivity of 84% and specificity of 73% for any traumatic intracranial injury [46].

Summary

Ophthalmologic complaints are a small but important proportion of emergency department visits. Familiarity with many important ophthalmologic procedures is an essential part of any emergency clinician's armamentarium, and may help to decrease morbidity associated with ophthalmologic emergencies.

References

[1] Blaivas M, Theodoro D, Sierzenski PR. A study of bedside ocular ultrasonography in the emergency department. Acad Emerg Med 2002;9(8):791–9.
[2] Kercheval DB, Terry JE. Essentials of slit lamp biomicroscopy. J Am Optom Assoc 1997; 48(11):1383–9.
[3] Broocker G. Chapter 15: the ophthalmic examination. In: Wolfson AB, Hendey GW, Hendry PL, ct al, editors. Harwood-Nuss' clinical practice of emergency medicine. 4th edition. Philadelphia: Lippincott, Williams and Wilkins; 2005. p. 112–7.
[4] Available at: http://www.academy.org.uk/lectures/eperjesi5.htm. Accessed August 2, 2007.
[5] Nemeth SC. Basic slit lamp techniques. J Ophthalmic Nurs Technol 1996;15(4):134–41.
[6] Blumenthal EZ, Serpetopolous CN. On focusing the slit lamp: part I. an inaccurate ocular setting—what is there to lose? Surv Ophthalmol 1998;42(4):351–4.
[7] Blumenthal EZ, Serpetopolous CN. On focusing the slit lamp: part II. "The fading-slit test"—verifying the ocular setting. Surv Ophthalmol 1998;42(4):355–7.
[8] Osuobeni EP, Oduwaiye KA. The effect of illumination-microscope angle on slit lamp estimate of the anterior chamber depth. Optom Vis Sci 2003;80(3):237–44.

[9] Dennis WR Jr, Dennis AM. Chapter 31: Eye emergencies. In: Stone CK, Humphries EH, editors. Current emergency diagnosis and treatment. 5th editon. Lange Medical Books/ McGraw-Hill; 2004.

[10] Knoop KJ, Dennis WR, Hedges JR. Opthalmologic procedures. In: Roberts MD, Hedges JR, editors. Clinical procedures in emergency medicine. 4th edition.

[11] Cullom Jr RD, Chang B, editors. The Wills eye manual: office and emergency room diagnosis and treatment of eye disease. 2nd edition. 1994.

[12] Baum J, Chaturvedi N, Netland PA, et al. Assessment of intraocular pressure by palpation. Am J Ophthalmol 1995;119(5):650–1.

[13] Beers MH, Porter RS, Jones, TV, et al, editors. The Merck manual of diagnosis and therapy—chapter 98: Approach to the ophthalmologic patient. 18th edition. 2006.

[14] Whitacre MM, Stein R. Sources of error with use of Goldmann-type tonometers. Surv Ophthalmol 1993;38(1):1–30.

[15] Schwartz GR, et al. Ocular foreign body removal. In: Principles & practice of emergency medicine. 4th edition. Copyright (c) 1999 Lippincott Williams & Wilkins.

[16] Coleman DJ, Lucas BC, Rondeau MJ, et al. Management of intraocular foreign bodies. Ophthalmology 1987;94:1647–53.

[17] Etherington RJ, Hourihan MD. Localisation of intraocular and intraorbital foreign bodies using computerized tomography. Clin Radiol 1989;40:610–4.

[18] De Juan E Jr, Sternberg P Jr, Michels RG. Penetrating ocular injuries: types of injuries and visual results. Ophthalmology 1983;90:1318–22.

[19] Calder L, Baladubramanian S, Stiell I. Lack of consensus on corneal abrasion management: results of a national survey. CJEM 2004;6(6):402–7.

[20] Donnenfeld ED, Selkin BA, Perry HD, et al. Controlled evaluation of a bandage contact lens and a topical non-steroidal anti-inflammatory drug in treating corneal abrasions. Ophthalmology 1995;102:979–84.

[21] Weaver CS, Terrell KM. Evidence-based emergency medicine. Update: do ophthalmic non-steroidal anti-inflammatory drugs reduce the pain associated with simple corneal abrasion without delaying healing? Ann Emerg Med 2003;41(1):134–40.

[22] Elkington AR, Khaw PT. ABC of eyes. Injuries to the eye. BMJ 1988;297(6641):122–5.

[23] Mukherjee P, Sivakumar A. Tetanus prophylaxis in superficial corneal abrasions. Emerg Med J 2003;20(1):62–4.

[24] Macedo Filho ET, Lago A, Duarte K, et al. Superficial corneal foreign body: laboratory and epidemiologic aspects. Arq Bras Oftalmol 2005;68(6):821–3.

[25] Fleiszig SM, Efron N, Pier GB. Extended contact lens wear enhances Pseudomonas aeruginosa adherence to human corneal epithelium. Invest Ophthalmol Vis Sci 1992;33(1):2908–16.

[26] Arbour JD, Brunette I, Boisjoly HM, et al. Should we patch corneal erosions? Arch Ophthalmol 1997;115:313–7.

[27] Wilson SA, Last A. Management of corneal abrasions. Am Fam Physician 2004;70(1):123–8.

[28] Newell SW. Management of corneal foreign bodies. Am Fam Physician 1985;31(2):149–56.

[29] Buttaravoli P, Stair T. Common simple emergencies. 2.12–Removal of dislocated contact lens. Available at: http://www.ncemi.org/cse/cse0212.htm. Accessed August 5, 2007.

[30] Ramponi DR. Eye on contact lens removal. Available at: http://findarticles.com/p/articles/mi_qa3689/is_200108/ai_n8985396. Accessed August 5, 2007.

[31] Kucklkorn R, Kottel A, Schrage N, et al. Poor prognosis of severe chemical and thermal eye burns: the need for adequate emergency care and primary prevention. Int Arch Occup Environ Health 1995;67(4):281–4.

[32] Cheh AI, Reensta-Buras WR, and Rosen C. Burns, ocular. Available at: http://www.emedicine.com/emerg/topic736.htm.

[33] Garcia GE. Management of ocular emergencies and urgent eye problems. Am Fam Physician 1996;53(2):565–74.

[34] Schrage, et al. Eye burns. Burn 2000;26:699.

[35] Langefeld S, Press UP, Frentz M, et al. Use of lavage fluid containing diphoterine for irriga-
     tion of eyes in first aid emergency treatment. Ophthalmologe 2003;100(9):727–31 [Article in
     German].
[36] Kompa S, Redbrake C, Hilgers C, et al. Effect of different irrigating solutions on aqueous
     humour pH changes, intraocular pressure and histological findings after induced alkali
     burns. Acta Ophthalmol Scand 2005;83(4):467–70.
[37] Saidinejad M, Burns MM. Ocular irrigant alternatives in pediatric emergency medicine.
     Pediatr Emerg Care 2005;21(1):23–6.
[38] Ikeda N, Hayasaka S, Hayasaka Y, et al. Alkali burns of the eye: effect of immediate copious
     irrigation with tap water on their severity. Ophthalmologica 2006;220(4):225–8.
[39] Jones JB, Schoenleber DB, Gillen JP. The tolerability of lactated Ringer's solution and BSS
     plus for ocular irrigation with and without the Morgan therapeutic lens. Acad Emerg Med
     1998;5(12):1150–6.
[40] Ernst AA, Thomson T, Haynes M, et al. Warmed versus room temperature saline solution
     for ocular irrigation: a randomized clinical trial. Ann Emerg Med 1998 Dec;32(6):676–9.
[41] Haddad C. Central retinal artery occlusion. Available at: http://www.eyeweb.org/CRAO.
     htm. Accessed August 5, 2007.
[42] Graham RH, Huang E, Kim DB, et al. Central retinal artery occlusion. Available at: http://
     www.emedicine.com/OPH/topic387.htm.
[43] Peak DA. Acute orbital compartment syndrome. Available at: http://www.emedicine.com/
     emerg/topic881.htm.
[44] Legome E, Pancu D. Future applications for emergency ultrasound. Emerg Med Clin North
     Am 2004;22:817–27.
[45] Blaivas M, Theodoro D, Sierzenski PR. Elevated intracranial pressure detected by emer-
     gency ultrasonography of the optic nerve sheath. Acad Emerg Med 2003;10(4):376–81.
[46] Tayal VS, Neulander M, Norton HJ, et al. Emergency department sonographic measure-
     ment of optice nerve sheath diameter to detect findings of increased intracranial pressure
     in adult head injury patients. Ann Emerg Med 2007;49(4):508–14.
[47] Tsung JW, Blaivas M, Cooper A, et al. A rapid noninvasive method of detecting elevated
     intracranial pressure using bedside ocular ultrasound: application to 3 cases of head trauma
     in the pediatric emergency department. Pediatr Emerg Care 2005;21(2):94–8.

ELSEVIER
SAUNDERS

Emerg Med Clin N Am
26 (2008) 35–55

EMERGENCY
MEDICINE
CLINICS OF
NORTH AMERICA

Diagnosis and Management of the Acute Red Eye

Ahmed R. Mahmood, MD, Aneesh T. Narang, MD*

*Department of Emergency Medicine, Boston Medical Center, Dowling 1 South,
1 Boston Medical Center Place, Boston, MA 02118, USA*

The red eye is a clinical problem encountered on a daily basis in most emergency departments. Fortunately, most causes are relatively benign and self-limiting; however, many conditions associated with high morbidity and that are potentially vision threatening may manifest as a red eye. The history should address the following essential components: the presence or absence of pain, foreign body sensation, and itching; the presence and type of discharge; photophobia; onset; visual disturbances; recent illnesses and trauma; and ophthalmologic history. The examination must include visual acuity, pupil shape and reactivity, a comparison between the pupils, the gross appearance of the sclera and conjunctiva, extraocular muscle function, and palpation for preauricular nodes. Often, evaluation of the affected eye requires measurement of intraocular pressure, fluorescein staining and a cobalt blue light, and a slit lamp evaluation [1].

Emergency physicians should be adept at recognizing high-risk features from the history and examination that would require urgent ophthalmologic referral and treatment. The differential diagnosis of the red eye is extensive. Some of the more common causes, including viral, allergic, and bacterial conjunctivitis, subconjunctival hemorrhage, episcleritis, scleritis, anterior uveitis, and acute angle-closure glaucoma (AACG), are discussed herein. Characteristic features of the history and examination as well as management and indications for ophthalmology consultation for each of these entities are described in detail.

Conjunctivitis

The most common cause of red eye is conjunctivitis. The term *conjunctivitis* refers to inflammation of the conjunctiva, a membrane that lines the

* Corresponding author.
E-mail address: atnarang@yahoo.com (A.T. Narang).

outer aspect of the globe (bulbar conjunctiva) and reflects back on itself to line the inner lids (the palpebral conjunctiva) [2]. Conjunctivitis is usually separated into broad categories based on the etiologic agent and time course of illness. The most common causes of acute conjunctivitis (less than 4 weeks) are allergic, viral, and bacterial. Common and distinguishing features of the various types of acute conjunctivitis are reviewed herein.

Allergic conjunctivitis, also known as hay fever conjunctivitis or seasonal allergic rhinoconjunctivitis, is the most common type of ocular allergy. This IgE-mediated reaction is usually, but not always, seasonal and may be seen with sensitivity to allergens such as dust or animal dander. The patient will almost always present with itching and may or may not have associated watery eyes and rhinorrhea. If there is no component of itching, allergic conjunctivitis is less likely, and another diagnosis should be sought. The family history often includes other forms of atopy such as asthma, eczema, or allergic rhinitis. On examination, the clinician will notice a global bilateral injection pattern that is equal in both eyes [1]. If there is a discharge, it may be clear and watery, such as in tears, or mucoid. Mild eyelid swelling may complete the clinical presentation. Similar presentations can be caused by dry eyes, contact lenses, and over-the-counter eye products, and these causes should be considered in the differential diagnosis [2].

As with the treatment of other forms of allergy, avoidance of triggers is paramount. The patient may use cold compresses, over-the-counter vaso-constrictors, or ocular non-steroidal anti-inflammatory agents (NSAIDs) to help reduce discomfort, redness, and swelling. Oral antihistamines can often help relieve many of the patient's symptoms. More specific therapy includes histamine-blocking drops such as olopatadine, pemirolast, or keto-tifen [1]. Topical mast cell stabilizers such as cromolyn sodium or lodoxa-mide can also be beneficial. Administering corticosteroids should only be done in consultation with an ophthalmologist [2].

Conjunctivitis can have a variety of infectious etiologies. Viral infections are among the most common forms of infectious conjunctivitis, with many types implicated, including adenovirus, herpes, mumps, and rubella. Be-cause the last two causes are rare, the more common presentations of ade-novirus and herpes virus are discussed herein. Adenovirus is the most likely etiologic agent of any viral conjunctivitis, with most of the common sero-types causing a mild follicular conjunctivitis. Common modes of transmis-sion for this viral-borne illness are the fingers, medical instruments, and swimming pool water. As such, it is responsible for community-wide epi-demics and is commonly found in schools, workplaces, and doctors' offices [2]. The patient will usually complain of irritation beginning in one eye and spreading to the other a few days later. This spread is not uncommon as the infection is transmitted via hand–eye contact. Some patients may have an associated upper respiratory tract infection. Common but nonspecific find-ings include preauricular lymphadenopathy, global conjunctival injection, watery discharge, and a follicular reaction of the inferior tarsal conjunctiva

(Fig. 1). Follicles are tiny, avascular, round, white or gray patches on the palpebral conjunctiva. They differ from papules, which are larger, include a tuft of blood vessels, and resemble cobblestones [3]. Pain and photophobia are not typically associated with most instances of adenoviral conjunctivitis. Likewise, blurred vision that does not clear on blinking may be an indication that another diagnosis should be considered [2].

Treatment for most cases of viral conjunctivitis includes supportive care such as artificial tears and cold compresses. Topical decongestants and topical steroids (in consultation with an ophthalmologist) may be prescribed if the ocular edema is severe. Because viral conjunctivitis is usually a benign and self-limiting condition, there is a low likelihood of secondary bacterial infection. Topical antibiotics such as erythromycin are not necessary; however, it is not inappropriate to prescribe antibiotics if the diagnosis is difficult to discern from bacterial conjunctivitis. Fortunately, there is little harm in using topical antibiotics for viral conjunctivitis [4]. Adenovirus has been found to have a 95% replication rate at 10 days, which drops to 5% at 16 days. The patient should be instructed to practice frequent hand washing for 2 weeks and should be reminded that personal items that may come in contact with the eyes, such as towels, should not be shared [1]. In most cases, viral conjunctivitis can be managed on an outpatient basis with elective referral to an ophthalmologist if there is no improvement within 7 to 10 days [5].

Depending on the serotype of adenovirus, the clinical presentation may include more than just a mild follicular conjunctivitis. Of the 47 adenoviral serotypes, many have a predilection for other mucosal surfaces in addition to the bulbar and palpebral conjunctiva. These serotypes can cause a clinically significant infection in the respiratory, genitourinary, or gastrointestinal tracts as well; hence, adenoviral conjunctivitis may be isolated or a feature of a systemic viral syndrome. Two of the more common syndromes

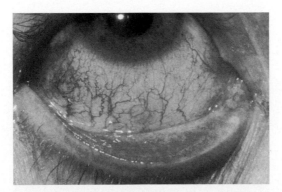

Fig. 1. Viral conjunctivitis. Note the global injection pattern. (*From* Boruchoff SA. Anterior segment disease: a diagnostic color atlas. Boston: Butterworth-Heinemann; 2001. p. 120; with permission.)

are pharyngoconjunctival fever and epidemic keratoconjunctivitis. Pharyngoconjunctival fever presents with an abrupt onset of high fever, pharyngitis, and bilateral follicular conjunctivitis. It is more common in children and can occur sporadically and in clusters. Schools during the winter and camps during the summer are common settings for this type of infection. Treatment is the same as for mild follicular conjunctivitis, with referral to ophthalmology if symptoms are unremitting after 1 week. Epidemic keratoconjunctivitis is frequently caused by serotypes 8, 19, and 37 and is associated with ocular pain and decreased visual acuity from corneal subepithelial infiltrates (Fig. 2). The infiltrates appear as 1- to 2-mm, grayish-white, "crumb-like" defects numbering up to 30 throughout the central and peripheral cornea. Visual acuity may drop by several lines on the Snellen chart. Edema, small petechial hemorrhages, and the formation of inflammatory pseudomembranes are other distinctive features of epidemic keratoconjunctivitis [3]. Treatment should consist of local care as outlined previously. Patients should receive follow-up with an ophthalmologist in 1 week to monitor for the development of keratitis, a complication of keratoconjunctivitis [6].

Herpes simplex virus (HSV) conjunctivitis is an example of another infection that may present as a conjunctivitis alone or as a more pervasive infection involving the cornea, eyelid, and skin. HSV conjunctivitis occurs at a higher rate in HIV-infected patients. This infection will usually present unilaterally and has many of the features of an adenovirus conjunctivitis, including a watery discharge and palpable preauricular nodes. Pain, burning, and a foreign body sensation associated with HSV conjunctivitis help distinguish it from most other forms of viral conjunctivitis. Other distinguishing features include episodic copious tearing and mildly decreased vision [3]. The first-line treatment for patients who have HSV conjunctivitis alone, without skin or corneal involvement, is cool compresses and topical antiviral medication for 10 to 14 days. Recommended medications are trifluridine 1% drops, five times per day, or vidarabine 3% ointment, five times

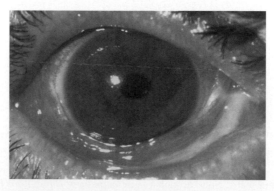

Fig. 2. Epidemic keratoconjunctivitis. (*From* Boruchoff SA. Anterior segment disease: a diagnostic color atlas. Boston: Butterworth-Heinemann; 2001. p. 132; with permission.)

per day. The patient should receive follow-up in 2 to 5 days to monitor for corneal involvement [7].

If HSV conjunctivitis also involves the skin (eg, HSV dermatitis of the eyelids) or is associated with photophobia or decreased vision, the clinician must be more aggressive with work-up and treatment. In these circumstances, corneal staining should be performed. On slit lamp examination, one may see pinpoint or dendritic lesions on the cornea using fluorescein staining and a cobalt blue light. The lesions may be confluent and geographic, or atypical. Classic skin findings include grouped pustules or vesicles on an erythematous base which progress to crusting. The patient may have a history of similar bouts of conjunctivitis, usually unilateral, suggesting remote HSV outbreaks. Stress, fever, trauma, or UV light can all trigger reactivation. In severe cases, uveitis, iritis, and increased intraocular pressure may be seen. Treatment consists of topical trifluridine 1% drops administered nine times per day and oral acyclovir, 400 mg orally five times daily for 7 to 10 days. If there is flare in the anterior chamber on slit lamp examination, one should consider the addition of a cycloplegic agent such as scopolamine 0.25% three times daily. The patient should undergo an ophthalmologic follow-up in 2 days to evaluate for response to treatment [7]. Steroids should not be prescribed for patients with HSV conjunctivitis because the risk for secondary infection and other complications from uncontrolled viral proliferation is increased [2].

Herpes zoster (HZV) ophthalmicus occurs when the varicella-zoster virus is reactivated in the ophthalmic division of the trigeminal nerve. This entity represents approximately 10% to 25% of all zoster cases. Although most cases of HZV ophthalmicus involve the skin only, serious ocular involvement can occur if the infection is reactivated in the nasociliary branch of the ophthalmic nerve (Fig. 3A, C). Herpes pustules at the tip of the nose (Hutchinson's sign) are thought to be a classic predictor of ocular involvement. Although patients with a positive Hutchinson's sign have twice the incidence of ocular involvement, one third of patients without the sign can experience ocular manifestations. A common complication of HZV infection is an injected and edematous conjunctiva, often with petechial hemorrhages. This conjunctivitis will usually resolve in 1 week unless secondary bacterial infection occurs. The use of topical antibiotics may help to prevent secondary infection, whereas cool compresses and lubrication drops can be used for comfort. In corneal involvement, HZV dendrites appear as a branching or "medusa-like" pattern with tapered ends in contrast to HSV dendrites, which often have terminal bulbs. This pattern can be viewed by Wood's lamp or slit lamp examination after fluorescein staining. These patients need preservative-free artificial tears every 1 to 2 hours and an ocular lubricant ointment nightly. An ophthalmologist should be consulted regarding systemic or topical antiviral agents; topical steroids are occasionally indicated depending on the ocular manifestations of HZV and should be prescribed only in consultation with ophthalmology [8].

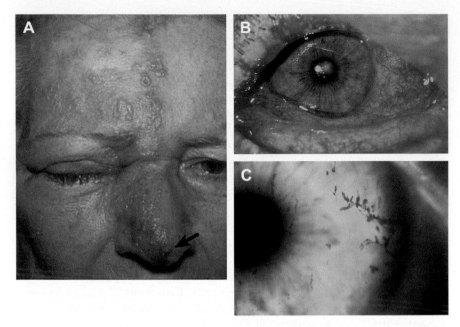

Fig. 3. (*A*) Herpes zoster in the distribution of the first division of the trigeminal nerve. Note the presence of Hutchinson's sign, a vesicle on the tip of the nose (*black arrow*). (*B*) Herpes zoster keratoconjunctivitis. (*C*) HZV dendrites have a "medusa-like" pattern. (*From* Boruchoff SA. Anterior segment disease: a diagnostic color atlas. Boston: Butterworth-Heinemann; 2001. p. 128–9; with permission.)

If the patient with HZV activation should have any ocular involvement, ophthalmologic follow-up should occur within 24 hours [8].

Bacterial conjunctivitis is a condition usually caused by gram-positive organisms, the most common being *Streptococcus pneumoniae* and *Staphylococcus aureus,* and gram-negative organisms such as *Haemophilus influenzae* [1]. The first two infections occur more often in children; the last afflicts mostly adults [2]. Bacterial conjunctivitis has a more abrupt onset than viral conjunctivitis and is also associated with tearing and ocular irritation. In bacterial conjunctivitis, the infection usually spreads to the contralateral eye within 48 hours [1]. The patient may complain of morning crusting and difficulty opening the eyelids [2]. This symptom results from a mucopurulent yellow-colored discharge that causes matting of the lids and lashes (Fig. 4). On examination, the red eye injection pattern of bacterial conjunctivitis is diffuse but often more pronounced at the fornices [1].

The definitive treatment for bacterial conjunctivitis is topical ophthalmic broad-spectrum antibiotics. Although it is usually a self-limiting disease, treatment shortens the course, reduces person-to-person spread, and lowers the risk of sight-threatening complications such as ulceration. Erythromycin and bacitracin/polymyxin B provide excellent broad-spectrum coverage against most pathogens found in adult and pediatric cases. Aminoglycosides

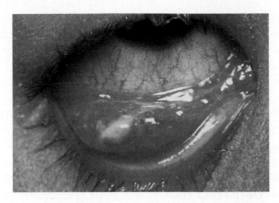

Fig. 4. Bacterial conjunctivitis. Note matting of the eyelashes caused by the mucoid and thick discharge. (*From* Boruchoff SA. Anterior segment disease: a diagnostic color atlas. Boston: Butterworth-Heinemann; 2001. p. 135; with permission.)

should not be used because they have relatively poor coverage of gram-positive organisms such as staphylococcus and streptococcus species. Ointment, which is less irritating, works best for children who also benefit from less frequent application and can tolerate the associated blurred vision well. Drops are recommended for adolescents and adults because they are easier to apply [2]. Most immunocompetent patients with uncomplicated cases of bacterial conjunctivitis should be seen in 3 to 4 days if there is no improvement in symptoms [9]. Bacterial conjunctivitis in young children or the debilitated should be managed conservatively and may need closer follow-up. It is wise to obtain cultures in these populations [2].

The contact lens user who has pain or redness should remove the lens immediately. After a work-up, if one suspects an infectious complication of contact lens use, the patient should discontinue lens wear. Smears and cultures, which are usually performed with ophthalmology consultation, should be obtained in patients who have an infectious corneal ulcer greater than 1 mm or when an unusual organism is suspected. Intensive antibiotic therapy should be initiated using topical fluoroquinolone, six to eight times per day, and a cycloplegic agent. The patient requires follow-up in 1 day [7].

Hyperacute conjunctivitis is a conjunctivitis caused by *Neisseria gonorrhoeae* and occurs most commonly in sexually active persons. Infection with *N meningitidis* is also known to cause hyperacute conjunctivitis but occurs less frequently and can only be differentiated from infection with *N gonorrhoeae* through laboratory testing. *N gonorrhoeae* is usually spread from genital-hand-eye contact in the young sexually active population, but neonates can acquire it from the birth canal. The infection will manifest in neonates 3 to 5 days postpartum with bilateral discharge [2].

Ocular *N gonorrhoeae* infection is abrupt in onset and produces copious amounts of purulent discharge that reforms quickly after wiping away. Marked conjunctival injection, conjunctival chemosis, lid swelling, globe tenderness through closed lids, and preauricular lymphadenopathy may all be found on physical examination (Fig. 5). Work-up should include immediate staining for gram-negative diplococci and special cultures for *Neisseria* sp. The infection may or may not be associated with a urethral discharge. In infants born to infected mothers, the infection may be localized to other organs (arthritis, meningitis, pneumonia) or may be disseminated (sepsis) [2].

Treatment for hyperacute conjunctivitis need not be complicated. The eye should be irrigated with saline solution. Selection of topical antibiotics is the same as for bacterial conjunctivitis. It is recommended that systemic antibiotics directed against *N gonorrhoeae* be initiated, because a large number of patients with *N gonorrhoeae* conjunctivitis also have concurrent venereal disease. Urgent referral is critical in *N gonorrhoeae* infection. In contrast to bacterial conjunctivitis, hyperacute conjunctivitis can have sight-threatening outcomes secondary to ulceration and perforation [2].

Ocular chlamydial infection leads to two forms of conjunctivitis depending on the serotype of the organism. Serotypes A through C cause trachoma, a chronic keratoconjunctivitis that is the most common form of preventable blindness in the world. Inclusion conjunctivitis is caused by serotypes D through K. Inclusion conjunctivitis is a common, primarily sexually transmitted disease that affects both newborns and adults. The incidence of inclusion conjunctivitis is higher than that of ocular *N gonorrhoeae* infection in newborns. Newborns acquire the infection in the birth canal and cervix and present with tearing, conjunctival inflammation, and eyelid swelling with moderate discharge starting from 5 to 12 days after birth. In adults, inclusion conjunctivitis is transmitted via genital secretions and may be a result of autoinoculation. The infection can be subacute or even chronic and is most common in young, sexually active persons aged 18 to 30 years. The adult patient will present with unilateral or bilateral redness, foreign body sensation, mucopurulent discharge, and preauricular adenopathy. Because as many as one half of affected adults will also have concurrent,

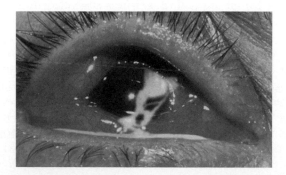

Fig. 5. Hyperacute conjunctivitis caused by *Neisseria* sp. Note the copious amounts of purulent discharge. (*From* Boruchoff SA. Anterior segment disease: a diagnostic color atlas. Boston: Butterworth-Heinemann; 2001. p. 136; with permission.)

possibly asymptomatic, cervical/urethral chlamydial infection, laboratory studies should be performed when inclusion conjunctivitis is suspected. A work-up for other sexually transmitted diseases such as syphilis and gonorrhea should also be considered because co-infection rates can be high [2].

In the adult, one should treat the sexual disease by prescribing azithromycin, 1 g orally for one dose, doxycycline, 100 mg orally twice daily, or erythromycin, 500 mg orally four times daily for 7 days for the patient and sexual partners. Topical erythromycin, tetracycline, or sulfacetamide ointment twice to three times daily for 2 to 3 weeks will help treat the ocular infection. Follow-up should be arranged with ophthalmology in 1 week [7]. In neonatal inclusion conjunctivitis, systemic antibiotics are commonly used in addition to topical antibiotics because this condition can be associated with otitis media and respiratory and gastrointestinal tract infections. Consultation with ophthalmology is essential because special cultures and stains may be required to direct treatment [2]. If no information regarding a specific organism is available during the initial visit, empiric therapy with erythromycin ointment four times daily and with erythromycin elixir, 50 mg/kg/d divided four times per day, may be initiated [7].

Chronic forms of conjunctivitis have many causes, such as contact lens use, prescription and over-the-counter eye drops, chlamydia, or molluscum contagiosum, as well as other less common causes. A history of collagen vascular disease or diuretic or antidepressant use raises the possibility of dry eyes as a cause of chronic conjunctivitis. Chronic unilateral conjunctivitis is a separate entity and has more causes. It presents a diagnostic dilemma even to the specialist. Possible diagnoses may include keratitis, nasolacrimal duct obstruction, occult foreign body, or ocular neoplasm. Referral is indicated in the case of chronic unilateral conjunctivitis [2].

Subconjunctival hemorrhage

Subconjunctival hemorrhage is caused by bleeding of the conjunctival or episcleral vessels deep to the conjunctiva into the subconjunctival space [10]. Subconjunctival hemorrhage can be spontaneous or related to trauma or systemic illness. When it is spontaneous, it is usually secondary to decreased lubrication of the eye [11].

The patient will usually present with a painless red eye that has no effect on his or her vision. It often causes alarm when the patient first notices it. There is no discharge associated with subconjunctival hemorrhage. The patient may recall a history of mild trauma or valsalva (such as coughing or vomiting). A history of anticoagulation therapy may also be elicited. The patient should be asked about a history of hypertension, diabetes, or any bleeding disorder because subconjunctival hemorrhage may be a presenting sign of any of these conditions [5].

On examination, subconjunctival hemorrhage appears as fresh red blood on a white sclera with clear borders and masks the conjunctival vessels

(Fig. 6). When evaluating a subconjunctival hemorrhage, one should consider staining the eye to rule out corneal injury if the history suggests it or if the patient has any type of pain associated with the subconjunctival hemorrhage [1]. If the subconjunctival hemorrhage is large and the injury occurred in the setting of trauma, there may be penetrating injury to the globe (globe rupture) that is obscured by the hemorrhage, requiring emergency ophthalmology consultation [7]. For minor subconjunctival hemorrhages, patient education and reassurance are the mainstays of treatment, and these patients do not need ophthalmology referral. Prescribing warm compresses and lubrication drops may help reduce recovery by 1 to 3 days. A high-profile subconjunctival hemorrhage will take approximately 10 to 14 days to resolve [1].

Episcleritis

The episclera is a thin membrane that covers the sclera and lies beneath the conjunctiva. Episcleritis is generally a benign inflammatory condition that involves only the superficial episcleral tissue and not the deep episcleral tissue that overlies the sclera. Most cases are idiopathic in nature and are commonly seen in young adults [12,13]. Episcleritis can be associated with systemic diseases such as rheumatoid arthritis, polyarteritis nodosa, systemic lupus erythematosus (SLE), inflammatory bowel disease, sarcoidosis, Wegener's granulomatosis, gout, HZV, or syphilis [13].

Episcleritis is usually characterized by a rapid onset of redness that may be associated with a feeling of grittiness and a dull headache. Vision is unaffected, and discharge, if present, is usually watery. On examination,

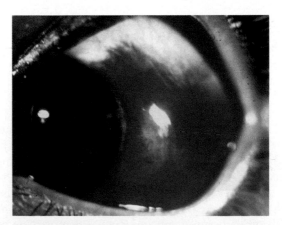

Fig. 6. Subconjunctival hemorrhage. The extravasated blood has completely obscured the sclera underneath. Note the slightly raised appearance of the affected area. (*From* Boruchoff SA. Anterior segment disease: a diagnostic color atlas. Boston: Butterworth-Heinemann; 2001. p. 147; with permission.)

focal areas of redness are usually observed rather than a diffuse process. White sclera may be seen between radially coursing dilated episcleral vessels [5]. The conjunctival and superficial episcleral vessels can be seen displaced outward from the sclera while the underlying deep episcleral plexus is not involved and lies flat against normal scleral tissue. This appearance is best observed using red-free light on slit lamp examination. Nodular episcleritis occurs with the presence of a tender scleral nodule and generally is more uncomfortable than simple episcleritis with a more prolonged course (Fig. 7). The engorgement of the superficial episcleral plexus gives the eye a distinct red or salmon hue, and there may be tenderness on palpation [12].

This condition is usually self-limiting and will resolve within 2 to 3 weeks even without intervention. Treatment may involve oral NSAIDs and should be referred electively to an ophthalmologist for outpatient evaluation. Topical anti-inflammatory agents and lubricants may also be helpful, but steroids should only be prescribed after consultation with an ophthalmologist [5,13].

Scleritis

Scleritis is defined as an inflammation of the sclera that may involve the cornea, adjacent episclera, and underlying uvea. The maximal involvement in scleritis is the deep episcleral plexus, which is displaced outward by the edematous swollen sclera. The classification of scleritis can be divided into anterior and posterior. Anterior scleritis is further subdivided into diffuse, nodular, or necrotizing. Diffuse anterior scleritis is characterized by extensive scleral edema and congestion of the scleral vessels with poorly defined margins. Nodular anterior scleritis is characterized by focal, often multiple well-defined nodules of scleral edema and congestion of scleral vessels distinct from its overlying inflamed episclera. Necrotizing anterior scleritis is

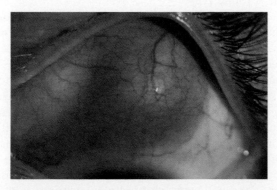

Fig. 7. Nodular episcleritis. Note the focal area of redness and dilated blood vessels. (*From* Boruchoff SA. Anterior segment disease: a diagnostic color atlas. Boston: Butterworth-Heinemann; 2001. p. 183; with permission.)

characterized by an avascular area of scleral necrosis and often by significant inflammation of the surrounding sclera. The sclera surrounding the
necrosis may also be devoid of any prominent inflammation, which is
seen in scleromalacia perforans, often associated with rheumatoid arthritis.
Posterior scleritis is characterized by involvement of the sclera posterior to
the insertion of the rectus muscles and may occur in association with anterior scleritis or in isolation [12].

Although most cases of scleritis are immune mediated, the disease can
also be triggered by infection, surgery, malignancy, or drugs. Approximately
39% to 50% of the cases are associated with a systemic disorder. The resulting scleral inflammation may be in part or completely secondary to the
immune-mediated response. A large number of connective tissue disorders
are associated with scleral disease; the most common is rheumatoid arthritis.
Wegener's granulomatosis is the most common vasculitis associated with
this condition. Other causes include relapsing polychondritis, SLE, polyarteritis nodosa, Reiter's syndrome, inflammatory bowel disease, and progressive systemic sclerosis. Approximately 5% to 10% of anterior scleritis is
infectious owing to viral, bacterial, fungal, or parasitic agents. Infectious
scleritis is more likely in the presence of infectious keratitis. Infectious scleritis should be suspected in patients with a history of accidental trauma,
ocular surgical procedures, or recurrent attacks of HSV or varicella-zoster
virus. Herpes zoster ophthalmicus was found in one review to be the most
common infectious cause of scleritis. Other common causes are syphilis, mil-
iary tuberculosis, HSV, *Pseudomonas aeruginosa*, Epstein-Barr virus, and
Coxsackie B5. A history of surgery has been shown to be a risk factor for
bacterial causes of scleritis. For instance, a patient with pterygium removal
may present months to years after surgery with bacterial scleritis, most often
owing to *Pseudomonas aeruginosa*. When a bacterial scleritis leads to a pyo-
genic infection, it can be a therapeutic challenge due to the avascularity of
the sclera. Fungal infections may remain undiagnosed for a long time before
the exact cause is found [12].

Patients who present with scleritis either already have a known underlying systemic disorder such as rheumatoid arthritis or present de novo. Scleritis may also be the sole initial presenting feature of a systemic disease, most
commonly rheumatoid arthritis [14]. Scleritis usually occurs in white, middle-aged women with a mean age of onset of 49 years, and female patients
account for 71% of all cases. The characteristic feature of scleritis is severe
pain that may involve the eye and orbit and radiate to the ear, scalp, face,
and jaw. It is usually dull, boring, and can be so severe that it often awakes
the patient from sleep or causes significant impairment in their daily activ-
ities. It may often be confused with other causes of headache, such as giant
cell arteritis, migraines, cerebral aneurysm, tic douloureux, and tumor [12].
It can also be associated with photophobia, tearing, and with pain on
accommodation [14]. Mild analgesics will often not relieve the pain,
although some patients may present with little or no discomfort due to

the use of NSAIDs before presentation. Patients who have posterior scleritis may present with reduced vision with or without pain [12].

Many features on the physical examination will aid in making the diagnosis. The redness may be focal or diffuse, unilateral or bilateral, and present with tenderness to palpation of the globe. Nodular anterior scleritis is characterized by a localized area of scleral edema in which distinct nodules reside. Nodules may be single or multiple and are tender to palpation. In scleritis, the vascular engorgement of the deep episcleral plexus gives the eye a characteristic bluish-violet discoloration, and the deep scleral vessels will not blanch in response to vasoconstrictor agents such as 2.5% to 10% phenylephrine or 1:1000 epinephrine (Fig. 8). This characteristic is in contrast to the blanching seen with conjunctival and superficial vessels in conjunctivitis and episcleritis [12]. The hallmark of scleritis is the presence of scleral edema and congestion of the scleral plexus, which may involve the superficial and deep vascular coats. In scleritis, the vascular architecture of the superficial episcleral plexus is disrupted by the presence of irregularly oriented vessels. In episcleritis, only the superficial episcleral plexus is congested, and its radial configuration is preserved. Avascular areas strongly imply the diagnosis of necrotizing scleritis. Slit lamp examination using red-free light is helpful in characterizing the pattern and depth of episcleral vascular engorgement. The sclera will often be edematous and may cause the slit lamp light beam to be displaced forward in the area of maximal swelling. Anterior uveitis, peripheral choroiditis with or without retinal detachment, uveal effusion, or disk edema can all be seen with posterior extension of scleritis and are not seen with episcleritis [14]. In isolated posterior scleritis, the eye may be white, but sometimes inflamed posterior sclera can be visualized in the extremes of gaze. Because there may be a paucity of physical examination findings, imaging is often necessary to make the diagnosis. Posterior scleritis can be delineated using B-scan ultrasonography and high-definition orbital MRI [12].

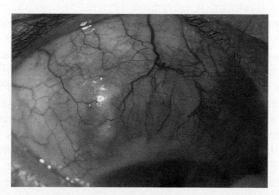

Fig. 8. Dilation of the deep episcleral vessels and a bluish discoloration of the eye in a patient with scleritis. (*From* Boruchoff SA. Anterior segment disease: a diagnostic color atlas. Boston: Butterworth-Heinemann; 2001. p. 183; with permission.)

In acute presentations of scleritis, blood work may include a complete blood count, electrolytes, tests of renal function, assays for acute phase reactants such as C-reactive protein, and evaluation of the erythrocyte sedimentation rate, and serologic testing to rule out and determine the degree of associated systemic conditions may be performed [12,14]. In cases of suspected infectious scleritis, serologies and conjunctival scrapings for smears and cultures are often obtained. If these tests are negative after 48 hours and the scleritis continues to progress, scleral or corneoscleral biopsy is essential. Tests may include rapid plasma reagin and microhemagglutination-*Treponema pallidum* in cases of suspected syphilis. A positive c-ANCA in a patient with scleritis is specific for Wegener's granulomatosis. Assays for rheumatoid factor for rheumatoid arthritis and for anti-nuclear antibody suggestive of SLE, rheumatoid arthritis, polymyositis, progressive systemic sclerosis, or mixed connective tissue diseases should also be performed. Ultrasonography, an orbital CT scan, fluorescein angiography, and high-definition orbital MRI may be required to confirm the diagnosis and to assess the extent of disease [14]. Although these tests are generally not done in the emergency room setting, the consulting ophthalmologist and primary care physician should be involved in expediting the work-up and delineating the etiology.

Making this diagnosis early is important owing to associated serious complications. In a study of 358 patients with scleritis, decreased vision occurred in 37%, anterior uveitis was present in 42%, peripheral ulcerative keratitis in 14%, glaucoma in 13%, and cataracts in 17%. Elevated intraocular pressure can develop in any patient with any type of scleritis, with the rate of glaucoma ranging from 9% to 22% in anterior scleritis. Greater visual loss is generally seen in patients with systemic disease, especially in rheumatoid arthritis, and is found to be independent of corneal complications and cataracts. Necrotizing scleritis also results in greater visual loss than in the non-necrotizing form [14].

The goal of treatment is to remove or treat the underlying cause but, most importantly, to control the inflammatory process and therefore reduce damage to the eye. Patients with posterior or necrotizing scleritis need more intensive and urgent therapy than patients with anterior non-necrotizing disease. Any scleritis associated with an underlying systemic disease usually requires more aggressive immunosuppressive therapy. Approximately one third of patients with anterior scleritis will respond to NSAIDs, one third to systemic corticosteroids, and the other third to more aggressive systemic immunosuppression [14]. The diagnosis of scleritis calls for a prompt referral to an ophthalmologist and initiation of an oral NSAID initially. Further management including topical or oral corticosteroids, other immunosuppressive agents, and possible surgical intervention should be done in conjunction with the primary care physician and ophthalmologist [12]. When timely outpatient evaluation is not possible or treatment is more urgent, admission may be required.

Uveitis

Uveitis can be defined as an inflammation of the iris (iritis), ciliary body (cyclitis), and choroid (choroiditis). Anterior uveitis, often called iridocyclitis, involves inflammation of the anterior portion of the uveal tract and usually affects young or middle-aged persons. Posterior uveitis includes vitritis, choroiditis, retinitis, chorioretinitis, or retinochoroiditis. Panuveitis or diffuse uveitis are the terms used to characterize both anterior and posterior involvement. There are multiple causes of uveitis, but uveitis can generally be characterized as inflammatory, traumatic, or infectious. Uveitis has been shown to be associated with the histocompatability antigen HLA B-27. In the United States and England, 30% to 70% of patients with anterior uveitis have this antigen. About half of these patients have an associated systemic disease such as ankylosing spondylitis, psoriatic arthritis, reactive arthritis, or inflammatory bowel disease. Many other systemic diseases may present with uveitis, including sarcoidosis, juvenile idiopathic arthritis, Behçet disease, Kawasaki disease, multiple sclerosis, and Wegener's granulomatosis [15].

Although infection is an uncommon cause of uveitis, it is important to rule it out before instituting immunosuppressive therapy. Parasitic (eg, toxoplasmosis), viral (cytomegalovirus, herpes viruses), bacterial (tuberculosis, Lyme disease), and treponemal (syphilis) agents could be responsible. Toxoplasmosis is a common cause of retinochoroiditis in normal and immunosuppressed patients and is responsible for as many as 25% of occurrences of posterior uveitis in the United States. Cytomegalovirus can cause posterior uveitis in immunocompromised individuals, particular in AIDS patients, but its incidence has decreased in the United States since antiretroviral therapy has become available. Tuberculosis was once the most common cause of choroiditis but is now found in less than 1% of all cases in the United States. Syphilis can cause both anterior and posterior uveitis, usually during the secondary or tertiary stages of infection. Traumatic iritis is commonly seen in the emergency department and is usually secondary to a direct blow from a blunt object [15].

Anterior uveitis often presents suddenly with a red and painful eye. Photophobia and conjunctival injection are often seen; sometimes blurred vision is present [1]. Patients generally complain of a deep aching pain that may radiate to the periorbital or temple area. It is worse with eye movement and during accommodation. On examination, hyperemia is prominent adjacent to the limbus (perilimbal or circumcorneal injection), in contrast to that seen in conjunctivitis in which inflammation tends be more prominent at a distance from the limbus (Fig. 9). Tearing may be present, but no purulent discharge is seen [16]. Generally, the pupil is constricted, may be irregular, and is sluggish in response to light in comparison with the uninvolved eye. On pupillary examination, the patient may have direct photophobia when light is directed into the affected eye, as well as consensual photophobia when light is shone on the unaffected eye. Consensual

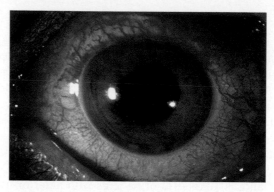

Fig. 9. Anterior uveitis. Note the perilimbal injection and the irregularly shaped pupil. (*Courtesy of* the University of Michigan Kellogg Eye Center, Ann Arbor, Michigan; with permission.)

photophobia can be a helpful distinguishing feature of anterior uveitis because it is not seen in other superficial causes of photophobia [1].

Posterior uveitis can cause "floaters" and visual changes but generally does not cause redness or significant pain. When the retina is involved, patients may complain of blind spots or flashing lights [15].

The diagnosis of uveitis is often confirmed by the presence of inflammatory cells and a proteinaceous flare in the anterior or posterior chambers of the eye on slit lamp examination. If inflammation is severe, leukocytes can settle in the anterior chamber and form a hypopyon, a white or yellowish accumulation of purulent material. This accumulation can sometimes be visible without the aid of magnification [5]. On slit lamp examination, deposits of white blood cells on the endothelium (keratitic precipitates) are often visualized, which is a hallmark of iritis. Small-to-medium keratitic precipitates are classified as nongranulomatous, whereas granulomatous (eg, sarcoid) keratitic precipitates are large [16]. Infectious uveitis can be difficult to diagnose and usually requires specific findings on a detailed ophthalmologic examination, specific serology testing, or, after uveitis, does not respond to anti-inflammatory therapy [15]. The diagnostic evaluation in patients suspected to have a systemic condition requires further testing. Patients with pulmonary complaints should undergo chest radiography or CT or both to assess for possible sarcoidosis. Radiographic images of the sacroiliac joints and HLA-B27 typing are helpful when considering a spondyloarthropathy as a diagnosis. Colonoscopy should be done in patients with gastrointestinal symptoms or heme-positive stools to assess for inflammatory bowel disease [15]. These tests rarely need to be done in the emergency room or inpatient setting as long as an expedited outpatient work-up can be performed.

Uveitis is best managed in collaboration with an ophthalmologist. Initiation of therapy in a timely fashion is critical because of the severe sight-threatening complications associated with uveitis, including cataracts, glaucoma, and retinal detachment. Corticosteroids are the mainstay of therapy in treating noninfectious causes [15]. Topical corticosteroids (eg, prednisolone acetate 1%) are used in anterior uveitis but are not helpful in posterior uveitis owing to poor penetration. This treatment may worsen this condition if there is a concern of an infectious etiology; therefore, it should only be prescribed after appropriate consultation with an ophthalmologist. Although cataracts can occur secondary to the inflammatory process, they are also a recognized complication of corticosteroids [15]. Mydriatic and cycloplegic agents are also often prescribed. Mydriatics (eg, phenylephrine HCl, hydroxyamphetamine HBr) are sympathomimetic agents used to prevent the formation of synechiae by pupillary dilation. A synechia is an adhesion where the iris adheres to either the cornea or lens. Although synechiae rarely cause visual problems, they can lead to secondary glaucoma. Parasympatholytic agents (eg, atropine sulfate, homatropine, cyclopentolate) produce both mydriasis and cycloplegia which block nerve impulses to the pupillary sphincter and ciliary muscle, reducing pain and photophobia [16]. Systemic corticosteroid therapy is usually reserved for bilateral disease that is refractory to local medication or for patients with significant ocular disability or retinitis. Other immunosuppressive medications may be used in steroid-dependent or refractory uveitis. In general, management of uncomplicated noninfectious uveitis can be done on an outpatient basis, but follow-up with an ophthalmologist should be arranged within 24 hours. Refractory cases or those secondary to an infectious cause often require admission and further diagnostic tests. Patients with suspected posterior uveitis who present with floaters or visual changes need urgent ophthalmology consultation [15].

Acute angle-closure glaucoma

AACG is a condition that develops when the peripheral tissue of the iris blocks the outflow of fluid from the anterior chamber, resulting in elevated intraocular pressure [1]. Mydriasis, such as in the low-light evening hours, can often worsen the condition as the accordion-like folds of the iris gather together into folds that cause obstruction. Mydriatic medications, systemic anticholinergics (eg, antihistamines or antipsychotics), and accommodation (ie, reading) can also cause pupillary block [7]. The patient with AACG will usually present with severe ocular pain, redness, a decrease in vision, and a pupil in mid-dilation [1]. Blurred vision, seeing halos around lights, and headache with nausea and vomiting may also be a part of the clinical presentation. Acute attacks may be self-limited and resolve spontaneously or may occur repeatedly. Patients who are elderly or far-sighted are at the highest risk for AACG because of enlargement of their lenses [7]. Because there are several other causes of a non-traumatic acute increase in intraocular pressure, such as glaucomatocyclitic crisis, inflammatory open-angle glaucoma, pigmentary glaucoma, and mechanical and postsurgical closure, the work-up should include a thorough history (family history, retinal problems, recent laser treatment or surgery, medications), a slit lamp examination, and measurement of intraocular pressure [7].

On physical examination, AACG will usually present with a global injection pattern. There may be tearing but no other discharge. Corneal edema may make the cornea appear "steamy" or "hazy." On slit lamp examination, there may be keratitic precipitates, anterior chamber cells and flare, posterior synechiae, and a shallow anterior chamber. A fundoscopic examination that reveals optic nerve cupping indicates the need for urgent treatment. Perhaps the most important feature is that, on penlight examination, the pupil will be mid-dilated and nonreactive (Fig. 10A, B). If the pupil reacts, the diagnosis should be reconsidered [1]. Normal intraocular pressure is less than 21 mm Hg. Patients with glaucoma have an intraocular pressure greater than that, and those with an intraocular pressure greater than 30 mm Hg require prompt treatment. Most emergency departments are fitted with at least one instrument to allow measurement of intraocular pressure. The emergency physician should be familiar with the tools available in his or her workplace. The most common instruments used in the emergency department for measuring intraocular pressure are the tonopen and Schiotz tonometer. Goldmann tonometry (applanation) may also be used. Other instruments include the MacKay-Marg tonometer. If infection is suspected, the clinician should be certain to use a sterile tip when using a contact tonometer. A simple and direct method to measure intraocular pressure is to gently press the globe through the eyelid while the patient is instructed to look down; the experienced practitioner may note differences in the "hardness" of one globe when compared with the other. Unfortunately, this method requires experience to gain accuracy, and most emergency physicians should use this only as a rough estimate [17].

Treatment for AACG mandates prompt and rapid transfer to an eye specialist. In the emergency department, 1 drop of 0.5% timolol can be administered, followed by another drop 5 minutes later. Topical steroids, such as 1%

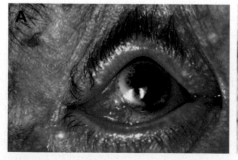
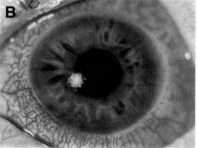

Fig. 10. (*A, B*) Acute angle-closure glaucoma. These close-ups reveal a global injection, a "hazy" appearance to the pupil, and a loss of iris structure. (Panel A is *from* Dayan M, Turner B, McGhee C. Lesson of the week: acute angle closure glaucoma masquerading as systemic illness. BMJ 1996;313:413–5; with permission; and Panel B is *from* Thiel R. Atlas of diseases of the eye, vol. I. New York: Elsevier; 1963. p. 255; with permission.)

prednisolone acetate, should be given every 15 to 30 minutes for four doses and then hourly [7]. Also, 1% topical apraclonidine or 0.15% or 0.2% topical brimonidine should be given for one dose [7]. Acetazolamide, a carbonic anhydrase inhibitor, can be given at a dose of 500 mg orally to help decrease the production of fluid. In cases of phakic pupillary block (in which there is a native, natural lens), pilocarpine, 1% to 2%, can be administered every 15 minutes for 2 minutes [7]. If vision has been compromised to detection of hand motion or worse, all topical medications not contraindicated, intravenous acetazolamide, and intravenous hyperosmotic fluid (such as mannitol) should be administered. Systemic symptoms such as pain and vomiting should be treated as appropriate with intravenous or oral medications. Definitive treatment includes peripheral iridotomy performed by either laser or incision. The fellow eye should receive a prophylactic iridotomy based on anatomy, because approximately one half of fellow eyes in patients with acute angle-closure will sustain acute attacks within 5 years [18]. The specialist may choose to delay definitive treatment until the inflammation has subsided.

Failure to recognize and treat AACG can result in excessive intraocular pressures that can damage the optic nerve and lead to visual loss. When evaluating a patient with migraine headache, it is prudent to document an eye examination and pupil reactivity because AACG can mimic migraine headache. One article highlights three cases in which the diagnosis of AACG was delayed or missed due to several factors that hindered appropriate and thorough evaluation. When patients are elderly, have disabilities such as dementia, deafness, or limited mobility, or have concurrent psychiatric or medical conditions, a thorough and directed history and physical (ie, using a slit lamp) may be problematic and challenging. In these cases, a high index of suspicion and a diligent work-up must be pursued when the presentation includes red eye, blurred vision, or headache [19].

Summary

The acutely red eye is a common complaint in the emergency department. Although most causes are benign and self-limiting, appropriate work-up and treatment can identify serious conditions and prevent significant morbidity such as blindness. As outlined herein, the emergency physician should obtain a relevant history and perform a thorough examination using the slit lamp and measurement of intraocular pressures when appropriate.

In general, patients who present with severe ocular pain, acute visual changes, corneal opacification, hypopyon, or blurred disk margins in the setting of a red eye warrant an aggressive search for serious causes and urgent ophthalmology referral. Topical analgesics should never be prescribed [5], and topical steroids should be initiated only after ophthalmology consultation. If the clinical presentation is concerning for scleritis and AACG, urgent consultation with the specialist for confirmation of diagnosis and initial management is recommended. Gonococcal conjunctivitis and posterior

Table 1
Common clinical findings in the acute red eye

Diagnoses	Pain	hyperemia	Foreign body sensation	Discharge	Itching	Photophobia	Onset	Pupil	Cornea	Vision	Threat to vision	Timing of consultation
Episcleritis	No	Focal	No	Tearing	No	No	Rapid	Not affected	Clear	Not affected	No	Electively
Scleritis	Yes	Focal or diffuse	No	No	No	Yes	Progressive	Not affected	Occasional peripheral opacity	Not affected	Yes	Urgent
Uveitis	Yes	Diffuse, perilimbal	No	Watery, minimal	No	Yes	Sudden	Constricted, sluggish to light	May be hazy	Blurred	Yes	Within 24 hours
Allergic conjunctivitis	No	Diffuse, toward fornices	Yes	Watery to mucoid	Yes	No	Progressive	Not affected	Clear	Not affected	No	Electively
Viral conjunctivitis	No[a]	Diffuse, toward fornices	Yes	Watery and clear	Mild	No[a]	Sudden with rapid progression	Not affected	Clear	Not affected	No[a]	Electively
Bacterial conjunctivitis	No	Diffuse, toward fornices	Yes	Mucopurulent	Mild	No	Sudden	Not affected	Clear	Not affected	No	Usually elective
Subconjunctival hemorrhage	No	Focal or diffuse	No	No	No	No	Acute	Not affected	Clear	Not affected	No	Usually elective
Acute angle-closure glaucoma	Yes	Diffuse, perilimbal	No	Tearing	No	Yes	Sudden, usually in evening	Mid-dilated, nonreactive	Hazy	Blurred, halos around lights	Yes	Urgent

[a] Can occur in patients with herpes zoster ophthalmicus.

uveitis associated with floaters also represent serious, sight-threatening conditions and similarly require urgent ophthalmology evaluation. Expeditious follow-up with the specialist will help ensure that the patient has as little permanent damage to their vision as possible. With this is mind, one should remember that most causes of red eye in the emergency department are self-limiting and can be treated supportively. In general, patients with benign etiologies may receive follow-up from their primary care physician or the ophthalmologist electively to monitor for treatment effectiveness and for complications. The key clinical features and the urgency of consultation for the various diseases are outlined in Table 1.

References

[1] Roscoe M, Landis T. How to diagnose the acute red eye with confidence. JAAPA 2006 2003;19(3)24–30.
[2] Morrow GL, Abbott RL. Conjunctivitis. Am Fam Physician 1998;57(4):735–46.
[3] Weber CM, Eichenbaum JW. Acute red eye: differentiating viral conjunctivitis from other, less common causes. Postgrad Med 1997;101(5):185–9.
[4] Hara JH. The red eye: diagnosis and treatment. Am Fam Physician 1996;54(8):2423–30.
[5] Leibowitz HM. The red eye. N Engl J Med 2000;343:345–51.
[6] Wirbelauer C. Management of the red eye for the primary care physician. Am J Med 2006; 119:302–6.
[7] Kunimoto DY, Kanitkar KD, Makar MS, editors. The Wills eye manual: office and emergency room diagnosis and treatment of eye disease. 4th edition. Philadelphia: Lippincott Williams & Wilkins; 2004. p. 61, 71, 91, 94, 98, 155, 179–81.
[8] Shaikh S, Ta CN. Evaluation and management of herpes zoster ophthalmicus. Am Fam Physician 2002;66(9):1723–30.
[9] Prepared by the American Academy of Ophthalmology Cornea/External Disease Panel Cornea/External Disease Panel Members. American Academy of Ophthalmology. Conjunctivitis, preferred practice pattern. San Francisco (CA): American Academy of Ophthalmology; 2003. Available at: www.aao.org/ppp. Accessed August 11, 2007.
[10] Roy FH. The red eye. Ann Ophthalmol 2006;38(1):35–8.
[11] Walling AD. Tips from other journals: when is red eye not just conjunctivitis? Am Fam Physician 2002;66(12):2299–300.
[12] Okhravi N, Odufuwa B, McCluskey P, et al. Scleritis. Surv Ophthalmol 2005;50(4):351–63.
[13] Sowka JW, Gurwood AS, Kabat AG. Episcleritis. Handbook of ocular disease management web site 2000. Available at: http://www.revoptom.com/HANDBOOK/sect2f.htm. Accessed August 4, 2007.
[14] Albini TA, Rao NA, Smith RE. The diagnosis and management of anterior scleritis. Int Ophthalmol Clin 2005;45(2):191–204.
[15] Hajj-Ali RA, Lowder C, Mandell BF. Uveitis in the internist's office: are a patient's eye symptoms serious? Cleve Clin J Med 2005;72(4):329–39.
[16] Nishimoto JY. Iritis. How to recognize and manage a potentially sight-threatening disease. Postgrad Med 1996;99(2):255–62.
[17] Knoop KJ, Dennis WR. Ophthalmologic procedures. In: Roberts JR, Hedges JR, editors. Clinical procedures in emergency medicine. 4th edition. Philadelphia: Saunders; 2004. p. 1241–79.
[18] American Academy of Ophthalmology. Primary angle closure, preferred practice pattern web site 2005. Available at: www.aao.org/ppp. Accessed August 5, 2007.
[19] Gordon-Bennett P, Ung T, Stephenson C, et al. Misdiagnosis of angle closure glaucoma. BMJ 2006;333(7579):1157–8.

ELSEVIER
SAUNDERS

Emerg Med Clin N Am
26 (2008) 57–72

EMERGENCY
MEDICINE
CLINICS OF
NORTH AMERICA

Ocular Infection and Inflammation

Jorma B. Mueller, MD[a],
Christopher M. McStay, MD[b],*

[a]*Emergency Medicine Residency, New York University/Bellevue Hospital Center,
462 First Avenue, New York, NY 10016, USA*
[b]*Department of Emergency Medicine, New York University/Bellevue Hospital Center,
462 First Avenue, New York, NY 10016, USA*

Managing the inflamed or infected eye in the emergency setting presents a diagnostic and therapeutic challenge to the emergency physician; the causes and prognoses range from benign, self-limited illness to organ-threatening pathology. A careful history, with attention to comorbid illnesses and time course, is paramount, as is knowledge of the complete ophthalmologic examination. Much of the organ morbidity is ameliorated with prompt therapy in the emergency department (ED) and by initiating ophthalmologic consultation.

Conjunctivitis

Inflammation of the bulbar (covering the globe of the eye) and tarsal (lining the orbit) conjunctiva can be caused by viral or bacterial infections, trauma, toxic exposure, or autoimmune disease. Patients will complain of redness, pruritis, and a foreign body sensation that is often associated with discharge. Awakening in the morning with eye crusting is a common complaint. Photophobia and visual loss should not be present. Physical examination will reveal injection of the conjunctiva associated with lid edema. Discharge may be scant or may range from stringy and fibrinous to copious and purulent. If bacterial conjunctivitis is expected, gram stain and culture of the discharge is often revealing and can guide initiation of therapy. Most conjunctivitis seen in the ED is of viral origin and is self limited. However, the emergency practitioner should be familiar with all causes because the clinical course of conjunctivitis can lead to significant morbidity, depending on the cause.

---

* Corresponding author.
E-mail address: chris.mcstay@med.nyu.edu (C.M. McStay).

0733-8627/08/$ - see front matter © 2008 Elsevier Inc. All rights reserved.
doi:10.1016/j.emc.2007.10.004   *emed.theclinics.com*

Viral conjunctivitis

Most cases of viral conjunctivitis are caused by adenoviridae, but entero-viruses and coxsackievirus may also be implicated. Conjunctivitis of viral origin is associated with significant redness and pruritis but should have less discharge than bacterial conjunctivitis. Chemosis and soft tissue swelling may be dramatic. The presence of preauricular lymphadenopathy, conjunc-tivitis, and a viral prodrome are classic and frequently present. Disease often becomes bilateral in the first 24 to 48 hours [1,2].

Viral conjunctivitis is contagious for almost 2 weeks; patients, family, and caretakers should be educated in appropriate infection-preventing measures, including hand washing. Treatment is symptomatic, with artificial tears, cold compresses, and vasoconstrictor-antihistamine combinations for severe pruritis.

Fever, lymphadenopathy, and conjunctivitis with concomitant pharyngi-tis constitute pharyngoconjunctival fever, caused by certain strains of adeno-viridae. It can have a prolonged course (up to 2 weeks) and resolves spontaneously. Preceding upper respiratory infection supports this diagnosis.

Epidemic keratoconjunctivitis is also caused by strains of adenoviridae (usually adenovirus type 8). It generally presents with thicker discharge and punctuate keratitis (corneal inflammation seen on fluorescein staining), and may result in conjunctival membrane formation with scarring. It has an even longer clinical course (up to 3 weeks) and corneal opacities may persist for months afterwards, affecting vision but ultimately resolving [1,2]. Consul-tation with an ophthalmologist is recommended to decide whether steroids are indicated based on the presence and extent of the corneal involvement (Fig. 1).

Bacterial conjunctivitis

The pathogens most commonly associated with bacterial conjunctivitis include staphylococci, streptococci, *N gonorrohae*, and *C trachomatis*. In

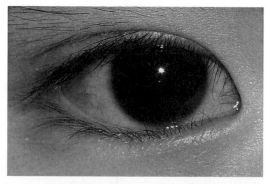

Fig. 1. Conjunctivitis in Kawasaki disease. (*Courtesy of* Christopher McStay, MD, New York, NY.)

contrast to viral conjunctivitis, discharge may be purulent, and crusting marked, typically with less pruritis. Patients who have bacterial pathogens may be more likely to report eye crusting that impedes opening each morning [3]. The process is more likely to be unilateral, but bilateral involvement does not rule out a bacterial cause. Acuity should be preserved and photophobia absent; presence of either photophobia or decreased visual acuity should raise concern for corneal involvement. In this setting, the practitioner should look for signs of keratoconjunctivitis on slit lamp examination. Corneal involvement portends a worse clinical course and is an indication for ophthalmologic consultation within the ED. Corneal opacification or hypopyon may indicate a keratitis, which could be vision threatening.

If a bacterial pathogen is suspected, treatment with topical drops (eg, quinolone, trimethoprim-polymyxin) should be initiated for 7 to 10 days. Erythromycin ointment may also be used and is preferred in pediatrics for easier compliance. In contact lens wearers, pseudomonal coverage is essential and a quinolone is first line. Most cases of bacterial conjunctivitis resolve spontaneously in a week to 10 days, but antibiotics limit the duration and severity of disease [4]. Delaying antibiotic therapy (by 1–3 days) while awaiting gram stain and culture results appears to cause little harm and may reduce inappropriate antibiotic usage [5]. Ophthalmologic or ED follow-up can be given, with antibiotic choice tailored to culture results. Supportive care, including warm compresses and eye irrigation, are also indicated and are of equal importance. Eye patching should be avoided.

A fulminant course of conjunctivitis in a young, sexually active patient or a neonate (24–48 hours postpartum) should raise the possibility of *N gonorrhae* as the causative organism (Fig. 2). Discharge is often thick, yellowish green, and associated with significant underlying chemosis. Concomitant and symptomatic genitourinary symptoms may be present, but their absence does not rule out the diagnosis. Untreated, corneal involvement leading to rupture and endophthalmitis can ultimately occur. The decision as to

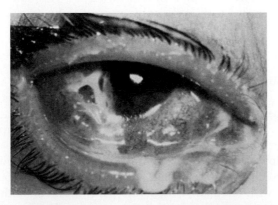

Fig. 2. Fulminant gonococcal conjunctivitis. (*From* Goldman L, Ausiello D, editors. Cecil textbook of medicine. 22nd edition. Philadelphia: Saunders (an imprint of Elsevier); 2004; with permission.)

whether to treat for gonococcal conjunctivitis is based on the history, fulminant course, and gram stain (chocolate agar cultures should also be sent). The practitioner should ask about sexual practices, partners, and symptoms [6]. Treatment is typically more aggressive, and hospital admission for intravenous and topical antibiotics may be warranted. For milder cases, one gram of ceftriaxone intramuscularly and appropriate coverage for concomitant Chlamydia infections (doxycycline or azithromycin) is indicated, in addition to ophthalmic antibiotics (bacitracin, erythromycin ointment). The high risk of corneal involvement warrants daily ophthalmologic follow-up. Sexual partners should seek appropriate medical care.

Neonatal conjunctivitis

In the neonatal period, conjunctivitis can occur and the causes are closely linked with postpartum age at presentation. Conjunctivitis in the first 36 hours postpartum is often chemically induced, caused by silver nitrate used to prevent maternal transmission of gonococcus, Chlamydia, and other bacteria. Almost all infants treated with silver nitrate will develop a transient conjunctivitis that resolves in 1 to 2 days. Silver nitrate drops have largely been replaced by topical erythromycin in the United States. Neonatal symptoms occurring 24 to 48 hours postpartum are often due to *N gonorrhoeae* and should be treated with intravenous penicillin, or intramuscular ceftriaxone or cefotaxime, in addition to saline washes. Topical antibiotics are also indicated; penicillin or erythromycin ointment should be used every 2 hours while discharge persists. Blood cultures and cerebrospinal fluid gram stain and culture are also recommended but are controversial. These patients should also be treated for concomitant Chlamydia infection [7]. Other bacterial causes often occur on days 2 through 5 postpartum and treatment should be guided by gram stain (erythromycin ointment for gram-positive organisms, gentamicin or tobramycin drops for gram-negative organisms). Chlamydial conjunctivitis often occurs on days 5 through 12 postpartum and should be treated with oral erythromycin for 2 weeks.

Episcleritis

Inflammation of the episclera and sclera may be difficult to distinguish. Because their causes and prognoses differ considerably, it is important to differentiate between the two. Both have significant association with systemic disease, so primary care or ophthalmologic follow-up is indicated, based on patient comorbidities and severity of symptoms.

Inflammation of the episclera, generally a benign, self-limited condition, presents as acute redness, tearing, pruritis, and foreign body sensation ("grittiness"), with minimal-to-moderate pain in one or both eyes. It typically occurs in young adults and may be recurrent. Examination will reveal dilated episcleral vessels and an overall injected appearance. The differential diagnosis also includes conjunctivitis, scleritis, keratitis, and glaucoma. A slit lamp examination should also be performed to rule out other common causes of ocular inflammation. A true change in acuity should prompt the clinician to consider other causes.

To differentiate episcleritis from conjunctivitis, topical anesthetic should be applied and, under slit lamp, the ocular surface probed with a cotton-tipped applicator. Conjunctival vessels will be highly mobile, whereas episcleral vessels should remain relatively fixed. In contrast to conjunctivitis, the findings are generally limited to one segment of the bulbar surface. Conjunctival involvement may also occur in episcleritis but should be focal [8,9]. The episcleral vessels should also blanch with application of a topical vasoconstrictor, which will help the clinician differentiate between episcleritis and scleritis.

Distribution of the findings may be simple or nodular. In simple disease, sectoral involvement of the episclera is generally seen, with only part of the episclera involved. Nodular densities with surrounding injection of the sclera vessels appear in nodular episcleritis.

Episcleritis is of idiopathic origin in two thirds of cases and generally improves after a week or so. Supportive treatment includes the use of artificial tears. The use of topical corticosteroids and nonsteroidal anti-inflammatory drugs has been suggested but both are controversial. A recent study found the duration and severity of symptoms the same with topical ketorolac and artificial tears. Patients treated with ketorolac were more likely to complain of stinging [10]. If treatment has failed by 2 weeks, ophthalmologic referral is indicated. In one third of cases, systemic disease is present. Evaluation for connective tissue, autoimmune vascular, or rheumatoid (more common in nodular subtypes) disease may be indicated. Rosacea and atopy are also commonly associated with episcleritis.

Inflammation of the sclera itself has a more insidious onset, more pronounced pain, and a greater number of complications and systemic associations (Fig. 3). It is most often idiopathic in origin, but patients may

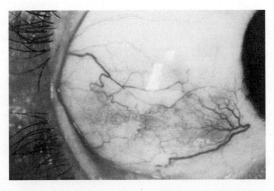

Fig. 3. Scleritis. (*From* Sen HN, Suhler EB, Al-Khatib SQ, et al. Mycophenolate mofetil for the treatment of scleritis. Ophthalmol 2003;110(9):1750–5; with permission.)

give a history of recent eye surgery, infection, new malignancy, or new drug therapy. Patients may describe the onset of progressive pain and visual deterioration over the course of days to weeks. Pain may radiate from the eye to the face and may be intense and boring in nature. Photophobia, tearing, and pain with ocular motion may be present. Patients may notice marked scleral swelling and globe tenderness if the anterior sclera is involved. On examination, swelling may be focal and limited to one part of the globe or may involve the entire visible sclera. The overlying episcleral and conjunctival vessels may be dilated and inflamed, making the diagnosis difficult. Engorgement of vessels with a surrounding violaceous hue is indicative of scleritis. Topical vasoconstrictors will blanch the conjunctival and episcleral vessels, but the sclera itself should remain swollen and inflamed. Findings adjacent to the cornea may also show a keratitis. Areas of necrosis should raise the possibility of an infectious cause of scleritis, including tuberculosis. Necrotizing scleritis will also reveal areas of capillary nonperfusion and represents an immediate threat to globe integrity [8,9].

In patients who do not have involvement of the anterior sclera, posterior scleritis is easily missed. Patients may have similar presenting symptoms and may also have proptosis. Alternatively, patients may present with minimal pain, complaining only of visual loss in a rare variant of necrotizing posterior scleritis. Concomitant, secondary uveitis, either anterior or posterior, is not uncommon and the ED practitioner can easily be fooled into thinking this is the primary diagnosis. Retinal detachment or other retinal pathology may also accompany posterior scleritis, but the painful nature of the condition should initiate a more thorough workup. Diagnosis by ultrasound is preferred. CT with intravenous contrast may be helpful in these cases and can show a thickened scleral component. MRI is also useful but is not routinely available in the ED [8,9,11].

One half of all cases of scleritis are associated with systemic disease. The most commonly associated disease is rheumatoid arthritis. Other associations include Wegener's granulomatosis, relapsing polychondritis, systemic lupus erythematosus, and polyarteritis nodosa. Workup for these conditions can begin in the ED or with the patient's primary care provider. All patients should have screening tests for syphilis. Tuberculosis and Hansen's disease can also cause a granulomatous scleritis.

Complications of scleritis include necrosis, scleral thinning, and visual loss. Treatment with oral indomethacin is the standard of care in patients who have active anterior scleritis. Necrotizing or posterior scleritis should be treated in concert with ophthalmologic consultation; treatment should include systemic and intraocular steroid injection. If disease is mild, with no tenting of the sclera, and with no secondary iritis or uveitis, treatment can be deferred, with close ophthalmologic follow-up. If an infectious cause is suspected (postsurgical patients, necrosis, immunocompromised hosts), treatment decisions should be made with an ophthalmologic consultant.

Antibiotic penetration into the sclera is generally poor, owing to its avascular nature [8,9].

Keratitis

Inflammation of the cornea with or without violation of its epithelium constitutes keratitis. Patients will present with an acutely red, painful eye and often complain of foreign body sensation, photophobia, tearing, and vision change. Infectious causes may be associated with secondary lid edema, conjunctival reaction, hypopyon, and anterior chamber reaction. Photophobia is due to ciliary spasm. Keratitis is most often viral or bacterial in origin, but exposure to intense ultraviolet light, chemicals, and contact lenses may be implicated. Contact lens use itself imparts a 10-fold risk of developing an infectious keratitis. Corneal abrasions may accompany (or mimic) a keratitis because of excessive rubbing or scratching of the affected eye. Prompt diagnosis, treatment, and identification of cause are paramount to prevent vision loss due to ulceration, necrosis, and scarring [12,13].

Patients should receive a full ophthalmologic examination. The presence of corneal opacification, ulceration, hypopyon, or other irregularities strengthen the diagnosis. Fluorescein staining is essential to evaluate for epithelial disruption, and its pattern can also help reveal the cause.

Viral keratitis

The herpesviridae (herpes simplex virus [HSV]-1, HSV-2, varicella zoster virus [VZV], Epstein-Barr virus [EBV], cytomegalovirus [CMV]) are the viral agents most commonly associated with keratitis. Their clinical presentations and treatments have considerable overlap.

HSV can present with ocular involvement in primary or recurrent infections. Primary infections often occur in neonates (by way of maternal delivery with active lesions) or at 6 months of age (by way of saliva), when maternal antibodies no longer protect the infant from HSV transmission. A follicular conjunctivitis with the presence of lid or periorbital vesicles should alert the clinician to HSV infection. Slit lamp examination may show staining of the cornea in a dendritic pattern. Ophthalmologic antivirals and systemic antivirals (acyclovir) should be initiated promptly. Corneal involvement may lag behind and persist after conjunctival and dermatologic involvement.

Most HSV pathology is caused by recurrent disease and may present without dermatologic findings. Patients may complain simply of eye pain, redness, and change in vision. Slit lamp examination should reveal a corneal ulcer with fluorescein uptake in a characteristic dendritic branching pattern that extends outward. Sometimes, the ulcer alone may stain with fluorescein, without staining of the advancing dendritic cells. In these cases, ophthalmologic consultation for rose bengal or other dye staining will reveal the pattern. Advanced or recurrent disease may lead to stromal (subepithelial corneal matrix) involvement with opacification, thinning, and edema present on slit lamp examination [14].

The cornea should be debrided of infected cells using a cotton applicator, starting with the ulcer. This procedure can be done by the ED practitioner or, preferably, by the ophthalmologic consultant. Pharmacologic treatment of HSV keratitis consists of ophthalmic antiviral drops (acyclovir or idoxuridine) or systemic antiviral medication (oral acyclovir). ED ophthalmologic consultation is indicated and close follow-up or admission is appropriate. Topical drops may be associated with corneal toxicity and could prolong healing, so some clinicians prefer oral agents. Some research suggests that topical ganciclovir gel may also be effective. Daily ophthalmologic follow-up or admission is indicated (Fig. 4) [14,15].

Reactivation of herpes zoster virus in the trigeminal distribution can cause significant ocular disease, including a keratitis. Zoster is often preceded by a viral prodrome of malaise, fever, headache, and neuralgia. Ocular and periorbital disease can then follow, with the conjunctiva, lid, and periorbital skin showing crops of vesicular lesions. The rash is typically unilateral, does not cross the midline, and involves only the upper portion of the lid. The presence of vesicular lesions on the tip of the nose (nasociliary branch of the ophthalmic division of trigeminal V1), or Hutchinson's sign, should prompt the clinician to evaluate the cornea for involvement. Disease can be marked and conjunctival vesicles with scarring can occur [16].

Corneal involvement usually occurs after other manifestations and may present after other symptoms have resolved, or separately from them. Fluorescein staining will reveal dendritic branching that is thicker and more rope-like than the lace-like pattern of HSV keratitis. Terminal bulbs, present in HSV keratitis, should be absent in VZV. Fluorescein uptake is much less pronounced on the VZV dendrites, so inspection under slit lamp must be

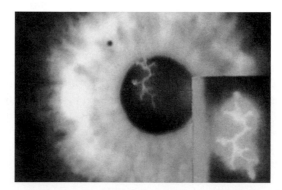

Fig. 4. HSV keratitis with characteristic dendritic pattern of staining. (*From* Goldman L, Ausiello D, editors. Cecil textbook of medicine. 22nd edition. Philadelphia: Saunders (an imprint of Elsevier); 2004; with permission.)

careful so as to avoid missing the lesions. Complications include uveitis and keratitis (even bacterial coinfection). Ophthalmologic consultation is indicated to start oral versus topical antivirals. Steroids are controversial and should not be started by the emergency practitioner [15,16].

EBV and CMV can also cause a keratitis, but this is much more likely in the immunocompromised host. A dendritic corneal branching pattern is often seen with EBV and the conjunctiva and soft tissue may be affected as in HSV infection. Diagnosis is made by way of polymerase chain reaction of infected cells. Supportive care is indicated; the use of systemic antivirals is controversial. In the ED, where it will be difficult to distinguish cause, starting the patient on oral acyclovir may be appropriate. CMV keratitis has been reported but is uncommon. Its corneal findings are almost identical to VZV [17].

Bacterial keratitis

The propensity to cause visual loss makes bacterial keratitis an ophthalmologic emergency. Its incidence is increasing in the setting of contact lens use. Most cases are caused by staphylococcal species, but in contact lens wearers, pseudomonas species may predominate. Both organisms have increased because of contact lens use; in the non–contact lens wearer, streptococcal species are common. In immunocompromised patients, *Moraxella catarrhalis* should be considered. Patients will complain of pain, tearing, and decreased vision. *N gonorrohae* and *C trachomatis* should be considered in the sexually active patient, particularly if conjunctivitis is present. Depending on the causative organism and the condition of the underlying cornea, physical examination may reveal a corneal ulcer, with or without surrounding stromal involvement. The overlying epithelium may be absent. The cornea will often be opacified and edematous, and hypopyon may be present. The surrounding conjunctiva may show injection with vessel dilatation [18].

Topical aminoglycosides, quinolones, or cephalosporins should be used, based on history and gram stain. If gram stain is unavailable or the causative organism is unlikely to be discovered in the ED, broad-spectrum coverage using two antibiotics should be initiated with rapid alternating of agent (eg, two drops aminoglycoside followed by two drops of cephalosporin every 5 minutes for the first hour followed by applications every 15 minutes to 1 hour around the clock). Alternatively, quinolone monotherapy may be effective. ED ophthalmologic consultation should be obtained and the patient admitted [18].

Keratitis due to light exposure

Prolonged exposure to ultraviolet light, or brief exposure to intense ultraviolet flashes, can produce a photokeratitis or photokeratoconjunctivitis of noninfectious origin. Patients may complain of eye pain, change in vision, and redness. The staining pattern is generally punctuated with some degree of corneal opacification. Ancillary signs of infection (purulent discharge, cellulitic changes) are generally absent. In punctuate keratitis due to welding exposure, symptoms begin hours after exposure. In patients who have had prolonged ultraviolet exposure (ie, snow blindness), time to onset may be variable [19]. Topical antibiotics are indicated to prevent bacterial superinfection.

Uveitis

Understanding the anatomy of the uvea is essential in diagnosing and treating the different forms of uveitis. The uvea is the middle eye. Anteriorly, this includes the iris and ciliary body, with the posterior reflection of these structures known as the choroid. Inflammation of the anterior structures presents with anterior chamber reaction and is easily seen and diagnosed in the ED. Inflammation of the anterior chamber (anterior uveitis) is a much more common presentation in the ED than middle or posterior involvement. Posterior involvement is synonymous with retinitis. Inflammation of the uveal structures can be a primary, idiopathic process, or can occur secondary to other ophthalmologic infections or inflammatory conditions.

Anterior uveitis

Patients who have anterior uveitis (commonly called iritis) can present with a remarkable range of complaints, from mild visual disturbance to severe pain and loss of vision. Approximately 50% of cases are considered idiopathic and the next most common cause is thought to be HLA-B27 associated. Patients typically present with eye pain, redness, decreased vision, photophobia, and headache. The symptoms may mimic glaucoma, which must be ruled out first by measuring intraocular pressure. When present, scleral injection and anterior chamber cells and flare make the diagnosis clear. The limbus is characteristically injected (known as ciliary flush) and the pupil is often constricted. In idiopathic anterior uveitis, small keratic precipitates may be present in the anterior chamber. Larger, granulomatous or clumpy precipitates should lead the physician to consider specific causes, including syphilis, toxoplasmosis, and tuberculosis. Hypopyon, when present, should prompt the clinician to think of HLA-B27–associated disease, and referral to a rheumatologist is appropriate [20].

In patients who have HIV, the antibiotic rifabutin and the antiviral cidofovir should be considered as possible causes. Both have been associated with anterior uveitis, and withdrawal of the drug, or reduction of the dose, is often enough to stop or reduce symptoms [21]. Anterior chamber reaction can also be secondary to many of the other conditions discussed in this article, including scleritis, episcleritis, and posterior segment disease. Autoimmune diseases, such as sarcoidosis, are also associated with anterior chamber reactions (Fig. 5).

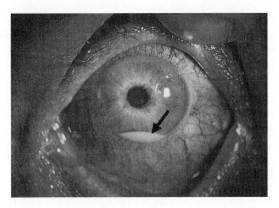

Fig. 5. Acute anterior uveitis with hypopyon (*arrow*). (*From* Munoz-Fernandez S, Martin-Mola E. Uveitis. Best Pract Res Cl Rh 2006;20(3):487–505; with permission.)

The ED workup will be dictated by the patient presentation. Individuals with only mild complaints without visual disturbance could be referred for ophthalmology follow-up. Those who have acute onset and severe symptoms may require more thorough testing in the ED, including chest radiography, angiotensin-converting enzyme, and syphilis and tuberculosis testing.

The common treatment for uncomplicated anterior uveitis is topical corticosteroid drops, which could potentially be started from the ED in conjunction with ophthalmology consultation. The addition of scopolamine or cyclopentolate drops may help decrease the pain associated with ciliary spasm. Disease that does not improve, or worsens, in the setting of steroid treatment should alert the practitioner to an infectious cause, particularly tuberculosis.

Intermediate uveitis

Patients who have blurry vision or floaters, mild pain, and redness but without elevated intraocular pressure or anterior chamber findings may have intermediate uveitis. Intermediate uveitis comprises inflammation of the anterior vitreous humor, the peripheral retina, or the pars plana ciliaris (the posterior aspect of the ciliary body). Examination will reveal anterior vitreous floaters and inflammatory cells, absence of anterior chamber cells, and snowbank-like exudates heaped at the inferior pars plana (in patients who have pars planitis). The diagnosis of pars planitis may be difficult to make because most ED practitioners are not familiar with scleral depression, which may be required to see the heaped exudates. Concomitant macular edema, cataract formation, or retinal detachment are the most common complications, in descending frequency. Disease is often bilateral and presents in patients in the first half of life; presentation in the elderly should raise the specter of human T-cell lymphoma virus–associated disease.

The association of uveitis with systemic disease should prompt investigation based on patient age and comorbidities. All patients who have not been evaluated for sarcoidosis should receive a chest radiograph as a screening test. Screening for syphilis is recommended. Its association with multiple sclerosis and Lyme disease has been documented. Still, most cases are idiopathic in origin.

Treatment should be initiated in concert with ophthalmologic consultation, and includes intraocular and systemic corticosteroids. Further ophthalmologic treatment is beyond the scope of the emergency physician.

Posterior uveitis and retinitis

Posterior uveitis and retinitis can be thought of interchangeably. The ED practitioner should be aware of the causes of acute retinitis. For the purposes of this article, retinitis pigmentosa and other slowly progressive causes of retinal deterioration are not discussed.

In the immunocompromised host (eg, patients who have AIDS, or who are on chemotherapy or receiving immunosuppressive treatment), progressive, painless vision loss should alert the practitioner to the possibility of CMV-induced retinitis. Patients may also complain of floaters and light flashes. CMV retinitis is a marker of profound immune suppression and rarely presents in AIDS patients unless the CD4 count is very low, but occasionally is the presenting symptoms of undiagnosed HIV infection [22]. Examination will generally reveal a necrotic retinitis with whitening. Hemorrhages may be present at the advancing edge of the lesion. Other causative organisms should be considered in the immunocompromised patient, including tuberculosis, toxoplasmosis, syphilis, and other herpesviridae. In the immunocompromised patient who has suspected CMV retinitis, acute or subacute visual loss does not preclude the diagnosis because retinal detachment is a well-described complication. Diagnosis of CMV retinitis warrants hospital admission and initiation of treatment with ganciclovir.

HSV and VZV can also cause a retinitis. Their pattern of retinal involvement and clinical presentation vary, depending on the host's immune status. In the immunocompromised host, HSV and VZV cause a rapidly progressive retinal necrosis without evidence of vasculitis and with minimal vitreous inflammatory changes. The pattern of retinal necrosis may be patchy and it may begin at the periphery, making diagnosis difficult for the ED practitioner. These viruses can also cause an acute retinal necrosis in the immunocompetent patient, with a marked vitritis and with a retinal vasculitic appearance. Eventually, retinal detachment occurs. Treatment for both is with intravenous acyclovir [23].

Hordeolum and chalazion

Patients who present complaining of acute onset of pain, focal swelling, and lid edema should be evaluated for hordeolum. A hordeolum represents

purulent infection of a cilium and adjacent gland with local abscess formation. They can be either present at the lid margin or contained in the lid itself. The resulting abscess can point toward either the mucosa (internal) or
the skin (external surface). They will generally swell and then ultimately resolve on their own within a week. Staphylococcal species are the most common causative organism. Cellulitis may accompany the hordeolum.
Treatment is conservative, with warm compresses several times a day for
10 minutes. If this fails, an incision and drainage may be performed.
Some sources cite the need for topical antibiotics to prevent local complications, but their use is controversial.

Chalazions are granulomatous inflammatory lesions present on the lid
that occur from obstruction of a sebaceous gland (Fig. 6) [24]. They may
arise acutely or persist and recur after initial formation. Clinically, they
are often indistinguishable from hordeolum and there is little reason to separate them. Indeed, a hordeolum may occur acutely in the setting of a chalazion. They may resolve spontaneously, similar to a hordeolum, with
a more sebaceous, waxy drainage. Recurrent chalazions need ophthalmologic referral for biopsy and evaluation for malignant origin [24].

Dacryocystitis

Acute infection of the lacrimal sac will present as pain, swelling, and erythema overlying the sac. Dacryocystitis is the result of obstruction of the
nasolacrimal duct and resultant purulent infection. Staphylococcal species
are the most common causative organisms. It is managed conservatively
initially with warm compresses and massage of the infected sac to encour-
age drainage of purulent material through the puncta. Oral and topical
antistaphylococcal antibiotics are also indicated. Prompt ophthalmologic

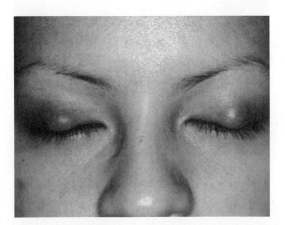

Fig. 6. Bilateral chalazion. (*From* Goldman L, Ausiello D, editors. Cecil textbook of medicine.
22nd edition. Philadelphia: Saunders (an imprint of Elsevier); 2004; with permission.)

140

MUELLER & MCSTAY

follow-up is indicated to evaluate for response to therapy. Patients who have signs of systemic illness should be hospitalized (Fig. 7).

In cases of impending rupture, incision and drainage are indicated, which, in the ED, should be done by an ophthalmologist, if possible. Aspiration with a high-gauge needle before incision and drainage should be performed and sent for culture. Incision and drainage is then performed in a vertical fashion, and purulent contents curetted. Prompt ophthalmologic referral is then indicated for follow-up and potential surgical intervention [24]. Acute dacryocystitis may progress to periorbital or orbital cellulites, depending on direction of spread and host factors. These patients should be managed as outlined in the next section.

Periorbital and orbital cellulitis

Infection of the periorbital and orbital soft tissues may represent extension of a primary infection, or may accompany other ocular pathology. Superficial anterior infection, with involvement limited by the ocular fascia, presents as upper or lower lid edema, pain, and warmth. Patients may have systemic symptoms (eg, fever), but change in vision should be absent and the pupil examination and intraocular pressures normal. Ocular range of motion should be essentially intact, with little pain. Treatment is with antistaphylococcal antibiotics, and selected cases may be managed in the outpatient setting. Amoxicillin-clavulanate or a suitable cephalosporin may be used (eg, cefpodoxime) [24,25].

Involvement of the orbital soft tissues is much more serious, with significant chance of permanent ocular damage and potentially fatal infectious consequences. Patients will present with marked swelling, pain, and edema,

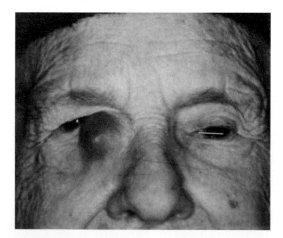

Fig. 7. Acute dacryocystitis. (*From* Goldman L, Ausiello D, editors. Cecil textbook of medicine. 22nd edition. Philadelphia: Saunders (an imprint of Elsevier); 2004; with permission.)

but symptoms will be more pronounced. Proptosis may be present, and the eye may exhibit an afferent papillary defect. Extraocular motion may be either limited or associated with pain. Intraocular pressure may be elevated because of external compression. CT is indicated to aid in diagnosis and to evaluate for abscess or soft tissue extension. Periorbital swelling should be evident on CT, and contrast enhancement may aid in abscess identification.

Most cases of orbital cellulitis represent an extension of sinusitis. Staphylococcal species are the most common pathogen, but other gram-positive organisms should be considered when starting antibiotics. Pseudomonas should also be considered in recently hospitalized, instrumented, or immunocompromised patients. The remaining cases are caused by primary infection of the lid or face, or by a foreign body. A recent case series in the pediatric population showed increasing presence of methicillin-resistant *Staphylococcus aureus* in orbital cellulitis, so vancomycin should be considered [24–26].

Ophthalmologic consultation and admission is indicated for cases of orbital cellulitis. The presence of proptosis, a dilated pupil, or vision loss portends a worse clinical course. Sinus drainage is often performed. Other complications, including cavernous sinus thrombosis and meningitis, have been described.

References

[1] Rubenstein JB, Jick SL. Cornea and external disease. In: Yanoff M, Duker JS, editors. Yanoff opthalmology. 2nd edition. Philadelphia: Mosby; 2004. p. 398–404.
[2] Kaufman HE. Treatment of viral diseases of the cornea and external eye. Prog Retin Eye Res 2000;19(1):69–85.
[3] Rietveld RP, ter Riet G, Bindels PJ, et al. Predicting bacterial cause in infectious conjunctivitis: cohort study on informativeness of combinations of signs and symptoms. BMJ 2004; 329:206–10.
[4] Sheikh A, Hurwitz B. Antibiotics versus placebo for acute bacterial conjunctivitis. Cochrane Database Syst Rev; 2006.
[5] Everitt HA, Little PS, Smith PW. A randomised controlled trial of management strategies for acute infective conjunctivitis in general practice. BMJ 2006;333:321–4.
[6] Wan WL, Farkas GC, May WN, et al. The clinical characteristics and course of adult gonococcal conjunctivitis. Am J Ophthalmol 1986;102:575–83.
[7] Woods CR. Gonococcal infections in neonates and young children. Semin Pediatr Infect Dis 2005;16(4):258–70.
[8] Jabs DA, Mudun A, Dunn JP, et al. Episcleritis and scleritis: clinical features and treatment results. Am J Ophthalmol 2000;130:469–76.
[9] Okhravi N, Odufuwa B, McCluskey P, et al. Scleritis. Surv Ophthalmol 2005;50:351–63.
[10] Williams CP, Browning AC, Sleep TJ, et al. A randomised, double-blind trial of topical ketorolac vs artificial tears for the treatment of episcleritis. Eye 2005;19:739–42.
[11] McCluskey PJ, Watson PG, Lightman S, et al. Posterior scleritis: clinical features, systemic associations, and outcome in a large series of patients. Ophthalmology 1999;106:2380–6.
[12] Keay L, Edwards K, Naduvilath T, et al. Microbial keratitis: predisposing factors and morbidity. Ophthalmology 2006;113:109–16.
[13] Titiyal JS, Negi S, Anand A, et al. Risk factors for perforation in microbial corneal ulcers in north India. Br J Ophthalmol 2006;90:686–9.

[14] Kaye S, Choudhary A. Herpes simplex keratitis. Prog Retin Eye Res 2006;25:355–80.
[15] Tabbara KF. Treatment of herpetic keratitis. Ophthalmology 2005;112:1640–1.
[16] Shaikh S, Ta CN. Evaluation and management of herpes zoster ophthalmicus. Am Fam Physician 2002;66(9):1723–30.
[17] McLeod SD. Infectious keratitis. In: Yanoff M, Duker JS, editors. Yanoff ophthalmology. 2nd edition. Philadelphia: Mosby; 2004. p. 466–91.
[18] Thomas PA, Geraldine P. Infectious keratitis. Curr Opin Infec Dis 2007;20(2):129–41.
[19] Cullen AP. Photokeratitis and other phototoxic effects on the cornea and conjunctiva. Int J Toxicol 2002;21(6):455–64.
[20] Gutteridge IF, Hall AJ. Acute anterior uveitis in primary care. Clinical Exp Optom 2007;90(2), 70–82.
[21] Bhagat N, Read RW, Rao NA, et al. Rifabutin-associated hypopyon uveitis in human immunodeficiency virus–negative immunocompetent individuals. Ophthalmology 2001; 108:750–2.
[22] Pertel P, Hirschtick R, Phair J, et al. Risk of developing cytomegalovirus retinitis in persons infected with the human immunodeficiency virus. J Acquir Immune Defic Syndr 1992;5: 1069–74.
[23] Ganatra JB, Chandler D, Santos C, et al. Viral causes of acute retinal necrosis syndrome. Am J Ophthalmol 2000;129:166–72.
[24] Wald ER. Periorbital and orbital infections. Pediatr Rev 2004;25(9):312–20.
[25] Starkey CR, Steele RW. Medical management of orbital cellulitis. Pediatr Infect Dis J 2001; 20:1002–5.
[26] McKinley SH, Yen MT, Miller AM, et al. Microbiology of pediatric orbital cellulitis. Am J Ophthalmol; 2007;144(4):497–501.

ELSEVIER
SAUNDERS

Emerg Med Clin N Am
26 (2008) 73–96

EMERGENCY
MEDICINE
CLINICS OF
NORTH AMERICA

Acute Monocular Visual Loss

Michael Vortmann, MD, Jeffrey I. Schneider, MD*

*Department of Emergency Medicine, Boston University School of Medicine, Boston Medical
Center, Dowling 1 South, 1 Boston Medical Center Place, Boston, MA 02118, USA*

Temporal arteritis

Temporal arteritis is a medium- and large-vessel vasculitis that affects the extracranial branches of the carotid artery. Its presentation can vary from that of a chronic headache to sudden monocular loss of vision. Confirmation of the diagnosis requires a temporal artery biopsy and the cornerstone of treatment is the administration of high-dose steroids. Sudden loss of vision attributable to temporal arteritis constitutes an ophthalmologic emergency; prompt recognition of the disorder and institution of therapy can prevent further vision loss in the affected eye or new visual deficits in the contralateral eye.

Epidemiology

Temporal arteritis is the most common primary vasculitis among the elderly with an annual incidence of approximately 18 per 100,000 in people older than 50 years. Peak incidence occurs between 70 and 80 years of age with a 2:1 female to male ratio. Of those affected, 88% are white [1]. Certain human leukocyte antigen (HLA) types have been found to entail an increased risk for developing temporal arteritis [2]. Although discussion of the relationship between temporal arteritis and polymyalgia rheumatica is beyond the scope of this article, individuals who have these same HLA types are at an increased risk for developing both of these disorders [2,3].

Etiology

Although the exact inciting event of temporal arteritis is poorly understood, and no causal relationship has been established, there is some evidence that infection may play a role, specifically parvovirus B19,

---

* Corresponding author.

E-mail address: jeffrey.schneider@bmc.org (J.I. Schneider).

0733-8627/08/$ - see front matter © 2008 Elsevier Inc. All rights reserved.
doi:10.1016/j.emc.2007.11.005   *emed.theclinics.com*

Mycoplasma pneumoniae, and *Chlamydia pneumoniae* [4,5]. CD4 cells, responding to an unknown antigen, migrate through all three layers of the affected artery and initiate an inflammatory cascade. This inflammation causes a reactive proliferation of the intimal layer of the artery, with resulting narrowing of the arterial lumen and ischemia distal to the lesion [6]. The occlusion of end-arteries to the eye, scalp, tongue, and muscles of mastication causes the blindness, jaw and tongue claudication, and scalp ischemia associated with the disease. The inflammation also produces cytokines, which are believed to be responsible for the frequent low-grade fever and constitutional symptoms, such as anorexia, malaise, and weight loss, that are often associated with the disease [7]. Thrombotic occlusion of the arteries, however, does not seem to play a role in the pathogenesis. Granulomatous inflammation forms giant cells in the classic pathologic lesion and gives the disease its alternate name, giant cell arteritis [6].

Clinical features

The most common clinical manifestation of temporal arteritis is headache, seen in two thirds of patients and generally located in the area of the temporal or occipital arteries [8,9]. Systemic symptoms, such as low grade fever, chills, malaise, anorexia, and weight loss, are present in one half of patients [8,10]. Other associated symptoms include jaw claudication, tongue pain, and mandibular pain [10]. Visual complaints are also common with partial or complete vision loss in one or both eyes occurring in up to 20% of patients as a presenting symptom of disease [9–12]. Amaurosis fugax precedes vision loss in 44% of affected individuals; diplopia and visual hallucinations are less common, but may also precede vision loss [11–13]. Thirty percent of patients have neurologic manifestations that may include mononeuropathies, peripheral polyneuropathies, and occasionally TIAs or strokes [14,15].

Physical examination should include temporal and occipital artery palpation searching for nodular or firm, tender arteries with overlying erythema. Joint examination may reveal polyarticular pain with movement or synovitis, especially of the shoulders and hip. This finding may suggest polymyalgia rheumatica, which is associated with temporal arteritis [16]. The eye examination should include visual acuity, assessment of pupils for an afferent pupillary defect, and a funduscopic examination to evaluate the retina and optic disks [17]. Typical funduscopic findings in those who have visual loss from temporal arteritis include pallor and edema of the optic disk with scattered cotton-wool patches and small hemorrhages (Fig. 1) [18]. Laboratory evaluation may reveal elevated C-reactive protein and erythrocyte sedimentation rate (ESR), a normocytic anemia, and a reactive thrombocytopenia. One may also see mild elevations in the liver enzymes [16].

A 2002 meta-analysis [19] that included 41 studies and more than 2600 patients evaluated the accuracy of history, physical examination, and ESR

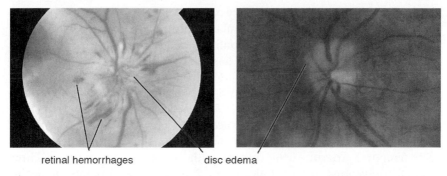

retinal hemorrhages   disc edema

Fig. 1. Giant cell arteritis. (*From* Kaiser PK, Friedman NJ, Pineda R, II. The Massachusetts Eye and Ear Infirmary illustrated manual of ophthalmology. 2nd edition. China: Saunders; 2004; with permission.)

in predicting a diagnosis of temporal arteritis. The only two historical features found to appreciably increase the likelihood of temporal arteritis were jaw claudication and diplopia. Other visual symptoms, including monocular vision loss, were not found to be helpful in distinguishing temporal arteritis from other causes of sudden vision loss.

On physical examination, the presence of any abnormality of the temporal artery (beading, prominence, tenderness) was most predictive of temporal arteritis. Conversely, the absence of any of these findings reduced the likelihood of the diagnosis substantially. Evidence of optic atrophy or any funduscopic abnormality was not helpful in establishing or eliminating the diagnosis, because the end result of retinal ischemia is common to many causes of sudden vision loss [19].

A normal ESR, defined as age in years divided by 2 for men, and age in years plus 10 divided by 2 for women, conferred a negative likelihood ration of 0.2. Any ESR of less than 50 conferred a reduced probability of having the disease. An ESR greater than 100, although increasing the likelihood of temporal arteritis, was less predictive than the previously described historical features and physical examination findings. Similarly, the mean ESR for patients who had biopsy-negative and biopsy-positive temporal arteries was not statistically different. CRP was not evaluated in the meta-analysis. Other laboratory abnormalities, such as anemia, were not helpful in distinguishing those who had temporal arteritis [19].

Diagnosis and treatment

Suspicion of temporal arteritis should trigger rheumatology and ophthalmology consultation, especially in the setting of acute vision loss. The criteria for diagnosis of temporal arteritis as defined by the American College of Rheumatology include: age greater than 50 years, new headache, temporal artery abnormality, ESR greater than 50, and abnormal findings on a temporal artery biopsy. The presence of three or more criteria conferred a sensitivity of 93.5% and a specificity of 91.2% for the diagnosis [20]. Characteristic giant cell granulomatous inflammation on temporal artery biopsy is considered the gold standard to confirm the diagnosis, however. Doppler ultrasound of the temporal arteries has been studied as a noninvasive adjunct to biopsy [21]. A sensitivity of 95% has been reported in biopsy-confirmed temporal arteritis when abnormalities in the structure of the arterial wall were discovered on ultrasound. The specificity is low, however, and a negative result cannot exclude the need for biopsy [22].

High-dose methylprednisolone is the first-line therapy in patients who have temporal arteritis who present with ocular manifestations. Three days of intravenous steroids followed by 2 years of oral prednisone beginning at 40 to 60 mg/d is a common suggested treatment course [16]. Patients who do not have ocular manifestations are started on oral prednisone without the methylprednisolone burst. Prednisone is gradually tapered in conjunction with monitoring ESR and CRP levels for change. Any increase in either halts any further reduction in prednisone level [18,23]. CRP has been shown to be more sensitive than ESR at diagnosis and during monitoring of relapse [24]. Various dosing protocols exist, but none have been prospectively validated.

Unfortunately, the visual loss associated with temporal arteritis is often permanent. In one retrospective study in patients who had biopsy-proven disease, central vision improvement after the initiation of steroid therapy was minimal, and was present in only 4% of patients [23]. Corticosteroids, however, do seem to prevent further vision loss; only 13% of those who had vision loss before diagnosis developed further vision loss after initiation of steroid therapy. Similarly, of those who had no visual complaints before steroid treatment, only 1% subsequently developed vision loss [11].

Optic neuritis

Optic neuritis is an acute demyelinating disorder of the optic nerve that typically presents as painful, monocular vision loss. Although most affected patients regain vision even without treatment, a substantial number subsequently develop multiple sclerosis (MS). Consequently, emergency physicians often enlist the help of ophthalmologists and neurologists in the management of these patients.

Epidemiology

Optic neuritis has an incidence of 6.4 per 100,000 with two thirds of cases occurring in women, generally between 20 and 40 years of age [25]. It is most common in northern latitudes (the United States and Northern Europe) and is more often diagnosed in white Americans than African Americans [25,26]. It is the presenting symptom in 15% to 20% of patients subsequently diagnosed with MS and occurs in one half of MS patients during the course of their illness [25,27,28]. In addition, 31% of patients who have optic neuritis have a recurrence within 10 years of their initial presentation [29].

Etiology

The inflammatory demyelination of the optic nerve is believed to be an autoimmune phenomenon characterized by systemic T-cell activation present at the onset of visual symptoms [30]. Although the specific mechanism is unknown, inflammatory cytokines are believed to play a role and B-cell activation against myelin basic protein may be seen in the cerebrospinal fluid of affected individuals [31]. The inflammatory response against the optic nerve results in edema and breakdown of the myelin sheaths and perivascular cuffing of the retinal vasculature [32]. Genetic susceptibility for optic neuritis is suspected based on higher incidences among certain HLA types [33].

Clinical features and diagnosis

Optic neuritis is a clinical diagnosis based on history and physical examination findings. The Optic Neuritis Treatment Trial [34] surveyed 448 patients who had optic neuritis about their visual symptoms and performed detailed visual assessments. Eye pain accompanied vision loss in 92% of patients. Vision loss was typically monocular and progressed rapidly over a period of hours to days. Even patients who had 20/20 vision at presentation had defects in their ability to perceive color and contrast; patients often described their vision as "blurry" or felt the color has been "washed out" [35].

Although physical examination findings may vary in optic neuritis, pain with eye movements and an afferent pupillary defect are almost universally present [34]. Even in those patients who have normal visual acuity, mild optic nerve dysfunction causes an asymmetry in the pupillary reflex that can be elicited by the swinging flashlight test [25]. Visual acuity in the affected eye can range from 20/20 to no light perception. Although central scotoma is the classic visual deficit, a wide variety of visual field cuts may occur [34]. Two thirds of patients have a normal funduscopic examination with retrobulbar optic neuritis. One third of patients have optic disk swelling, blurring of disk margins, and swollen veins caused by optic nerve inflammation as it terminates in the retina (Fig. 2) [34].

Although the diagnosis of optic neuritis is often made on clinical grounds, gadolinium-enhanced MRI can help confirm the diagnosis and risk-stratify patients who are likely to develop MS. Optic nerve inflammation can be demonstrated in 95% of patients who have optic neuritis on gadolinium-enhanced MRI [36–38]. The imaging may also demonstrate oval-shaped lesions in the periventricular white matter that suggest MS [39]. In one study, the risk for MS 10 years after the first episode of optic neuritis was 56% versus 22% in those who did not have lesions [40]. This information may be useful for consulting ophthalmologists and neurologists and may guide the initial therapy of affected patients.

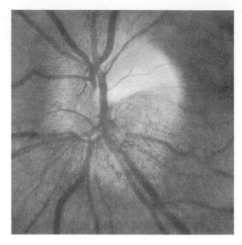

Fig. 2. Optic neuritis. (*From* Kanski JJ. Clinical Diagnosis in Ophthalmology. China: Mosby Elsevier; 2006; with permission.)

Treatment

Visual acuity in optic neuritis generally improves without treatment over the course of several weeks [29]. Treatment is focused on hastening the return of vision, preventing recurrences, and reducing the incidence of MS. In a study that randomized affected patients to either high-dose intravenous methylprednisolone or oral prednisone (or placebo), those who were given the methylprednisolone demonstrated a more rapid return to normal vision [41] and a lower risk for recurrent optic neuritis. The differences in visual acuity were not significant at 2 years follow-up, however. Oral prednisone was associated with an increased risk for recurrent optic neuritis compared with placebo. Methylprednisolone delayed the onset of MS compared with placebo at 2 years, but this advantage did not persist beyond this time frame [41]. According to the American Academy of Neurology, although corticosteroids may hasten the return of vision after initial presentation, there is no compelling evidence for long-term benefit for patients who have optic neuritis [42].

Several randomized trials have demonstrated that interferon beta 1a and interferon beta 1b may reduce the development of MS in patients who have optic neuritis [25,39,43,44]. Although this is typically started at the onset of symptoms, the initiation of this therapy is probably beyond the scope of emergency physicians and should only be done in conjunction with an involved neurology consultant.

Central retinal artery occlusion

Central retinal artery occlusion (CRAO) generally causes abrupt, painless loss of vision that can be permanent unless blood flow to the retina is restored before the onset of irreversible ischemic damage. The retina is perfused by the retinal artery, a branch of the ophthalmic artery that arises from the internal carotid artery. The ophthalmic artery enters the orbit along with the optic nerve at which point the retinal artery branches off, enters the cerebrospinal space, and travels within the optic nerve where it provides blood flow to the central retina and optic nerve. In some patients, additional perfusion of the central retina (including the macula) is provided by the cilioretinal artery, an anatomic variant that allows for the preservation of central vision in some who have CRAO.

Epidemiology

Although the true incidence of CRAO is unknown, most estimates are that it occurs in between 1 to 10 in 100,000 individuals [45]. Risk factors for the development of CRAO are similar to those of other cardiovascular diseases, namely increasing age, hypertension, hypercholesterolemia, diabetes, elevated homocysteine levels, and tobacco use. Some studies have described an increased incidence in males, whereas others have failed to demonstrate a difference in disease prevalence in one sex over the other [46–48].

Etiology

CRAO and other strokelike syndromes share a final common pathway: interruption of blood flow to distal tissues. Although several causes of CRAO are described later, the most common are atherosclerotic disease of the ipsilateral carotid artery [49] and propagation of cardiogenic emboli to the retinal artery [50]. Several studies have suggested factors such as patient age and ethnicity may play a role in the distribution of these causes. For example, whites are more likely to have carotid disease [49], whereas those less than 40 years of age are more likely to have a cardiogenic embolus as the source of their symptoms [50], and patients older than age 70 are more likely to have temporal arteritis as the basis of their CRAO [49].

Carotid artery atherosclerosis

Atherosclerotic disease of the carotid artery is believed to be the most common source of emboli resulting in the disruption of retinal artery blood flow. Although the data are largely from small case series, the prevalence of carotid artery disease in those who have CRAO is generally believed to be 10% to 25%, although there is literature suggesting rates as high as 70% [49,51–55]. Additionally, CRAO in the setting of carotid disease may portend an increased risk for stroke; for this reason, carotid endarterectomy is often recommended in this setting [55].

Cardiogenic embolism

Between 2% and 20% of patients who have CRAO have a cardiac source of embolus [54,56]. These patients tend to be younger in age, and there may be aspects of their history that should alert the clinician to consider this as a possible cause, including: a history of congenital heart disease, rheumatic heart disease, myocardial infarction, endocarditis, or the presence of a cardiac tumor or murmur [57]. Chronic anticoagulation may be warranted for patients who have a cardiogenic source of embolus.

Other causes

Although carotid artery atherosclerosis and cardiogenic embolism represent the cause of most cases of CRAO, there are several other causes reported in the literature. These can be divided broadly into other vascular disease processes (carotid artery dissection [58], radiation injury of the retinal artery [59], Moyamoya disease [60], arterial vasospasm, and migraine) [61], hematologic disorders (sickle cell disease) [62], disorders resulting in hypercoagulable states (antiphospholipid syndrome, factor V Leiden mutation [63], protein S deficiency [64], and protein C deficiency) [65], and autoimmune/inflammatory conditions (giant cell arteritis [66], lupus [67], polyarteritis nodosa [68], and Wegener granulomatosis) [69]. There are case reports of all of these causes of CRAO; no large cohort studies have been published.

Clinical features

The visual loss associated with central retinal artery occlusion is generally painless, monocular, and dramatic, often leaving the affected individual with only a small area of unaffected vision. The symptoms may be less severe, however, if the retina is also perfused by a ciolioretinal artery (15% of patients in one series) [70]. Similarly, the blindness may be transient, or the patient may have "stuttering" symptoms if an embolus moves along the vascular tree and eventually dissolves before causing complete vessel occlusion [71].

On funduscopic examination, the ischemic retina initially appears white and the macula classically is described as having a "cherry red spot" where the retinal epithelium is thinner and the retinal pigment epithelium and choroidal vasculature appear more prominent and can be seen more easily (Fig. 3). In those who have a cilioretinal artery, there may be an area of normal-appearing retina surrounded by an ischemic, pale retina. The actual embolus may be visible in as many as 40% of patients who have CRAO [72]. The clinician may see shiny, iridescent cholesterol plaques, grayish platelet deposits, or bright white calcium fragments. There is generally a complete or relative afferent papillary defect. Finally, funduscopic examination may reveal a characteristic "boxcarring" in the retinal veins and arteries as serum separates from the Rouleau stacking of red blood cells.

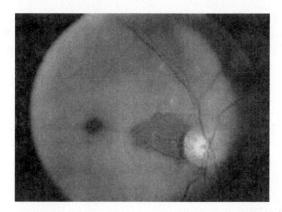

Fig. 3. Central retinal artery occlusion. (*From* Wipf JE, Paauw DS. Ophthalmologic emergencies in the patient with diabetes. Endocrinol Metab Clin N Am 2000;29(4):813–29; with permission.)

Diagnosis and treatment

The diagnosis of central retinal artery occlusion is made on clinical grounds in combination with characteristic eye ground findings. It is a true ocular emergency; retinal ischemia lasting longer than 240 minutes may lead to massive irreversible vision loss [73], whereas restoration of blood flow within 100 minutes may preserve a patient's vision [74]. Although many of those who have occlusion of a branch retinal artery may regain normal vision, spontaneous visual recovery in those who have CRAO is rare and the literature of this population is largely limited to case reports. In one case series, only 35% of patients recovered vision that was better than 20/100 [75], whereas in another series of 73 CRAOs, there were only four instances in which final visual acuity was better than counting fingers [70]. Visual acuity at presentation is believed to be predictive of eventual acuity after the acute CRAO.

Although there is literature documenting and describing the debilitating effects of CRAO, there is a relative paucity of literature examining and comparing the effectiveness of several different treatments. Given the poor outcomes of those afflicted with CRAO, however, several potential therapies have been advocated. Although some of the more conservative treatments are within the practice scope of emergency medicine, patients who have suspected CRAO should receive emergent ophthalmologic consultation and evaluation.

Although many of the therapies vary in their invasiveness and risk, all share a common goal of restoring blood flow to an ischemic retina. As mentioned previously, spontaneous resolution (ie, the embolus dissolving or moving on from the ophthalmic circulation) is relatively uncommon, occurring in 1% to 8% of cases [45]. Initial therapies involved attempts by patients or clinicians to manually dislodge the embolus by massaging the eyeball over a closed lid. It is believed that this may also augment aqueous outflow and retinal perfusion may increase with relief of the digital pressure [76,77].

Other therapies have aimed to increase ocular perfusion pressure by decreasing intraocular pressure, which may be accomplished by performing anterior chamber paracentesis [78]; giving intravenous diuretics, such as acetazolamide [79] or mannitol [45]; using enhanced external counterpulsation (a procedure in which air-filled cuffs are applied to the vascular bed of the lower extremities during diastole) [80]; or performing a trabeculectomy [81], in which a fistula is created between the anterior chamber and the subconjunctival space.

Some have suggested treating affected patients with vasodilators with the hope of increasing retinal blood flow or perhaps even dislodging the culprit embolus. The use of agents such as nitrates [45], rebreathing carbon dioxide [82], and inhaling carbogen (95% oxygen and 5% carbon dioxide) [78] have been met with mixed results because systemic vasodilatation may result, causing a reduction in systemic blood pressure and a subsequent decrease in retinal perfusion. Others have advocated for alternative forms of medical therapy, including various platelet inhibitors, anticoagulants, aqueous formation inhibitors, hyperosmotics, and corticosteroids.

A more aggressive approach involves the use of lytic agents in the treatment of CRAO. Using principles adapted from the use of thrombolytics in acute myocardial infarction and ischemic stroke, some have advocated for its use in CRAO. Any benefits, however, must be weighed against the risk for life-threatening complications (ie, hemorrhage, especially intracranial) in what is a debilitating, but not necessarily life-threatening, disease. Several reports involving various agents, including urokinase and recombinant tissue plasminogen activator (rt-PA), given both systemically and locally are reported in the literature. A 2000 meta-analysis provides the best summary of these data (although it examines only 16 studies, all of which were retrospective and nonrandomized and included a total of only 100 patients). The authors concluded that local intra-arterial fibrinolysis offered a "marginally better visual outcome than conservative forms of management" [83]. Similarly, a 2005 Cochrane review suggested that "there is currently not enough evidence to decide which, if any, interventions for acute nonarteritic central retinal artery occlusion would result in any beneficial or harmful effect. Well-designed randomized controlled trials are needed to establish the most effective treatment" [84].

In summary, although a wide variety of medical and surgical treatments for CRAO have been used, none have been prospectively shown to have more than a limited or marginal benefit. There are few, if any, randomized controlled trials of these therapies, and there has been little advancement in the treatment of this disorder in the last 20 years.

Central retinal vein occlusion

There is much overlap in the epidemiology, causes, clinical features, and diagnosis and treatment between central retinal artery and vein occlusion. Below, critical similarities and differences are highlighted.

Epidemiology

Retinal vein occlusion (RVO) is the second most common retinal vascular disorder behind diabetic retinopathy [85]. Prevalence reports vary, largely depending on whether the data are taken from a hospital- or population-based sample. The prevalence of RVO in hospital-based studies generally ranges from 0.3% to 1.6% [86,87], whereas a large Israeli population-based study reported a 4-year incidence of retinal vein occlusion of 2.14 cases per 1000 of general population older than 40 years and 5.36 cases per 1000 of general population older than 64 years [88]. An Australian population-based study reported a 1.6% 10-year incidence of RVO in those older than 60 years [89].

Etiology

Since the initial description of RVO in the medical literature in 1854, several different classification systems have been used. Typically, RVO is first divided into that affecting a central vein (CRVO) and that affecting a branch vein (BRVO). Central vein occlusion is further divided into ischemic and nonischemic types.

BRVO is believed to result in large part from factors related to the anatomic relationship between the retinal vein and artery as they pass through the region of the lamina cribrosa. In this area, the structures share an adventitial sheath and are in close proximity to each other. This factor, in combination with degenerative changes in the wall of the vein and artery, leads to a narrowing of the vein lumen and subsequently to stasis and thrombosis. Ischemic RVO can also occur in any other area of the retina where the arteries and veins cross [90]. Many of the risk factors for the development of BRVO are similar to those of CRAO, and include hypertension [87,91,92], diabetes [87,91,93], cerebrovascular disease [91,92], cardiovascular disease [94], increased body mass index [94], dyslipidemia [94], thyroid disease [91], peptic ulcer disease [91], glaucoma [95], and hyperhomocysteinuria [96]. On ophthalmologic examination, those who have focal arteriolar narrowing or arteriovenous nicking are also more likely to develop RVO [89].

CRVO, however, is believed to occur because of clots present in the main draining vein of the retina. Depending on clot burden, collateral circulation, and perfusion of the retina, it is divided into ischemic and nonischemic types. In nonischemic CRVO, the vascular lesion is generally more proximal, allowing for collateral circulation to provide some blood flow to the retina. Consequently, visual loss is by and large less severe and debilitating.

In addition, in those eyes that have nonischemic disease, examination may reveal stasis of blood within the veins as opposed to frank thrombosis [90].

Clinical features

In those who have ischemic RVO, the visual loss is often dramatic and is frequently noted on awakening one morning. The persistent blurring may be preceded by episodes of amaurosis fugax in some patients. Conversely, non-ischemic RVO may be relatively asymptomatic and may only be noted on routine ophthalmologic examination. Visual symptoms, when present, may be limited to a vague blurring of central vision with sparing of the peripheral vision and are often worse in the morning and improve gradually over the course of the day [90]. In one study, the final visual acuity was 20/400 or worse in 87% of those who had ischemic RVO, whereas it was 20/30 or better in 57% of those who had nonischemic disease [97]. As with CRAO, long-term visual acuity in those who have ischemic RVO is largely determined by visual acuity at presentation [98].

Diagnosis and treatment

Although the formal diagnosis of RVO and the differentiation between the ischemic and nonischemic varieties is beyond the clinical scope of most emergency medicine physicians, one should be able to appreciate several of the clinical aspects of RVO mentioned earlier, along with some typical findings on funduscopic examination.

The funduscopic examination classically reveals retinal hemorrhages (which may be mild or severe), dilated and tortuous retinal veins, edema of the optic disc, and small areas of yellow-white discoloration of the retina ("cotton wool spots"), which are indicative of local retinal ischemia (Fig. 4). When retinal hemorrhages are severe, and cover much of the fundus, the

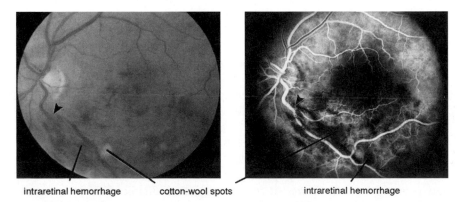

intraretinal hemorrhage   cotton-wool spots   intraretinal hemorrhage

Fig. 4. Branch retinal vein occlusion Arrows represent sites of branch retinal vein occlusion. (*From* Kaiser PK, Friedman NJ, Pineda R, II. The Massachusetts Eye and Ear Infirmary illustrated manual of ophthalmology. 2nd edition. China: Saunders; 2004; with permission.)

clinician may see the classic "blood and thunder" appearance of the retina (Fig. 5).

RVO is generally a self-limited disease (the retinopathy may resolve over weeks to years), but the complications of the disorder can be severe. Although there is little that an emergency medicine physician can do acutely for affected patients, referral to a specialist is of paramount importance. In addition to making a formal diagnosis, ophthalmologists should differentiate between ischemic and nonischemic disease, a distinction that has important ramifications in the complications that may be anticipated. Specifically, those who have ischemic disease are at a higher risk for developing ocular neovascularization, which may result in severe vision loss. A detailed discussion of this complication is beyond the scope of this article.

As with CRAO, various therapeutic strategies have been used with varying levels of success. Interventions, such as anticoagulation, lytic agents, hemodilution, hyperbaric oxygen, surgical decompression, and systemic and intravitreal steroids, are all reported in the literature. A recent meta-analysis reported that although hemodilution seemed to be of some benefit in some trials, and panretinal photocoagulation may improve visual acuity in those who have neovascularization, there is "limited level I evidence for any intervention to improve visual acuity in patients with RVO" [99]. Most studies are case reports, retrospective, do not have a control group, or involve very small numbers of patients.

Retinal detachment

Epidemiology

Retinal detachment is a relatively uncommon affliction of the eye, affecting approximately 1 to 2 in 10,000 people per year [100,101], or about 1 in

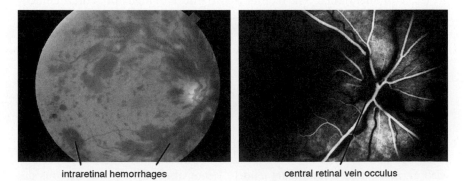

intraretinal hemorrhages   central retinal vein occulus

Fig. 5. Central retinal vein occlusion. (*From* Kaiser PK, Friedman NJ, Pineda R, II. The Massachusetts Eye and Ear Infirmary illustrated manual of ophthalmology. 2nd edition. China: Saunders; 2004; with permission.)

300 people over the course of their lifetime [102]. Risk factors for the development of retinal detachment include increasing age [103], previous cataract surgery [104], focal retinal atrophy, myopia [105], trauma [106], diabetic retinopathy, family history of retinal detachment, uveitis, and prematurity [107].

Etiology

Although the pathogenesis of retinal detachment can be divided into three subtypes, all share a common final pathway: separation of the retina from the underlying retinal epithelium. In the first type, exudative retinal detachment, there is accumulation of serous or hemorrhagic fluid in the subretinal space, generally as a result of systemic conditions, such as severe acute hypertension, sarcoid, or cancer. In the second type, tractional retinal detachment, previous trauma from infection, surgery, inflammation, or hemorrhage results in fibrotic tissue that can provide traction on the retina resulting in detachment [107–109].

The third type, rhegmatogenous detachment, is the most commonly encountered. In this form of retinal detachment, age-related changes in the vitreous humor cause it to liquefy and shrink away from the back of the eye (termed posterior vitreous detachment). In turn, the vitreous may pull the retina from its underlying epithelial layer. Although patients who have posterior vitreous detachment often only experience bothersome floaters in their peripheral vision, more dramatic vision loss can occur if a retinal tear or flap occurs. As the vitreous pulls away from the retina, the vitreous is able to enter the subretinal space and create a plane of dissection. As more vitreous enters this space, more retina is separated from its underlying epithelial layer. As the detachment grows, so does the patient's visual field deficit. Most rhegmatogenous detachments, if left untreated, expand to eventually include the macula, impacting central visual acuity [107–109].

The aforementioned risk factors for the development of retinal detachment all result in either changes in the makeup of the vitreous or in alterations in the normal anatomy or shape of the eyeball, resulting in retinal traction and forces that tend to pull the retina from the epithelium layer it normally covers.

Clinical features

The hallmark complaint of those who have vitreous detachment is the presence of floaters. Characteristically described as dots, cobwebs, lines, or strings in the visual field, the floaters of vitreous detachment (especially with an associated retinal tear) tend to occur abruptly. As the vitreous detachment progresses to retinal detachment, patients may describe visual field loss. This loss generally begins at the periphery (where the retina is the thinnest), and over hours to weeks may spread toward the central visual field axis. Other ocular complaints such as pain, tearing, redness, and drainage are typically associated with conditions other than retinal detachment.

Diagnosis and treatment

Funduscopic examination with a direct ophthalmoscope is generally not sufficient to rule out the diagnosis of retinal detachment. The narrow field of view provided by the instrument does not allow one to see the peripheral aspects of the retina where tears are more frequently seen. Although the clinician may see an abnormal red reflex or occasionally the classic white billowing retinal separation, and indirect examination in a dilated eye by an ophthalmologist is often necessary (Fig. 6) [110].

A central tenet in the treatment of retinal detachment is its initial prevention. Risk factor modification and education of susceptible patients is crucial. For example, those who have severe myopia should be encouraged to wear protective lenses when playing sports, and those who undergo cataract surgery should receive specific instructions about worrisome symptoms and reasons to return to care. Similarly, those who have known vitreous detachment or are at risk for developing the finding should be followed closely. Fortunately, only 1% to 2% of such patients have a retinal break. If vitreous hemorrhage is present, however, this risk increases to 70% [111]. If identified, retinal tears can be treated with cryotherapy or laser therapy, which serve to create a scar at the site of the tear and prevent fluid from entering the subretinal space. Success rates (ie, the prevention of retinal detachment) are greater than 95% with this technique [112].

Surgical repair of retinal detachments, typically done by a retinal specialist, also has high success rates. More invasive therapies, such as scleral buckling and posterior vitrectomy, post success rates of nearly 90% [113,114], whereas less invasive therapies, such as pneumatic retinopexy, may be performed in an office setting in select cases [115]. Retinal detachment surgery

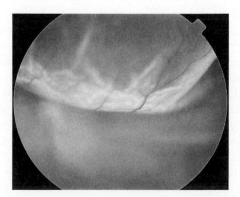

Fig. 6. Retinal detachment. (*From* Kanski JJ. Clinical diagnosis in ophthalmology. China: Mosby Elsevier; 2006; with permission.)

generally fails because of the growth of scar tissue on the retina in the weeks following repair [116]. This phenomenon, termed proliferative vitreoretinopathy, is also amenable to surgery, although success rates are not as high and resulting visual acuity is often poor [117].

If repair is technically successful, visual acuity is often restored to predetachment levels. Critical in determining eventual visual outcome is the presence or absence of macular involvement in the tear, and if it is involved, the duration and extent of its involvement. For this reason, those who have preserved central acuity should be referred for immediate surgery [118,119].

Retinal vasculitis

Retinal vasculitis is characterized by inflammation of the blood vessels of the retina. It may be primarily ocular and limited to the orbit or may be associated with various autoimmune and infectious systemic diseases. Retinal vasculitis typically presents as a painless decrease in vision and is diagnosed clinically by funduscopic examination; ancillary fluorescein angiography and laboratory testing may be used to define the degree of involvement and diagnose associated conditions. Treatments include local and systemic immunosuppressive regimens and treatment of the underlying disorder.

Epidemiology and etiology

Retinal vasculitis may be caused by infectious or systemic inflammatory conditions or may be restricted solely to the retina. Retinal vasculitides associated with primary ocular disorders include idiopathic retinal vasculitis, birdshot retinochoroidopathy, Eales disease, and pars plantaris syndrome [120].

Autoimmune causes of retinal vasculitis include systemic lupus erythematosus (SLE), Behçet disease, sarcoidosis, Wegener granulomatosis, polyarteritis nodosa (PAN), HLA-B27 associated conditions, and inflammatory bowel disease (IBD). Various inflammatory ocular conditions may occur as part of these diseases. In SLE, retinal involvement, including vasculitis, is seen in 3% to 30% of patients [121,122]. Severe decreases in vision correlate with decreased survival and are likely related to uncontrolled systemic inflammation [121,123–125]. Similarly, 80% of those who have Behçet disease have ocular involvement [126]. Those who have skin lesions and arthritis have an increased risk for visual loss, generally resulting from recurrent vasoocclusive disease from retinal vein vasculitis [127]. Of those patients who have sarcoidosis, 20% to 25% have ocular disease [128,129], and 7% of those have posterior segment involvement (a subset of which includes retinal vasculitis) [129]. In Wegener granulomatosis ocular involvement occurs in 30% to 60% with significant vision loss in 8%. Retinal vasculitis is rare, however [130,131]. There are ocular findings in 10% to 20% of patients who have PAN. Anterior segment findings are most common but retinal veins may also be affected [132]. In HLA-B27 associated conditions, anterior uveitis is most common; posterior segment disease occurs in 4% to 17%. Of those who have posterior segment disease, 24% have retinal vasculitis [133–135]. Retinal vasculitis is uncommon in IBD and has only been observed in case reports with Crohn disease [136].

Infectious causes of retinal vasculitis include toxoplasmosis, syphilis, tuberculosis, and several viruses, including varicella (VZV), herpes simplex (HSV), and cytomegalovirus (CMV). Toxoplasmosis is responsible for 25% of cases of posterior uveitis in the United States. The resulting vitreous inflammation often induces localized retinal vasculitis [137]. Ocular tuberculosis is an uncommon manifestation of extrapulmonary TB seen in approximately 1% of patients [138,139]. Similarly, retinal vasculitis in syphilis is rare, but may be seen in the secondary or tertiary stages [140]. HSV and VZV retinal vasculitis are seen in immunocompromised chemotherapy patients, and those who are congenitally infected [141]. CMV retinal vasculitis is seen in those who have HIV and low CD4 counts.

Clinical characteristics

Those who have retinal vasculitis typically present with a painless decrease in vision but may also report blind spots or floaters. More subtle symptoms, such as changes in color vision and changes in the perceived shape of an object, may occur with involvement of the macula [141].

Slit lamp examination reveals cells in the vitreous body [141]. Funduscopic examination may reveal characteristic "vascular sheathing," the accumulation of inflammatory cells on vessel walls manifested as an area of retinal pallor paralleling the vessel lumen. This finding is more common in peripheral vessels, and there may be segments of unaffected arterioles. The increased vessel permeability that leads to vascular sheathing predisposes patients to vitreous hemorrhage and macular edema that may also be seen [120].

Diagnosis and treatment

Retinal vasculitis is diagnosed clinically based on a dilated funduscopic examination in conjunction with consultation from an ophthalmologist. A history and physical should be performed with specific attention to associated findings seen in the various systemic inflammatory and infectious conditions described above and should direct laboratory and radiographic testing. A detailed review of the clinical presentation of the various disorders is beyond the scope of this article.

Regardless of the cause of the retinal vasculitis, fluorescein angiography (injection of fluorescein in the retinal artery percutaneously to delineate the retinal vasculature) is a commonly used ancillary test. It can help define the extent of disease and aid in narrowing the differential diagnosis of causative disorders. Angiography typically demonstrates perivascular staining that results from increased vascular permeability and is the visual correlate of vascular sheathing on funduscopic examination. Areas of nonperfused retina may also be detected as dark patches on the angiogram [142].

In addition to angiography, focused laboratory and radiographic assessment is still indicated even in the absence of historical or examination findings that suggest an associated condition. According to a study performed by the National Eye Institute, only 1% of patients initially diagnosed with idiopathic retinal vasculitis developed subsequent systemic disease after 4 years of follow-up. The authors recommend a CBC, urinalysis, ESR, syphilis and HIV serologies, and a chest radiograph in the absence of indications for additional testing, but caution against low-yield indiscriminate laboratory testing [120].

Treatment of retinal vasculitis generally includes an immunosuppressive regimen that may be topical, intraorbital, or systemic. Systemic corticosteroids are often the cornerstone of treatment, but regimens may also include methotrexate, azathioprine, cyclosporine, and other immunosuppressive agents, depending on the cause of the vasculitis. Important exceptions are retinal vasculitides associated with infectious causes, wherein treatment is based on correcting the underlying infection. Corticosteroids are used adjunctively in CMV, VZV, HSV, and toxoplasmosis to reduce inflammation. [140]. The decision to initiate treatment of retinal vasculitis should be made in conjunction with ophthalmology consultation, in addition to infectious disease and rheumatology consultation if appropriate.

Summary

In summary, there are several causes of acute monocular vision loss, some of which are discussed here, that require prompt recognition by the emergency physician. Although the initial diagnosis is made by the emergency department clinician, a prompt, and at times emergent, referral to an ophthalmologist may be necessary.

References

[1] Salvarani C, Gabriel SE, O'Fallon WM, et al. The incidence of giant cell arteritis in Olmsted County, Minnesota: apparent fluctuation in a cyclic pattern. Ann Intern Med 1995;123(3): 192–4.
[2] Weyand CM, Hunder NN, Hicok KC, et al. HLA-DRB1 alleles in polymyalgia rheumatica, giant cell arteritis, and rheumatoid arthritis. Arthritis Rheum 1994;37(4): 514–20.
[3] Haworth S, Ridgeway J, Stewart I, et al. Polymyalgia rheumatica is associated with both HLA-DRB1*0401 and DRB1*0404. Br J Rheumatol 1996;35(7):632–5.

[4] Elling P, Olsson AT, Elling H. Synchronous variations of the incidence of temporal arteritis and polymyalgia rheumatica in different regions of Denmark: association with epidemics of Mycoplasma pneumoniae infection. J Rheumatol 1996;23(1):112–9.

[5] Gabriel SE, Espy M, Erdman DD, et al. The role of parvovirus B19 in the pathogenesis of giant cell arteritis: a preliminary evaluation. Arthritis Rheum 1999;42(6):1255–8.

[6] Weyand C, Goronzy JJ. Medium and large vessel vasculitis. N Engl J Med 2003;349(2): 160–9.

[7] Weyand CM, Tetzlaff N, Bjornsson J, et al. Disease patterns and tissue cytokine profiles in giant cell arteritis. Arthritis Rheum 1997;40(1):19–26.

[8] Salvarani C, Macchioni PL, Tartoni PL, et al. Polymyalgia rheumatica and giant cell arteritis: a 5 year epidemiologic and clinical study in Reggio Emilia, Italy. Clin Exp Rheumatol 1987;5(3):205–15.

[9] Huston KA, Junder GG, Lie JT, et al. Temporal arteritis: a 25 year epidemiologic, clinical, and pathologic study. Ann Intern Med 1978;88(2):162–7.

[10] Calamia KT, Hunder GG. Clinical manifestations of giant cell (temporal) arteritis. Clin Rheum Dis 1980;6:389–403.

[11] Aiello PD, Trautmann JC, McPhee TG, et al. Visual prognosis in giant cell arteritis. Ophthalmology 1993;100(4):550–5.

[12] Gonzales-Gay MA, Blanco R, Rodriguez-Valverde V, et al. Permanent visual loss and cerebrovascular accidents in giant cell arteritis: predictors and response to treatment. Arthritis Rheum 1998;41(8):1497–504.

[13] Nesher G, Nesher R, Rozenman Y, et al. Visual hallucinations in giant cell arteritis: association with visual loss. J Rheumatol 2001;28(9):2046–8.

[14] Caselli RJ, Junder GG, Whisnant JP. Neurologic disease in biopsy-proven giant cell (temporal) arteritis. Neurology 1988;38(3):352–9.

[15] Caselli RJ, Daube JR, Junder GG, et al. Peripheral neuropathic syndromes in giant cell (temporal) arteritis. Neurology 1988;38(5):685–9.

[16] Unwin B, Williams C, Gilliland W. Polymyalgia rheumatica and giant cell arteritis. Am Fam Physician 2006;74(9):1547–54.

[17] Spiera R, Spiera H. Inflammatory disease in older adults. Cranial arteritis. Geriatrics 2004; 59(12):25–9.

[18] Salvarani C, Cantini F, Boiardi L, et al. Polymyalgia rheumatica and giant cell arteritis. N Engl J Med 2002;347(4):261–71.

[19] Smetana GW, Shmerling RH. Does this patient have temporal arteritis? JAMA 2002; 287(1):92–101.

[20] Hunder GG, Bloch DA, Michel BA, et al. The American College of Rheumatology 1990 criteria for the classification of giant cell arteritis. Arthritis Rheum 1990;33(8):1122–8.

[21] Schmidt W. Doppler sonography in rheumatology. Best Pract Res Clin Rheumatol 2004; 18(6):827–46.

[22] Reinhard M, Schmidt D, Hetzel A. Color-coded sonography in suspected temporal arteritis-experiences after 83 cases. Rheumatol Int 2004;24(6):340–6.

[23] Hayreh SS, Zimmerman B, Kardon R. Visual improvement with corticosteroid therapy in giant cell arteritis. Report of a large study and review of literature. Acta Ophthalmol Scand 2002;80(4):355–67.

[24] Hayreh SS, Podhajsky PA, Rama R, et al. Giant cell arteritis: validity and reliability of various diagnostic criteria. Am J Ophthalmol 1997;123(3):285–96.

[25] Balcer LJ. Clinical practice. Optic neuritis. N Engl J Med 2006;354(12):1273–80.

[26] Phillips PH, Newman NJ, Lynn MJ. Optic neuritis in African Americans. Arch Neurol 1998;55(2):186–92.

[27] Arnold AC. Evolving management of optic neuritis and multiple sclerosis. Am J Ophthalmol 2005;139:1101–8.

[28] Frohman EM, Frohman TC, Zee DS, et al. The neuro-ophthalmology of multiple sclerosis. Lancet Neurol 2005;4(2):111–21.

[29] Beck RW, Gal RL, Bhatti MT, et al. Visual function more than 10 years after optic neuritis: experience of the Optic Neuritis Treatment Trial. Am J Ophthalmol 2004;137(1):77–83. [Erratum in: Am J Ophthalmol 2004 Apr;137(4):following 793. Am J Ophthalmol 2004 Aug;138(2):following 321].

[30] Roed H, Frederiksen J, Langkilde A, et al. Systemic T-cell activation in acute clinically isolated optic neuritis. J Neuroimmunol 2005;162(1–2):165–72.

[31] Soderstrom M, Link H, Xu Z, et al. Optic neuritis and multiple sclerosis: anti-MBP and anti-MBP peptide antibody-secreting cells are accumulated in CSF. Neurology 1993; 43(6):1215–22.

[32] Lightman S, McDonald WI, Bird AC, et al. Retinal venous sheathing in optic neuritis. Its significance for the pathogenesis of multiple sclerosis. Brain 1987;110(Pt 2):405–14.

[33] Frederiksen JL, Madsen HO, Ryder LP, et al. HLA typing in acute optic neuritis. Relation to multiple sclerosis and magnetic resonance imaging findings. Arch Neurol 1997;54(1): 76–80.

[34] Optic Neuritis Study Group. The clinical profile of acute optic neuritis: experience of the Optic Neuritis Treatment Trial. Arch Ophthalmol 1991;109(12):1673–8.

[35] Cole SR, Beck RW, Moke PS, et al. The national eye institute visual function questionnaire: experience of the ONTT. Invest Ophthalmol Vis Sci 2000;41(5):1017–21.

[36] Rizzo JF III, Andreoli CM, Rabinov JD. Use of magnetic resonance imaging to differentiate optic neuritis and nonarteritic anterior ischemic optic neuropathy. Ophthalmology 2002;109(9):1679–84.

[37] Rocca MA, Hickman SJ, Bo L, et al. Imaging the optic nerve in multiple sclerosis. Mult Scler 2005;11(5):537–41.

[38] Kupersmith MJ, Alban T, Zeiffer B, et al. Contrast-enhanced MRI in acute optic neuritis: relationship to visual performance. Brain 2002;125(Pt 4):812–22.

[39] CHAMPS Study Group. Interferon beta-1a for optic neuritis patients at high risk for multiple sclerosis. Am J Ophthalmol 2001;132(4):463–71.

[40] Beck RW, Trobe JD, Moke PS, et al. High- and low-risk profiles for the development of multiple sclerosis within 10 years after optic neuritis: experience of the Optic Neuritis Treatment Trial. Arch Ophthalmol 2003;121(7):944–9.

[41] Beck RW, Cleary PA, Anderson MM Jr, et al. A randomized, controlled trial of corticosteroids in the treatment of acute optic neuritis. N Engl J Med 1992;326(9): 581–8.

[42] Kaufman DI, Trobe JD, Eggenberger ER, et al. Practice parameter: the role of corticosteroids in the management of acute monosymptomatic optic neuritis: report of the Quality Standards Subcommittee of the American Academy of Neurology. Neurology 2000; 54(11):2039–44.

[43] Jacobs LD, Beck RW, Simon JH, et al. Intramuscular interferon beta-1a therapy initiated during a first demyelinating event in multiple sclerosis. N Engl J Med 2000;343(13): 898–904.

[44] Comi G, Filippi M, Barkhof F, et al. Effect of early interferon treatment on conversion to definite multiple sclerosis: a randomised study. Lancet 2001;357(9268):1576–82.

[45] Rumelt S, Dorenboim Y, Rchany U. Aggressive systematic treatment for central retinal artery occlusion. Am J Ophthalmol 1999;128:733–8.

[46] Cugati S, Wang JJ, Rochtchina E. Ten-year incidence of retinal emboli in an older population. Stroke 2006;37:908–10.

[47] Wong TY, Klein R. Retinal arteriolar emboli: epidemiology and risk of stroke. Curr Opin Ophthalmol 2002;13(3):142–6.

[48] Cahill MT, Stinnett SS, Fekrat S. Meta-analysis of plasma homocysteine, serum folate, serum B12, and thermolabile MTHFR genotype as risk factors for retinal vascular occlusive disease. Am J Ophthalmol 2003;136(6):1136–50.

[49] Ahuja RM, Chaturvedi S, Eliott D, et al. Mechanisms of retinal artery occlusive disease in African American and Caucasian patient. Stroke 1999;30:1506–9.

[50] Greven CM, Slusher MM, Weaver RG. Retinal arterial occlusions in young adults. Am J Ophthalmol 1995;120(6):776–83.

[51] Sharma S, Brown GC, Pater JL, et al. Does a visible retinal embolus increase the likelihood of hemodynamically significant carotid artery stenosis in patients with acute retinal artery occlusion? Arch Ophthalmol 1998;116(12):1602–6.

[52] Sheng FC, Quinones-Baldrich W, Machleder HI, et al. Relationship of extracranial carotid occlusive disease and central retinal artery occlusion. Am J Surg 1986;152(2): 175–8.

[53] Merchut MP, Gupta SR, Naheedy MH. The relation of retinal artery occlusion and carotid artery stenosis. Stroke 1988;19(10):1239–42.

[54] Babikian V, Wijman CA, Koleini B, et al. Retinal ischemia and embolism. Etiologies and outcomes based on a prospective study. Cerebrovasc Dis 2001;12(2):108–13.

[55] Douglas DJ, Schuler JJ, Buchbinder D, et al. The association of central retinal artery occlusion and extracranial carotid artery disease. Ann Surg 1988;208(1):85–90.

[56] Appen RE, Wray SH, Cogan DG. Central retinal artery occlusion. Am J Ophthalmol 1975; 79(3).374–81.

[57] Sharma S, Naqvi A, Sharma SM, et al. Transthoracic echocardiographic findings in patients with acute retinal arterial obstruction. A retrospective review. Arch Ophthalmol 1996; 114(10):1189–92.

[58] Mokhtari F, Massin P, Paques M, et al. Central retinal artery occlusion associated with head or neck pain revealing spontaneous internal carotid artery dissection. Am J Ophthalmol 2000;129(1):108–9.

[59] Evans LS, Van de Graaf WB, Baker WH, et al. Central retinal artery occlusion after neck irradiation. Am J Ophthalmol 1992;114:224–5.

[60] Chace R, Hedges TR. Retinal artery occlusion due to Moyamoya disease. J Clin Neuroophthalmol 1984;4(1):31–4.

[61] Katz B. Migrainous central retinal artery occlusion. J Clin Neuroophthalmol 1986;6(2): 69–75.

[62] Mansi IA, Alkhunaizi AM, Al-Khatti AA. Bilateral central retinal artery occlusion secondary to sickle cell disease. Am J Hematol 2000;64:79–80.

[63] Rumelt S, Rehany U. Central retinal artery occlusion associated with primary antiphospholipid syndrome. Eye 1999;13(part 5):699–700.

[64] Greven CM, Weaver RG, Owen J, et al. Protein S deficiency and bilateral branch retinal artery occlusion. Ophthalmology 1991;98(1):33–4.

[65] Nelson ME, Talbot JF, Preston FE. Recurrent multiple-branch retinal arteriolar occlusions in a patient with protein C deficiency. Graefes Arch Clin Exp Ophthalmol 1989;227(5): 443–7.

[66] Mohan K, Gupta A, Jain IS, et al. Bilateral central retinal artery occlusion in occult temporal arteritis. J Clin Neuroophthalmol 1989;9(4):270–2.

[67] Read RW, Chong LP, Rao NA. Occlusive retinal vasculitis associated with systemic lupus erythematosus. Arch Ophthalmol 2000;188:588–9.

[68] Soloman SM, Soloman JH. Bilateral central artery occlusions in polyarteritis nodosa. Ann Ophthalmol 1978;10(5):567–9.

[69] Mirza S, Raghu Ram AR, Bowling BS. Central retinal artery occlusion and bilateral choroidal infarcts in Wegener's granulomatosis. Eye 1999;13(pt 3a):374–6.

[70] Brown GC, Shields JA. Cilioretinal arteries and retinal artery occlusion. Arch Ophthalmol 1979;97(1):84–92.

[71] Werner MS, Latchaw R, Baker L, et al. Relapsing and remitting central retinal artery occlusion. Am J Ophthalmol 1994;188:393–5.

[72] Savino PJ, Glaser JS, Cassady J. Retinal stroke. Is the patient at risk? Arch Ophthalmol 1977;95(7):1185–9.

[73] Hayreh SS, Zimmerman MB, Kimura A, et al. Central retinal artery occlusion. Retinal survival time. Exp Eye Res 2004;78(3):723–36.

[74] Hayreh SS, Weingeist TA. Experimental occlusion of the central artery of the retina. Retinal tolerance time to acute ischaemia. Br J Ophthalmol 1980;64(11):818–25.

[75] Stone R, Zink H, Klingele T, et al. Visual recovery after central retinal artery occlusion: two cases. Ann Ophthalmol 1977;9(4):445–50.

[76] Ffytche TJ. A rationalization of treatment of central retinal artery occlusion. Trans Ophthalmol Soc U K 1974;94(2):468–79.

[77] Nielsen NV. Treatment of acute occlusion of the retinal arteries. Acta Ophthalmol 1979; 57(6):1078–113.

[78] Atebara NH, Brown GC, Cater J. Efficacy of anterior chamber paracentesis and carbogen in treating acute nonarteritic central retinal artery occlusion. Ophthalmology 1995;201(12): 2029–34.

[79] Rassam SM, Patel V, Kohner EM. The efficacy of acetazolamide on the retinal circulation. Eye 1993;7(part 5):697–702.

[80] Werner D, Michalk F, harazny J, et al. Accelerated reperfusion of poorly perfused retinal areas in central retinal artery occlusion and branch retinal artery occlusion after a short treatment with enhanced external counterpulsation. Retina 2004;24:541–7.

[81] Harvey PA, Winder S, Talbot JF. Trabeculectomy for central retinal artery occlusion. Eye 2000;14(part 2):256–7.

[82] Harino S, Grunwald JE, Petrig BJ, et al. Rebreathing into a bag increases human retinal macular blood velocity. Br J Ophthalmol 1995;79(4):380–3.

[83] Beatty S, Au Eong KG. Local intra-arterial fibrinolysis for acute occlusion of the central retinal artery: a meta-analysis of the published data. Br J Ophthalmol 2000;84:914–6.

[84] Fraser S, Siriwardena D. Interventions for acute non-arteritic central retinal artery occlusion. Cochrane Database of Systematic Reviews 2002;1:CD001989.

[85] Bananrjee S. A review of developments in the management of retinal diseases. J R Soc Med 2006;99:125–7.

[86] Wong TY, Larsen EK, Klein R, et al. Cardiovascular risk factors for retinal vein occlusion and arteriolar emboli: the atherosclerosis risk in communities & cardiovascular health studies. Ophthalmology 2005;112:540–7.

[87] Mitchell P, Smith W, Chang A. Prevalence and associations of retinal vein occlusion in Australia: the Blue Mountains Eye Study. Arch Ophthalmol 1996;114:1243–7.

[88] David R, Zangwill L, Badarna M. Epidemiology of retinal vein occlusion and its association with glaucoma and increased intraocular pressure. Ophthalmologica 1988;197(2): 69–74.

[89] Cugati S, Wang JJ, Rochtchina E, et al. Ten year incidence of retinal vein occlusion in an older population. The Blue Mountain Eye Study. Arch Ophthalmol 2006;124:726–32.

[90] Hayreh SS. Retinal vein occlusion. Indian J Ophthalmol 1994;42:109–32.

[91] Hayreh SS, Zimmerman B, McCarthy MJ, et al. Systemic diseases associated with various types of retinal vein occlusion. Am J Ophthalmol 2001;131:61–77.

[92] Elman MJ, Bhatt AK, Quinlan PM, et al. The risk for systemic vascular diseases and mortality in patients with central retinal vein occlusion. Ophthalmology 1990;97:1543–8.

[93] Eye Disease Case-Control Study Group. Risk factors for central retinal vein occlusion. Arch Ophthalmol 1996;114:545–54.

[94] Eye Disease Case-Control Study Group. Risk factors for branch retinal vein occlusion. Am J Ophthalmol 1993;116:286–96.

[95] Hayreh SS, Zimmerman MB, Beri M, et al. Intraocular pressure abnormalities associated with central and hemicentral retinal vein occlusion. Ophthalmology 2004;111: 133–41.

[96] Janssen MC, den Heijer M, Cruysberg JR, et al. Retinal vein occlusion: a form of venous thrombosis or a complication of atherosclerosis? A meta-analysis of thrombophilic factors. Thromb Haemost 2005;93:1021–6.

[97] Zegarra H, Gutman FA, Conforto J. The natural course of central retinal vein occlusion. Ophthalmology 1979;86:1931–42.

[98] Shahid H, Hossain P, Amoaku WM. The management of retinal vein occlusion: is interventional ophthalmology the way forward? Br J Ophthalmol 2006;90:627–39.

[99] Mohamed Q, McIntosh RL, Saw SM, et al. Interventions for central retinal vein occlusion: an evidence-based systematic review. Ophthalmology 2007;114(3):507–19, 524.

[100] Algvere PV, Jahnberg P, Textorius O. The Swedish retinal detachment register. I. A database for epidemiological and clinical studies. Graefes Arch Clin Exp Ophthalmol 1999;237: 137–44.

[101] Rowe JA, Erie JC, Baratz KH, et al. Retinal detachment in Olmsted County, Minnesota, 1976 through 1995. Ophthalmology 1999;106:154–9.

[102] Haimann MH, Burton TC, Brown CK. Epidemiology of retinal detachment. Arch Ophthalmol 1982;100:289–92.

[103] Flood MT, Balazs EA. Hyaluronic acid content in the developing and aging human liquid and gel vitreous. Invest Ophthalmol Vis Sci 1977;16(Suppl):67.

[104] Javitt JC, Street DA, Tielsch JM, et al. National outcomes of cataract extraction. Retinal detachment and endophthalmitis after outpatient cataract surgery. Cataract Patient Outcomes Research Team. Ophthalmology 1994;101:100–5.

[105] Schepens CL, Marden D. Data on the natural history of retinal detachment. Further characterization of certain unilateral nontraumatic cases. Am J Ophthalmol 1966;61:213–26.

[106] Delori F, Pomerantzeff O, Cox MS. Deformation of the globe under high-speed impact: its relation to contusion injuries. Invest Ophthalmol 1969;8:290–301.

[107] Gariano RF, Kim CH. Evaluation and management of suspected retinal detachment. Am Fam Physician 2004;69:1691–8.

[108] Ghazi NG, Green WR. Pathology and pathogenesis of retinal detachment. Eye 2002;16: 411–21.

[109] Zayit-Soudry S, Moroz I, Loewenstein A. Retinal pigment epithelial detachment. Surv Ophthalmol 2007;52:227–43.

[110] Shingleton BJ, O'Donoghue MW. Blurred vision. N Engl J Med 2000;343(8):556–62.

[111] Benson WE. Retinal detachment: diagnosis and management. 2nd edition. Philadelphia: Lippincott; 1988. p. 4.

[112] Smiddy WE, Flynn HW Jr, Nicholson DH, et al. Results and complications in treated retinal breaks. Am J Ophthalmol 1991;112:623–31.

[113] Campo RV, Sipperley JO, Sneed SR, et al. Pars plana vitrectomy without scleral buckle for pseudophakic retinal detachments. Ophthalmology 1999;106:1811–5.

[114] Saw SM, Gazzard G, Wagle AM, et al. An evidence-based analysis of surgical interventions for uncomplicated rhegmatogenous retinal detachment. Acta Ophthalmol Scand 2006;84: 606–12.

[115] Tornambe PE, Hilton GF. Pneumatic retinopexy. A multicenter randomized controlled clinical trial comparing pneumatic retinopexy with scleral buckling. The Retinal Detachment Study Group. Ophthalmology 1989;96:772–83.

[116] Machemer R, Aaberg TM, Freeman HM, et al. An updated classification of retinal detachment with proliferative vitreoretinopathy. Am J Ophthalmol 1991;112:159–65.

[117] Vitrectomy with silicone oil or perfluoropropane gas in eyes with severe proliferative vitreoretinopathy: results of a randomized clinical trial. Silicone Study Report 2. Arch Ophthalmol 1992;110:780–92.

[118] Hassan TS, Sarrafizadeh R, Ruby AJ, et al. The effect of duration of macular detachment on results after the scleral buckle repair of primary, macula-off retinal detachments. Ophthalmology 2002;109:146–52.

[119] Das T. Guidelines for the management of rhegmatogenous retinal detachment. Indian J Ophthalmol 1993;41:37–40.

[120] George R, Walton R, Whitcup S, et al. Primary retinal vasculitis. Systemic associations and diagnostic evaluation. Ophthalmology 1996;103(3):384–9.

[121] Gold D, Morris D, Henkind P. Ocular findings in systemic lupus erythematosus. Br J Ophthalmol 1972;56(11):800–4.

[122] Dunn JP, Noorily SW, Petri M, et al. Antiphospholipid antibodies and retinal vascular disease. Lupus 1996;5(4):313–22.

[123] Lanham JG, Barrie T, Kohner EM, et al. SLE retinopathy: evaluation by fluorescein angiography. Ann Rheum Dis 1982;41(5):473–8.

[124] Stafford-Brady FJ, Urowitz M, Gladman D, et al. Lupus retinopathy: patterns, associations, and prognosis. Arthritis Rheum 1988;31(9):1105–10.

[125] Hall S, Buettner H, Luthra HS. Occlusive retinal vascular disease in systemic lupus erythematosus. J Rheumatol 1984;11(6):846–50.

[126] Mishima S, Masuda K, Izawa Y, et al. Behcet's disease in Japan: ophthalmologic aspects. Trans Am Ophthalmol 1979;77:225–79.

[127] Sakamoto M, Akazawa K, Nishioka Y, et al. Prognostic factors of vision in patients with Behcet disease. Ophthalmology 1995;102(2):317–21.

[128] Siltzbach LE, James DG, Neville E, et al. Course and prognosis of sarcoidosis around the world. Am J Med 1974;57(6):847–52.

[129] Jabs D, Johns C. Ocular involvement in chronic sarcoidosis. Am J Ophthalmol 1986;102(3):297–301.

[130] Hoffman G, Kerr G, Leavitt R, et al. Wegener's granulomatosis: an analysis of 158 patients. Ann Intern Med 1992;116(6):488–98.

[131] Spalton D, Graham E, Page N, et al. Ocular changes in limited forms of Wegener's granulomatosis. Br J Ophthalmol 1981;65(8):553–63.

[132] Morgan C, Foster C, D'Amico D, et al. Retinal vasculitis in polyarteritis nodosa. Retina 1986;6(4):205–9.

[133] Rodriguez A, Akova Y, Pedroza-Seres M, et al. Posterior segment ocular manifestations in patients with HLA-B27 associated uveitis. Ophthalmology 1994;101(7):1267–74.

[134] Rothova A, Buitenhuis H, Meenken C, et al. Uveitis and systemic disease. Br J Ophthalmol 1992;76(3):137–41.

[135] Mapstone R, Woodrow J. HLA-27 and acute anterior uveitis. Br J Ophthalmol 1975;59(5):270–5.

[136] Ruby A, Jampol L. Crohn's disease and retinal vascular disease. Am J Ophthalmol 1990;110(4):349–53.

[137] Henderly D, Gentsler A, Smith R, et al. Changing pattern of uveitis. Am J Ophthalmol 1987;103(2):131–6.

[138] Dutt A, Moers D, Stead WW. Short-course chemotherapy for extrapulmonary tuberculosis: nine years' experience. Ann Intern Med 1986;104(1):7–12.

[139] Donahue H. Ophthalmic experience in a tuberculosis sanatorium. Am J Ophthalmol 1967;64(4):742–8.

[140] Park SS, Friedman A. Infectious causes of posterior uveitis. In: Alberts D, Jakobiec F, editors. Principles and practice of ophthalmology. Philadelphia: WB Saunders; 2000. p. 1236–49.

[141] Lang GK. Retinal inflammatory disease. In: Lang GK, editor. Ophthalmology. New York: Thieme; 2000. p. 346–53.

[142] Alexander A, Sherman J, Horn D. Fundus fluorescein angiography: a summary of theoretical concepts and clinical applications. J Am Optom Assoc 1979;50(1):53–63.

ELSEVIER
SAUNDERS

Emerg Med Clin N Am
26 (2008) 97–123

EMERGENCY
MEDICINE
CLINICS OF
NORTH AMERICA

Trauma to the Globe and Orbit

Sharon P. Bord, MD*, Judith Linden, MD

*Department of Emergency Medicine, Boston University Medical Center,
One Boston Medical Center Place, Dowling 1 South, Boston, MA 02118, USA*

Trauma to the eye represents approximately 3% of all emergency department visits in the United States. Rapid assessment and examination following trauma to the eye is crucial. A thorough knowledge of potential injuries is imperative to ensure rapid diagnosis, to prevent further damage to the eye, and to preserve visual capacity. Although the eye represents only 0.3% of the total surface area on the human body, loss of vision in one or both eyes has been classified as a 24% or 85% whole-person impairment or disability, respectively [1].

History and physical examination

The general principles of the routine ocular examination also pertain to an examination in the setting of trauma, but certain aspects of the examination deserve special attention. Triage and registration personnel should be instructed regarding the urgency of eye injuries and of the need for simultaneous treatment and triage. One always should "take a step back" when considering eye injuries and assess the entire patient. Life- or limb-threatening injury should be addressed initially. In addition, concomitant injury to the brain, spinal cord, or facial bones is common and should be ruled out in the appropriate setting. Historical details should include the timing, mechanism, and location of injury. If there is penetrating trauma, one should learn the energy and type of material involved; organic matter has a higher rate of infection, and metal sometimes can cause a reaction in the vitreous. In pediatric eye trauma, obtaining a history can be difficult; reluctance of the caregiver to provide basic historical information should raise concern for abuse [2]. Visual symptoms such as change in vision, floaters, flashing lights, pain, discharge, or diplopia should be noted. Prior ocular

* Corresponding author.
 E-mail address: sharonbord@gmail.com (S.P. Bord).

doi:10.1016/j.emc.2007.11.006

history such as previous visual impairment, tetanus status, and surgical history should be recorded. In addition one should ascertain if protective eyewear was used.

Physical examination should be performed in a systematic manner to avoid missed injury. The examination can be accomplished in an external to internal fashion. Throughout the examination, care should be taken to avoid placing pressure on the globe, because pressure can cause herniation of intraocular contents if the globe is ruptured. Initially, one should examine the head, scalp, face, and periorbital tissues to assess for lacerations, lid edema, foreign bodies, or sensory deficits (such as infraorbital hypoesthesia in the setting of orbital blowout fractures). Tenderness to palpation around the orbital rim or step-offs should be noted as well. One should look for exophthalmos, enophthalmos, or deformity of the external eye structures. Visual acuity should be tested before manipulation of the eye. Both near and far vision of each eye should be tested separately, with the other eye occluded if possible. Visual acuity should be measured with the patient wearing spectacle correction or using a pinhole occluder if spectacles are not available. A Snellen eye chart or standardized near reading card should be used. Any written material or an intravenous bottle may be used. If the patient is unable to read, one can assess vision by having the patient count the examiner's displayed fingers, detecting hand motion, and indicating light perception or lack of light perception. The conjunctivae should be examined for blood, chemosis (swelling), foreign bodies, and exposed tissue. Examination of the cornea should include fluorescein staining under cobalt blue light to look for irregularities and foreign bodies. Next, the internal structures, including the iris and pupil, should be inspected, noting size, shape, symmetry, and reaction to light. In addition to direct pupillary response, one should assess consensual response using the "swinging flashlight" test. When an afferent pupillary defect is present, both pupils will dilate when the affected eye is exposed to the light source. This defect should be differentiated from pharmacologic or traumatic mydriasis, which is more specifically poor pupillary constriction and is more evident in bright settings. In mydriasis the pupil of the nonaffected eye constricts briskly. Intraocular pressure measurements help differentiate glaucomatous etiologies from other causes of a red painful eye with decreased visual acuity. Elevated intraocular pressure measurements also may indicate the need for emergent procedures such as canthotomies. Devices that can measure intraocular pressure are adequate; even palpation on an anesthetized cornea can give useful diagnostic information. Fundoscopy should be performed, first noting the presence of a red reflex. Decreased intensity of the red reflex may indicate the presence of a cataract, vitreous hemorrhage, or a large retinal detachment. Slit-lamp examination should be performed when possible to assess for injury to the anterior chamber, cornea, iris, and lens. If a slit-lamp examination cannot be performed, examination with a penlight may be used to look for visible hyphema, obvious laceration, or a shrunken-appearing globe.

Imaging techniques

Plain films

Plain film radiographs of the orbits and sinuses are rarely used for diagnosis in orbital trauma. When performed, various views can provide information regarding the orbits and sinuses, such as the presence of an orbital wall or facial bone fracture or opacification of the sinuses. The conventional Caldwell's and Waters' views have moderate sensitivity in detecting orbital fractures: 73% to 78% for fractures of the orbital floor, 71% for fractures of the medial orbital wall, and 64% for fractures of the ethmoid-maxillary plate [3].

CT scan

The CT scan is considered the reference standard imaging modality in the diagnosis of mid-face fracture and orbital trauma. Orbital fractures are commonly missed in patients who have concomitant head trauma, making it imperative that one maintain a high suspicion for orbital injury [4]. The advent of thin-slice helical CT with coronal reconstructions has demonstrated improved image quality and reduced radiation to the lens [5]. The sensitivity of CT scan for orbital fractures ranges from 79% to 96%, with a lower sensitivity when evaluating the infraorbital rim [6]. Vegetable or organic foreign bodies, which increase the risk of endophthalmitis, may not be visualized on CT scan.

Ultrasound

Ocular ultrasound can be a useful tool for the emergency physician when evaluating trauma to the eye. Trauma frequently results in considerable soft tissue swelling, making it difficult to retract the lids and examine the eye fully. Ultrasound can evaluate noninvasively for lens dislocation, globe rupture, retrobulbar hemorrhage, intraocular foreign body, and retinal detachment (Fig. 1). Visualization of periorbital gas on ultrasound may prompt the physician to evaluate further for orbital fracture if not previously considered [7]. One study reported that ocular ultrasound performed by emergency physicians had a sensitivity of 100% and a specificity of 97.2% for identifying ocular pathology [8]. Care should be taken to place minimal pressure on the lid when performing the study, especially if globe rupture has not yet been ruled out. Ultrasound is contraindicated if there is high suspicion of rupture.

MRI

MRI is of limited usefulness in the acute stages of ocular trauma and should not be performed if there is any concern that a metallic intraocular foreign body is present. If there is concern regarding an organic foreign body, MRI may help further differentiate this foreign body from soft tissues when compared with a CT scan.

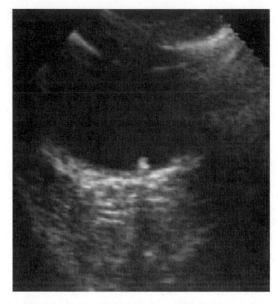

Fig. 1. Ultrasound demonstrating intraocular foreign body. (*Courtesy of* Andreas Dewitz, MD, Boston, MA.)

Blunt trauma to the orbit

Periorbital tissues

Contusion

Periorbital contusion and swelling may be the most prominent initial features in patients presenting to the hospital following trauma to the orbit. The appearance of the ecchymosis and swelling can be dramatic and make examination of the orbit challenging (Fig. 2). The emergency physician always must attempt to examine the structures underlying the swollen

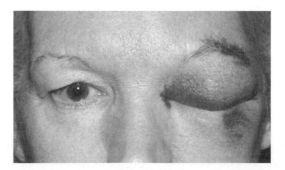

Fig. 2. Contusion of the eye and adnexa. (*From* Boruchoff SA. Anterior segment disease: a diagnostic color atlas. Philadelphia: Elsiever; 2001. p. 204; with permission.)

eyelids. Examination of the underlying tissue may be aided with a Desmarres retractor, which will help avoid global pressure and damage to underlying structures. It is important to keep in mind that periorbital contusion may indicate related significant injury (eg, bilateral raccoon eyes may indicate basilar skull fracture). A study of 600 patients who had sustained significant head trauma found that 58.3% of patients who had isolated blepharohematoma on examination were found to have an orbital fracture on CT scan [9]. Treatment includes head elevation, cold compresses, and reassurance. Complete resolution typically takes 2 to 3 weeks.

Orbital fractures

Orbital wall fractures were first termed "blowout' fractures" in 1957 by Converse and Smith. Orbital blowout fractures are those that occur within the bony orbit, usually along the medial walls and/or the floor, but the orbital rims are intact. There are three proposed theories regarding the mechanism of a blowout fracture. The first is the hydraulic theory, which postulates that when orbital pressure is increased, the globe decompresses through the weakest part of the orbit. The globe-to-wall contact theory was postulated in 1943 by Raymond Pfeiffer. This theory states that when the globe becomes displaced posteriorly in trauma, it strikes the wall, causing a fracture. The third theory, proposed by Le Fort and Lagrange in 1917, is that of buckling: the posterior movement of the orbital rim causes fracture along the medial wall or floor of the orbit [10].

Blowout fractures account for approximately 11% of fractures involving the orbit [11]. Following a blowout fracture, contents may herniate into the maxillary sinus (with orbital floor fractures), or into the ethmoid sinus (with medial wall fracture). A blowout fracture should be suspected when a patient presents with trauma to the globe and soft tissue swelling. Patients may complain of swelling following nose blowing, diplopia, or epistaxis. On examination one may find periorbital ecchymosis, subcutaneous emphysema, restricted extraocular movements, enophthalmos or exophthalmos, ptosis, or anesthesia in the distribution of the infraorbital nerve. The most common limitation in extraocular movements is restriction of upward gaze caused by the entrapment of the inferior rectus muscle. Muscle contusion or cranial nerve disruptions also may be the cause of abnormal extraocular motility, however (Fig. 3). Decreased sensation thought to be related to infraorbital nerve injury can be verified further by testing sensation on the ipsilateral upper gum. It is of utmost importance to remember to inspect the entire globe, because associated injury may occur in 10% to 25% of patients who have orbital floor fractures [11].

The diagnosis of orbital fractures is made most often using CT scan. Although rarely performed, plain-film radiographs of the orbits and sinuses may demonstrate the classic teardrop sign, which may signify orbital contents herniating into the maxillary sinus. In addition one can see air fluid levels or opacification of the sinuses that may indicate a blowout fracture.

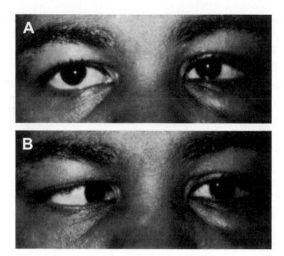

Fig. 3. Decreased extraocular movement. (*Courtesy of* D. Wagner, MD, Washington, DC.)

CT scan of the orbits is extremely sensitive for identifying fractures. In addition ultrasound is a promising tool that can be used to identify orbital fractures. Periorbital gas seen on ultrasound may indicate an underlying orbital fracture [7].

Orbital fractures are not considered an ophthalmologic emergency unless there is visual impairment or globe injury. Surgical repair is indicated for patients who have persistent diplopia or cosmetic concerns (enophthalmos) and in general is not performed until swelling subsides 7 to 10 days following injury [12].

Patients should be discharged with instructions to use ice compresses and should be cautioned to avoid nose blowing and Valsalva maneuvers and to sneeze with their mouths open. The routine use of prophylactic antibiotics following orbital fracture is controversial and may not be indicated in all cases [13]. Orbital cellulitis is a rare complication following orbital fracture. Risk factors for developing orbital cellulitis include fracture adjacent to an infected sinus and nose blowing. Prophylactic antibiotics are recommended if adjacent sinusitis is present [14].

Patients should be instructed to return if they experience intense eye pain, changes in vision, proptosis, or a tense globe. These complaints should raise concern for compressive orbital emphysema or retrobulbar hemorrhage.

Retrobulbar hemorrhage

Traumatic hemorrhage into the retrobulbar space may result in acute visual loss [15]. Hemorrhage into the potential space surrounding the globe may occur following blunt trauma because of injury to the orbital vessels. It is important to remember that the orbit is an enclosed space bound laterally and posteriorly by bony walls, superiorly and inferiorly by the orbital septa, and anteriorly by the globe and inelastic orbital septum. In a small series of patients nondisplaced fractures of the orbital walls were found to be associated with retrobulbar hematoma [16]. This condition is rare following displaced fractures, however, because the blood will decompress into the sinuses [17]. Hemorrhage can lead to an acute increase in intraorbital pressure, which then is transmitted to the optic nerve and globe, resulting in central retinal artery occlusion and optic nerve ischemia. Clinical signs and symptoms include proptosis, limitation of extraocular movements, visual loss, afferent pupillary defect, and increased intraocular pressure. Diagnosis can be confirmed by CT scan, but treatment never should be delayed while waiting for imaging.

Early recognition and decompression is key to preserving vision and warrants emergent ophthalmologic consultation. Treatment of increased intraocular pressure can be attempted with topical beta-blockers or intravenous mannitol or carbonic anhydrase inhibitor. Lateral canthotomy can be a vision-saving procedure and is indicated in patients who have a history of trauma and marked periorbital edema with visual loss, severe proptosis, diffuse subconjunctival hemorrhage, or an afferent papillary defect. Lateral canthotomy is performed by applying a small, straight clamp to the lateral canthus, aiming inferiorly and laterally toward the conjunctival sac after local anesthesia administration (lidocaine 1% with epinephrine). The clamp is left in place for 15 seconds to 2 minutes. After removal of the clamp there is an impression in the tissue. A 1-cm incision is made along this impression using iris scissors. If pressures remain elevated, the lateral canthal tendon should be transected as well by aiming scissors inferolaterally. Transecting the inferior lateral canthal tendon should result in the lower lid pulling easily away from the lid margin (Fig. 4). Despite the decompression of high intraorbital pressure, usually only a small amount of blood is expressed with the release of the hematoma.

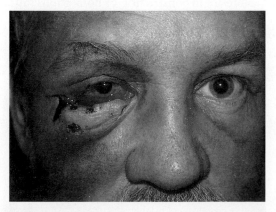

Fig. 4. Orbit following lateral canthotomy. Note the lower lid pulling easily away from lid margin. (*Courtesy of* John Lee, MD, Boston, MA.)

Anterior chamber

Traumatic hyphema

Traumatic hyphema is caused by disruption of blood vessels in the iris or ciliary body causing blood to extravasate into the anterior chamber (Fig. 5). Hyphemas are classified from grade 0 to 4, based on the percentage of the anterior chamber that is filled with blood. Microhyphemas are grade 0 and represent circulating red blood cells that can be detected only by slit-lamp examination. The grading system then progresses from grades 1 (less than one fourth to one third of the anterior chamber) through 4 (total anterior chamber filled with blood). An "eight-ball hyphema" refers to an anterior chamber that is entirely filled with a black-appearing clot. Hyphema may occur after blunt or penetrating trauma, and more than 50% have been documented as being sports related [1].

In traumatic hyphema, it is important to obtain a complete past medical history specifically addressing bleeding disorders such as hemophilias and Von Willebrand's disease and hemoglobinopathies such as sickle cell anemia or sickle trait. Patients also should be questioned regarding the use of medications that may affect coagulation, including warfarin and aspirin. The symptoms of hyphema include pain, photophobia, and blurring of vision. Lethargy or somnolence can be associated with isolated traumatic hyphemas but always should raise concern for a concomitant head injury. On examination one frequently can see a hyphema on gross inspection with the patient sitting upright (causing the blood to layer in the aqueous fluid). In addition slit-lamp examination should be performed to assess for associated injury and further quantify the hyphema. Traumatic miosis or mydriasis may be present as well and should be differentiated from an afferent papillary defect. This distinction can be done by the swinging flashlight test, as described elsewhere in this issue. An afferent papillary defect will cause paradoxical dilatation in the affected eye and the unaffected eye, whereas traumatic mydriasis will result in constriction of both pupils (although limited in the affected eye). An afferent pupillary defect should raise concern for an optic nerve or posterior pole injury.

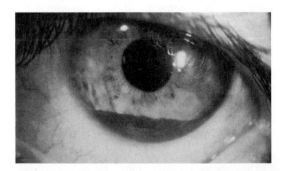

Fig. 5. Hyphema. (*Courtesy of* D. Wagner, MD, Washington, DC.)

The most common complication of hyphema is rebleeding, which occurs 2 to 5 days following injury when the initial clot retracts and loosens. Rebleeding occurs in approximately 22% of patients [1]. Rebleeding is more common in those who have visual acuities of 20/200 on presentation, initial hyphema of more than one third of the anterior chamber, more than 1 day's delay in obtaining medical attention, and elevated intraocular pressure at initial presentation [1,18]. Other complications include corneal blood staining (in approximately 5% of patients), elevated intraocular pressure, and synechiae formation between the iris and the cornea or the lens posteriorly. Elevated intraocular pressure facilitates corneal blood staining. As the pressure in the anterior chamber increases, the ability of the corneal endothelial cells to transport fluid out of the stroma is impaired. The cornea swells, and the endothelium becomes leaky, forming gaps large enough for the hemoglobin to enter the corneal stroma. Patients who have sickle cell anemia or who are trait positive have a higher rate of complications associated with hyphema. The acidic and hypoxic nature of the anterior chamber leads to sickling of the red blood cells, which can cause increased intraocular pressure and decreased aqueous humor output. Patients who have a history of sickle cell trait have rates of rebleeding up to 64% [1].

Treatment for hyphema should be directed at minimizing secondary hemorrhage and reducing the incidence of secondary glaucoma. Recent literature indicates that hospitalization versus outpatient management, moderate ambulation versus strict bed rest, or treatment with unilateral or bilateral eye patches has no significant effect on the incidence of secondary hemorrhage or final visual outcome [1]. In addition, outpatient treatment has been shown to be cost effective [19]. Hospitalization has been recommended for patients who have rebleeding, elevated intraocular pressure, positive sickle cell trait or anemia, hyphemas greater than 50%, or decreased vision, for noncompliant patients, and in suspected child abuse. The disposition of these patients always should be discussed with an ophthalmologist. Patients who are discharged from the hospital must undergo daily examinations by an ophthalmologist to assess for increased size of hyphema or other complications.

Supportive therapy includes elevation of the head to 30° while at rest. In addition, eye patching with a metal shield provides protection from further ocular injury and often is recommended until the hyphema resolves. The shield must have holes or be made of clear plastic so that patients can monitor their vision, because decreased vision is the earliest symptom of rebleeding. Topical application of cycloplegics has not been shown to have significant therapeutic effects but can increase patient comfort and facilitate the examination of the posterior segment. Topical corticosteroids have been shown to reduce intraocular inflammation and decrease the incidence of secondary hemorrhage [20]. Topical and systemic antifibrinolytics, such as aminocaproic acid (ACA) and tranexamic acid (not available in United States), have been shown to decrease secondary hemorrhage significantly [18]. Aminocaproic acid is an antifibrinolytic agent that prevents the conversion of plasminogen to plasmin and therefore delays clot dissolution and theoretically decreases the risk of rebleeding. Studies have shown that topical ACA is as effective as systemic ACA and avoids the side effects typically associated with administration such as nausea, vomiting, and hypotension [1]. These agents should be avoided in pregnant patients, patients who have renal or hepatic dysfunction, or those at risk for thromboembolic disease. Intracameral tissue plasminogen activator currently is under investigation and is reserved for large clots of prolonged duration or malignant elevation of intraocular pressure. In addition, elevated intraocular pressure (> 24 mm Hg) can be treated with topical beta-blockers and carbonic anhydrase inhibitors such as acetazolamide. Acetazolamide lowers pH, causing increased sickling, and should be avoided in pediatric patients or those who have sickle cell trait or anemia. Methazolomide is the preferred agent in this situation [21]. Mannitol may be administered for severely elevated intraocular pressure (> 35 mm Hg). Nonsteroidal anti-inflammatory medications and aspirin should be avoided because of the increased risk of rebleeding. Surgery usually is reserved for delayed complications such as corneal staining and persistently elevated intraocular pressures but often is performed early in patients who have sickle cell anemia or trait.

Subconjunctival hemorrhage

Subconjunctival hemorrhage is caused by the rupture of small subconjunctival blood vessels. Although patients may report a prior sneezing or coughing episode or a Valsalva maneuver, some patients may have no recollection of the preceding events. Patients often seek care because of the dramatic appearance. On examination a painless, smooth, bright-red area is noted over the bulbar conjunctiva and is sharply demarcated at the limbus. Visual acuity should be normal. If there is preceding blunt or penetrating trauma, underlying scleral penetration should be considered. Pain on extraocular movements and bloody chemosis also should prompt suspicion for injury to the globe. Subconjunctival hemorrhage should always be distinguished from chemosis: a hemorrhage is flat and smooth, whereas chemosis presents as erythema with edema, and the area is raised. Bilateral or recurrent subconjunctival hemorrhage may require a work-up for bleeding diathesis. Treatment of subconjunctival hemorrhage consists of reassurance and local cold compresses for 24 hours. Subconjunctival hemorrhages heal spontaneously in 2 to 4 weeks.

Injury to the iris and ciliary body

Traumatic iridocyclitis (uveitis)

Blunt injury to the globe may contuse and inflame the iris and ciliary body, resulting in ciliary spasm. Patients may complain of photophobia, blurred vision, and eye pain. Examination reveals conjunctival injection, specifically ciliary flush, cells, and flare in the anterior chamber and a small, poorly dilating pupil. Cells and flare are best seen in the slit lamp with high magnification and very bright light. This condition is self limited; symptomatic treatment consists of paralyzing the iris and ciliary body with long-acting cycloplegic agents such as homatropine 5% for a period of 7 to 10 days. If there is no improvement after 5 to 7 days, prednisolone acetate 1% may be used to decrease inflammation in consultation with an ophthalmologist. Topical steroids should be withheld in patients who have a corneal epithelial defect. Resolution typically occurs within 1 week.

Traumatic mydriasis and miosis

Blunt injury to the orbit may damage the iris sphincter. Bruising and irritation of the sphincter leads to constriction of the pupil (miosis). Small tears to the sphincter muscle may result in dilatation or mydriasis. In the setting of significant head trauma and altered mental status, one must rule out a cranial nerve palsy and brain herniation. Treatment is supportive, and the condition often resolves spontaneously.

Iridodialysis

Traumatic iridodialysis is a tearing of the iris root from the ciliary body leading to formation of a "secondary pupil" (Fig. 6). This injury may also cause a hyphema. Large tears can be a cause of monocular diplopia. Urgent ophthalmologic consultation is warranted when iridodialysis causes a hyphema or decreased visual acuity. Surgical repair may be indicated for persistent monocular diplopia.

Acute glaucoma

Acute glaucoma can occur following trauma. The underlying pathophysiology is narrowing of the anterior chamber or disruption of outflow of

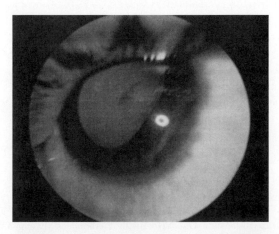

Fig. 6. Iridodialysis. (*Courtesy of* D. Wagner, MD, Washington, DC.)

aqueous humor, either secondary to red blood cells (hyphema), formation of a trabecular meshwork scar, or lens dislocation. Posttraumatic glaucoma is associated with advanced patient age, lens injury, poor baseline visual acuity, and inflammation of the anterior chamber [22]. Patients who have these characteristics should be followed closely by an ophthalmologist to assess for development of glaucoma. Acute rises in intraocular pressure should be treated aggressively with miotics (contraindicated in eyes following cataract surgery or lens extraction), topical drops including beta-blockers, alpha agonists, prostaglandin analogues, acetazolomide, or mannitol.

Injury to the lens

Subluxation and dislocation

Blunt trauma to the eye results in a sudden compressive deformation of the globe, displacing the cornea and anterior sclera posteriorly with a compensatory expansion of the globe in the equatorial direction. This trauma can result in damage to the lens zonule fibers, which are responsible for holding the lens in place, causing lens dislocation or subluxation. Following complete disruption of the lens zonules, the lens may dislocate posteriorly or, less commonly, into the anterior chamber (Fig. 7). Diagnosis of this injury is based on history and physical examination. Symptoms include blurring of the vision or monocular diplopia and distortion when the lens remains partially in the visual axis. The lens may be visualized when displaced into the anterior chamber or may be viewed after pupillary dilatation when dislocated posteriorly. Iridodonesis, a tremor of the iris after rapid eye movements, may be a helpful finding associated with posterior dislocations [23]. An anteriorly dislocated lens may cause acute angle closure glaucoma, which may be a vision-threatening complication. Predisposing factors for lens dislocation include Marfan's syndrome, homocystinuria, and spherophakia [23]. Lens subluxations and dislocations should be referred to an

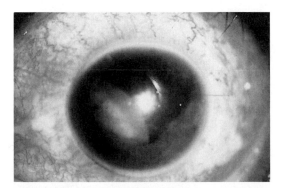

Fig. 7. Traumatic lens dislocation. (*From* Harlan JB, Pieramici DJ. Evaluation of patients with ocular trauma. Ophthalmol Clin North Am 2002;15:159; with permission.)

ophthalmologist for surgical repair. Repair should be performed on an emergent basis if the lens is obstructing the flow of aqueous humor, leading to elevated intraocular pressure.

Cataract formation

The stroma of the lens normally are sequestered in a relatively dehydrated environment by the lens capsule. If the lens capsule is disrupted by either blunt or penetrating trauma, the stroma may absorb fluid, swell, and become cloudy (Fig. 8), obstructing the outflow of aqueous humor and leading to acute glaucoma. Traumatic cataracts may occur acutely or develop over weeks to months. Bilateral cataracts may develop after lightning strike or electrical injury [24]. There is no effective prevention, and definitive treatment requires lens replacement.

Globe injury

Globe rupture

Globe rupture always should be considered when evaluating a patient who has sustained blunt trauma or a penetrating injury, because it is a major cause of monocular blindness. More than 90% of these injuries are preventable, with trauma from violent behavior accounting for a large portion [25]. Ruptures are most common at the insertions of the intraocular muscles or at the limbus, where the sclera is thinnest. Diagnosis of a ruptured globe can be obvious if intraocular contents are visualized, but occult rupture can be difficult to diagnose. Critical signs and symptoms include decreased visual acuity, severe bullous subconjunctival hemorrhage (involving 360° of the bulbar conjunctiva), a deep or shallow anterior chamber, and limitation of extraocular motility. Other signs include low intraocular pressure (although pressure may be normal or increased), an irregularly shaped pupil (peaked toward the wound), iridodialysis, exposed uveal tissue (which appears brownish-red), or vitreous hemorrhage (Fig. 9).

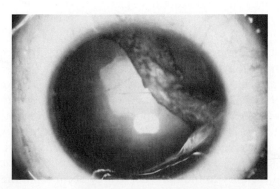

Fig. 8. Traumatic cataract and iridodialysis. (*From* Harlan JB, Pieramici DJ. Evaluation of patients with ocular trauma. Ophthalmol Clin North Am 2002;15:159; with permission.)

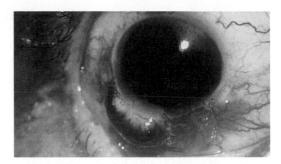

Fig. 9. Ruptured globe. (*From* Kanski JJ. Clinical diagnosis in ophthalmology. Philadelphia: Mosby Elsevier; 2006.)

Once the diagnosis of globe rupture is made or suspected, further manipulation of the globe should be deferred. Treatment includes emergent ophthalmologic consultation, placement of a protective eye shield, antiemetics (to avoid further increasing intraocular pressure during a Valsalva maneuver), analgesics, and systemic antibiotics to prevent endophthalmitis. Any maneuver that may increase intraocular pressure should be avoided. A CT scan should be obtained to evaluate for the presence of orbital and intraocular foreign bodies. CT scan evaluation alone is only 75% sensitive for diagnosis of globe rupture and therefore should be used as a complement to physical findings [26]. Ultrasonography and indirect ophthalmoscopy may be helpful in further evaluation but should be deferred to the ophthalmologist. The administration of succinylcholine for airway management is controversial. There have been anecdotal reports of expulsion of intraocular material with succinylcholine use, but more recent case studies do not support this finding [27]. The current recommendation for patients who require rapid airway management with concomitant penetrating ocular injury is rapid-sequence intubation with succinylcholine following pretreatment with a nondepolarizing and sedating agent.

Globe luxation

Luxation of the globe is a rare condition that results from an extreme form of trauma. Many years ago it was thought to be caused by gouging during fights and historically has been a complication of forceps delivery in obstructed labor [28]. Now it is seen more commonly after great forces are applied to the head in an anteroposterior direction (eg, in a motor vehicle crash), but there have been case reports documented in which luxation was caused by penetrating trauma. The most commonly injured and avulsed extraocular muscle is the medial rectus. The status of the optic nerve is clinically important. Injury to the optic nerve may occur from the forward propulsion of the globe with traction on the nerve or may be related to a sudden rise in intraocular pressure.

Acute care consists mainly of protecting the eye from further damage. This protection can be accomplished with a cup or other hard protective device. In addition, early reduction with topical anesthesia can be attempted, because it will minimize the amount of traction placed on the optic nerve. Globe reduction may not be possible in the emergency department because of the swelling of the eyelids and surrounding tissues, necessitating intraoperative reduction under general anesthesia [28]. Spontaneous and voluntary globe luxation has been reported during the insertion of contact lenses and may be more common in diseases that cause proptosis such as Grave's disease and orbital tumors. Calming the patient and having the patient relax the eyelids will make it easier for spontaneous repositioning to occur.

Posterior segment

Vitreous hemorrhage

Vitreous hemorrhage occurs when blood enters the normally avascular vitreous space, which is filled with a clear gelatinous material. This space is bordered anteriorly by the lens, posteriorly and laterally by the retina, and laterally by the ciliary body. Although most causes of vitreous hemorrhage are nontraumatic (diabetic retinopathy, sickle cell disease, posterior vitreous detachment, retinal vein occlusion, leukemia), trauma accounts for 12% to 31% (depending on study population) and is the most common cause of vitreous hemorrhage in younger patients [29,30]. Vitreous hemorrhages can be associated with retinal tears, avulsed retinal veins, or subarachnoid hemorrhage. Vitreous hemorrhages in an infant should prompt consideration of shaken baby syndrome, admission, and an in-depth search for other traumatic injuries. Vitreous hemorrhages may be associated with traumatic and atraumatic subarachnoid hemorrhage (Terson's syndrome). The theory is that increasing intracranial pressure results in increased retinal vein pressures, causing rupture and vitreous hemorrhage [31]. Patients who have Terson's syndrome have a poorer prognosis than patients who have subarachnoid hemorrhage without vitreous hemorrhage.

Symptoms of vitreous hemorrhage include floaters (small hemorrhage), cobwebs, shadows, a smoky haze, or loss of vision (larger hemorrhage). Physical examination may reveal a decreased or absent light reflex, loss of fundus detail, or floating debris but may be normal in the undilated eye. An indirect fundoscopic examination should be performed if the direct examination is normal. In the preretinal hemorrhages of shaken baby syndrome, layering of blood with a meniscus may be seen on the retina.

Traumatic vitreous hemorrhage mandates emergent ophthalmologic consultation, because 11% to 44% of vitreous hemorrhages are associated with retinal tears [32]. Ultrasound may be helpful if the fundus is obscured. Discharge instructions include limited physical activity and head elevation when sleeping. Nonsteroidal anti-inflammatory drugs and aspirin should be avoided, unless the benefit outweighs the risk (ie, in patients who have unstable angina or other clinical indications). Definitive treatment depends on the underlying cause and may include laser, cryotherapy, or scleral buckling in cases of retinal detachment. Most hemorrhages resolve spontaneously within a few weeks to months.

Chorioretinal injury

Trauma is the most common cause of retinal detachment in children and is responsible for about 10% of detachments in the general population [33]. Symptoms of retinal tears or detachments include floaters from bleeding and flashing lights from stimulation of retina neurons. Isolated tears and detachments do not cause pain. Visual field defects or decreased visual acuity may be present as well. Retinal detachment generally progresses slowly following injury, occurring weeks to months later. Fundoscopic examination may reveal a hazy, gray membrane of the retina billowing forward (Fig. 10), but small peripheral tears may not be visualized on direct ophthalmoscopy. Indirect ophthalmoscopy should be performed on every patient in whom the diagnosis of retinal detachment or tear is being considered. Approximately one third of retinal detachments are not diagnosed until at least 6 weeks after trauma [34].

Management of retinal tears or detachment begins with urgent ophthalmologic consultation. Treatment consists of either head elevation or supine positioning, depending on whether the tear is superior or inferior. Surgical correction consists of scleral buckling, pars plana vitrectomy, or photocoagulation. The timing of surgical correction is based on the size of the retinal detachment and the degree of macular involvement.

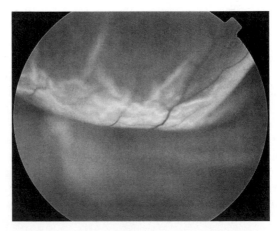

Fig. 10. Retinal detachment. (*From* Kanski JJ. Clinical diagnosis in ophthalmology. Philadelphia: Mosby Elsevier; 2006.)

Commotio retina

Commotio retina, also known as "Berlin's edema," may occur after recent blunt ocular trauma. Studies have demonstrated this injury to be present in 9% to 14% of blowout fractures [11]. The term "commotio retina" literally means retinal contusion in Latin and is caused by disruption of the retinal photoreceptors. The term "Berlin's edema" is actually a misnomer, because no edema is present (Fig. 11). Patients may complain of decreased visual acuity or may be asymptomatic if the macula is not involved. Examination reveals a confluent area of retinal whitening. Blood vessels can be seen distinctly below the whitened area. Commotio retina can occur anywhere on the retina, but it usually is maximal in the area opposite the traumatic blow. There is no specific treatment for this condition, because it usually resolves spontaneously in approximately 2 weeks. Serial examination is necessary to ensure that retinal tear or detachment has not occurred.

Penetrating ocular injury

Periorbital tissues

Conjunctival lacerations

Lacerations of the bulbar conjunctiva are commonly associated with intraocular foreign bodies or underlying sclera perforation, so a ruptured globe must be ruled out. Conjunctival lacerations may be seen as a conjunctival defect, exposure of Tenon's capsule, or orbital fat. Slit-lamp examination can help differentiate superficial from deep lacerations. Small, superficial lacerations (< 1 cm) require no suturing and generally heal rapidly. Lacerations that are greater than 1 cm may be repaired by an

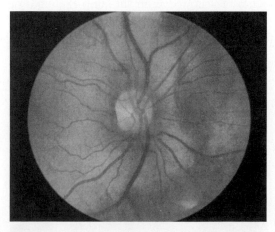

Fig. 11. Commotio retina is visualized as a patchy, gray-white opacification of the retina. (*Courtesy of* D. Wagner, MD, Washington, DC.)

ophthalmologist using 6-0 to 8-0 absorbable suture. Treatment with prophylactic antibiotic ointment or drops is recommended for all patients who have
conjunctival lacerations [35].

Laceration of the eyelid

Lacerations of the eyelid should prompt concern for a penetrating globe
injury or foreign body. Emergency physicians can manage simple horizontal
or oblique partial-thickness lid lacerations. Closure should be performed
with interrupted 6-0 or 7-0 nylon sutures. Sutures should be removed in 3
to 5 days. Lacerations that require immediate referral to an ophthalmologist
for repair include those that involve the lid margins, the canalicular system,
or the levator or canthal tendons, loss of tissue, or lacerations through the
orbital septum. A laceration through the orbital septum should be suspected
if orbital fat protrudes through the wound [35].

Globe injury

Corneoscleral laceration and puncture wounds

Signs of corneal perforation include loss of anterior chamber depth,
blood in the anterior chamber, and a teardrop-shaped pupil caused by iris
prolapse through the corneal laceration. Small corneal lacerations may be
difficult to diagnose. If corneal laceration is suspected, one must inspect
the entire cornea while taking care to not put excessive pressure on the
globe. Corneal lacerations occur most often on the inferior aspect of the
globe because of Bell's phenomenon, the reflex upward rotation of the globe
during blinking in response to potential foreign body penetration. Suspicion
that aqueous humor is leaking from the wound can be confirmed by Seidel's
test, which is performed by applying fluorescein dye over the area of concern
and noting a stream of yellow dye on slit-lamp examination (Fig. 12).

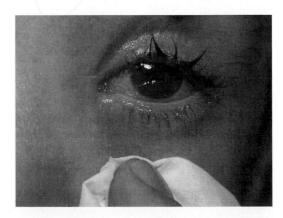

Fig. 12. Corneal laceration following repair. (*Courtesy of* John Lee, MD, Boston, MA.)

Once a laceration is suspected, a protective cover should be placed on the eye, and prophylactic antibiotics should be administered. Ophthalmologic consultation should be obtained when there is concern for a full-thickness laceration. Partial-thickness lacerations that are not widened can be treated with cycloplegics, topical antibiotics, and a pressure patch. Lacerations that require repair are performed in the operating room.

Intraocular foreign body

An intraocular foreign body is present in 18% to 41% of open globe injuries. The diagnosis should be suspected based on history [36]. Hammering (especially of metal on metal) is the most common mechanism, responsible for 60% to 80% of cases (Figs. 13 and 14). In developed countries this type of injury now occurs more commonly in the home than in the workplace. It is crucial to identify the material of the foreign body because it will influence treatment decisions. Specifically, iron-containing foreign bodies can cause siderosis, brownish discoloration of the iris, and yellow cataracts, and copper may lead to cheilosis, a rapidly developing sterile endophthalmitis. Lead-containing products may cause lead poisoning if left in place.

An intraocular foreign body should be considered strongly in penetrating globe injuries. Visual acuity generally is decreased, but normal visual acuity does not rule out the presence of a foreign body. Additional warning signs on examination consist of localized corneal edema, hemorrhage over the sclera, a nonsurgical hole in the iris, or a cloudy lens. CT has largely replaced plain-film radiography in the diagnosis of an intraocular foreign

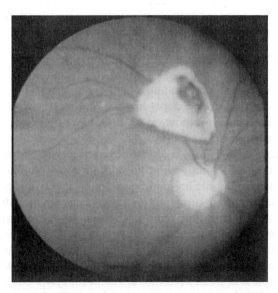

Fig. 13. Intraocular foreign body located near the retina. (*Courtesy of* D. Wagner, MD, Washington, DC.)

bodies did not increase the rate of endophthalmitis if systemic and topical antibiotics were administered [42]. Definitive treatment consists of vitrectomy in addition to antibiotics. Topical or systemic corticosteroid therapy is controversial. Early recognition and prompt treatment of Bacillus infection increases the chances of improved visual outcome.

Sympathetic ophthalmia

Sympathetic ophthalmia is an inflammation that occurs in the uninjured (sympathizing) eye weeks to decades following the initial insult to the injured eye. It also may occur following uncomplicated intraocular surgery. It is thought to be caused by an autoimmune response to the release of the uveal contents into the vitreous humor of the injured eye. This release of tissue leads to autoimmune destruction in the uninjured eye, potentially causing severe bilateral vision loss. Sympathetic ophthalmia is rare, occurring in 0.2% to 1% of patients following trauma and in 0.001% of patients following surgical procedures. Symptoms are similar to a nongranulomatous uveitis with blurry vision, photophobia, decreased visual acuity, and tearing. Examination may reveal keratic precipitates, papillitis, and subretinal exudates. These exudates may coalesce at the posterior pole, producing an area of exudative retinal detachment and, over time, scarring of the posterior pole. Treatment consists of high-dose oral corticosteroids. If the inflammation cannot be controlled, other immunosuppressive agents, including cyclosporine, chlorambucil, or azathioprine, may be used. Sympathetic ophthalmia can be prevented if the hopelessly injured eye with no visual potential is enucleated within 14 days of trauma. The role of enucleation following development of sympathetic ophthalmia is controversial and should be based on the visual acuity of the injured eye. It remains unclear if enucleation of the injured eye improves prognosis of the sympathizing eye. If the eye retains some visual function, it probably should not be removed.

Burns

Acid and alkali exposure

Chemical burns are worrisome because of their ability to affect multiple ocular structures profoundly and potentially cause blindness. Alkali-containing agents, such as oven and drain cleaners (potassium hydroxide), lime in plaster (calcium hydroxide), fertilizers and sparklers (ammonium hydroxide), and high-concentration bleach (sodium hypochlorite), are particularly damaging because they are both lipophilic and hydrophilic and can penetrate cell membranes rapidly (Fig. 16). Deployment of airbags causes release of sodium hydroxide, which can lead to an alkaline chemical keratitis [34]. Ocular damage results from saponification of cell membranes and cell death along with destruction of the extracellular matrix. Acidic agents, such as hydrofluoric acid (used in industrial etching and alkylation of high-octane gasoline), battery acid (sulfuric acid), and hydrochloric acid, generally cause

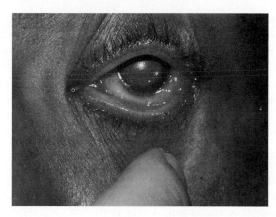

Fig. 16. Eye following alkaline exposure. (*Courtesy of* John Lee, MD, Boston, MA.)

less damage than alkaline agents because many corneal proteins bind acid and act as a buffer. The coagulated tissue functions as a barrier and prevents further penetration of the acid.

The Roper-Hall classification of chemical burns can be used; for simplicity, however, burns can be classified as mild-to-moderate burns and severe burns. The most important differentiating feature is limbal and corneal ischemia. On examination of mild-to-moderate burns one can see focal areas of conjunctival chemosis and hyperemia as well as mild eyelid edema and anterior chamber reaction. First- and second-degree burns may be noted on the periocular skin. Severe burns are characterized by conjunctival blanching and pallor [43]. Corneal edema or opacification can make it difficult to evaluate the anterior chamber. Early sequelae of chemical burns occurring 1 to 3 days after exposure include elevated intraocular pressure caused by damage of the trabecular meshwork and corneal edema. Long-term complications include perforation, scarring, and neovascularization of the cornea, adhesions of the lids to the globe (symblepharon), glaucoma, cataract, and retinal damage.

Treatment should be initiated immediately after exposure by irrigating the eyes with copious amounts of fluid, preferably saline or lactated Ringer's solution, for at least 30 minutes. A Morgan lens may be used if there is no particulate material. (See the article entitled "Eye Exposures" in this issue for a discussion of eye irrigation techniques, including the Morgan lens). Five to 10 minutes after completing irrigation, litmus paper should be placed in the inferior cul de sac. Irrigation is continued until a neutral pH, 7.0 to 7.4, is reached. pH is measured before adding topical anesthetic to the eye, because most anesthetics have an acidic pH and may lower the measured pH artificially. Foreign body removal, by sweeping the fornices with a cotton swab, should be performed as well, with special attention to the conjunctival fornices, because material that is crystallized may cause a persistently elevated pH. Additional treatment consists of cycloplegia (using scopolamine 0.25%), topical antibiotic ointment, and topical steroids if significant inflammation of the cornea or anterior chamber is present. Phenylephrine should be avoided because it causes vasoconstriction. If elevated intraocular pressure is noted, anti-glaucoma medications such as acetazolamide should be initiated. Oral vitamin C (ascorbic acid) stimulates collagen production and therefore has a theoretical benefit [43]. These patients require close follow-up, and some may require hospital admission for further irrigation or monitoring.

Miscellaneous irritants, solvents, and detergents

Unknown exposures should be treated initially as though they were an acid or alkali exposure. The eye should be irrigated immediately. Detergents generally cause only a mild conjunctival irritation, but more irritating substances can cause denudation of the cornea and inflammation of the anterior chamber. After the eye is thoroughly irrigated, it should be treated like a corneal abrasion with topical erythromycin ointment. Exposure to aerosol products may lead to intraocular foreign body from the propellant. Compounds that are found in personal protective devices such as mace and pepper spray are treated in the same fashion as other chemical injuries.

Special consideration should be given to cyanoacrylate adhesive ("superglue") exposure. These glues are rapid setting and harden quickly on contact with moisture. If the eyelids are glued together, an attempt should be made to separate them with gentle traction. Lids that are sealed shut in normal anatomic position that cannot be separated with gentle traction can be left alone, allowing time for the super glue to dissolve over the next few days. Misdirected lashes and hardened glue may cause corneal defects and irritation. These defects should be treated like corneal abrasions. Attempts to dissolve the adhesive with other agents should be avoided. Ophthalmologic consultation should be obtained for these exposures [43].

Thermal burns

Thermal burns are more frequently seen on the eyelids than on the globe because of reflex blinking and Bell's phenomenon. Superficial burns may be treated with irrigation and topical antibiotic ophthalmic ointment. Second- or third-degree burns of the eyelid warrant ophthalmologic consultation. Although patients frequently cover the face, hot liquid splashes and cigarettes ashes may cause a superficial corneal epithelial injury and are treated like a corneal abrasion. There have also been documented cases of air bag–related thermal burns caused by failure of the inflation mechanism [34].

UV keratitis

Exposure to UV light can occur from tanning booth exposure, from high-altitude environments, or from welding. The UV light causes direct corneal epithelial damage. Patients give a history of exposure approximately 6 to 10 hours before developing symptoms. Symptoms include moderate-to-severe ocular pain, foreign body sensation, red eye, tearing, photophobia, and blurred vision. Examination reveals decreased visual acuity and diffuse punctate lesions on fluorescein staining, with a sharp demarcation at the lower lid where the eye was protected. Treatment consists of cycloplegic drops, topical antibiotic ointment, and oral analgesics.

Prevention

Wearing protective eyewear often can prevent injuries to the globe. A study of patients in the US military who had sustained eye injury found that only a small percentage of them were wearing protective glasses at the time of injury [37,42]. In addition, many sports-related eye injuries could be prevented by wearing the recommended protective equipment. Air bag deployment, although associated with a 20% reduction in the incidence of fatal and severe injuries after frontal and near-frontal automobile collisions, increases the risk of orbital fractures or other ocular trauma [44].

Acknowledgment

The authors thank Dr. John Lee for his expert manuscript review and comments.

References

[1] Brandt MT, Haug R. Traumatic hyphema: a comprehensive review. J Oral Maxillofac Surg 2001;56:1462–70.
[2] Harlan JB, Pieramici DJ. Evaluation of patients with ocular trauma. Ophthalmol Clin North Am 2002;15:153–61.
[3] Iinuma T, Hirota Y, Ishio K. Orbital wall fractures. Conventional views and CT. Rhinology 1994;32(2):81–3.
[4] Holmgren E, Dierks E, Homer L, et al. Facial computed tomography use in trauma patients who require a head computed tomogram. J Oral Maxillofac Surg 2004;62(8):913–8.
[5] Lakits A, Prokesch R, Scholda C. Orbital helical computed tomography in the diagnosis and management of eye trauma. Ophthalmology 1999;106:2330–5.
[6] Jank S, Deibl M, Strobl H, et al. Intrarater reliability in the ultrasound diagnosis of medial and lateral orbital wall fractures with a curved array transducer. J Oral Maxillofac Surg 2006;64(1):68–73.
[7] McIlrath ST, Blaivas M, Lyon M. Diagnosis of periorbital gas in ocular ultrasound after facial trauma. Am J Emerg Med 2005;23:517–20.
[8] Blaivas M, Theodoro D, Sierzenski P. A study of bedside ultrasonography in the emergency department. Acad Emerg Med 2002;9(8):791–9.
[9] Exadaktylos A, Sclabas GM, Smolka K, et al. The value of computed tomographic scanning in the diagnosis and management of orbital fractures associated with head trauma: a prospective, consecutive study at a level I trauma center. J Trauma 2005;58(2):336–41.
[10] Kreidl K, Kim D, Mansour S. Prevalence of significant intraocular sequelae in blunt ocular trauma. Am J Emerg Med 2003;21(7):525–8.
[11] He D, Blomquist P, Ellis E. Association between ocular injuries and internal orbital fractures. J Oral Maxillofac Surg 2007;65(4):713–20.

[12] Burnstine AU. Clinical recommendations for repair of orbital facial fractures. Curr Opin Ophthalmol 2003;14(5):236–40.

[13] Martin B, Ghosh A. Antibiotics in orbital floor fractures. J Emerg Med 2003;20(1):66.

[14] Simon GJB, Bush S, Selva D, et al. Orbital cellulitis: a rare complication after orbital blow-out fracture. Ophthalmology 2005;112(11):2030–4.

[15] Vasallo S, Hartstein M, Howard D, et al. Traumatic retrobulbar hemorrhage: emergent decompression by lateral canthotomy and cantholysis. J Emerg Med 2001;22(3):251–6.

[16] Gerbino G, Ramieri GA, Nasi A. Diagnosis and treatment of retrobulbar haematomas following blunt orbital trauma: a description of eight cases. Int J Oral Maxillofac Surg 2005; 34(2):127–31.

[17] Popat H, Doyle PT, Davies SJ. Blindness following retrobulbar haemorrhage—it can be prevented. Br J Oral Maxillofac Surg 2007;45(2):163–4.

[18] Rahmani B, Jahadi H, Rajaeefard A. An analysis of risk for secondary hemorrhage in traumatic hyphema. Ophthalmology 1999;106:380–5.

[19] Shiuey Y, Lucarelli MJ. Traumatic hyphema: outcomes of patient management. Ophthalmology 1998;105:851–5.

[20] Crouch ER Jr, Crouch ER. Management of traumatic hyphema: therapeutic options. J Pediatr Ophthalmol Strabismus 1999;36:238–50.

[21] Recchia F, Saluja R, Hammel K. Outpatient management of traumatic microhyphema. Ophthalmology 2002;109(8):1465–70.

[22] Girkin C, McGwin G, Morris R, et al. Glaucoma following penetrating ocular trauma: a cohort study of the United States eye injury registry. Am J Ophthalmol 2005;139(1):100–5.

[23] Netland K, Martinez J, LaCour O, et al. Traumatic anterior lens dislocation: a case report. J Emerg Med 1998;17(4):637–9.

[24] Lee MS, Gunton KB, Fischer D, et al. Ocular manifestations of remote lightning strike. Retina 2002;22(6):808–10.

[25] Rahman I, Maino A, Devadson D, et al. Open globe injuries: factors predictive of poor outcome. Eye 2006;20:1336–41.

[26] Joseph D, Pieramici D, Beauchamp N. Computed tomography in the diagnosis and prognosis of open-globe injuries. Ophthalmology 2000;107:1899–906.

[27] Vachon C, Warner D, Bacon D. Succinylcholine and the open globe: tracing the teaching. Anesthesiology 2003;99(1):220–3.

[28] Bajaj M, Pushker N, Naniwal S, et al. Traumatic luxation of the globe with optic nerve avulsion. Clin Experiment Ophthalmol 2003;31:362–3.

[29] Rabinowitz R, Yagev R, Shoham A, et al. Comparison between clinical and ultrasound findings in patients with vitreous hemorrhage. Eye 2004;18(3):253–6.

[30] Dana MR, Werner MS, Viana MA, et al. Vitreous hemorrhage. Ophthalmology 1993; 100(9):1380–2.

[31] McCaron MO, Alberts MJ, McCaron P. A systematic review of Terson's syndrome: frequency and prognosis after subarachnoid hemorrhage. J Neurol Neurosurg Psychiatry 2004;75(3):491–3.

[32] Spraul CW, Grossniklaus HE. Vitreous hemorrhage. Surv Ophthalmol 1997;42(1):3–39.

[33] Pieramici DJ. Vitreoretinal trauma. Ophthalmol Clin North Am 2002;15:225–35.

[34] Duma S, Kress T, Porta D, et al. Airbag-induced eye injuries: a report of 25 cases. J Trauma 1996;41(1):114–9.

[35] Brunette DD. Ophthalmology. In: Marx JA, Hockberger RS, Walls R, editors. Rosen's emergency medicine: concepts and clinical practice, vol 2. 6th editionPhiladelphia: Mosby; 2006. p. 1044–52.

[36] Mester V, Kuhn F. Intraocular foreign bodies. Ophthalmol Clin North Am 2002;15:235–42.

[37] Thach A, Ward T, Dick J, et al. Intraocular foreign bodies during Operation Iraqi Freedom. Ophthalmology 2005;112(10):1829–33.

[38] Fulcher T, McNab A, Sullivan T. Clinical features and management of intraorbital foreign bodies. Ophthalmology 2002;109(3):494–500.

[39] Long J, Tann T. Orbital trauma. Ophthalmol Clin North Am 2002;15:249–53.

[40] Essex R, Yi Q, Charles P, et al. Post-traumatic endophthalmitis. Ophthalmology 2004; 111(11):2015–22.

[41] Danis RP. Endophthalmitis. Ophthalmol Clin North Am 2002;15:243–8.

[42] Colyer M, Weber E, Weichel E, et al. Delayed intraocular foreign body removal without endophthalmitis during operations Iraqi Freedom and Enduring Freedom. Ophthalmology 2007;114(8):1439–47.

[43] The Wills eye manual. In: Rhee D, Pyfer M, editors. Philadelphia: Lippincott, Williams & Wilkins; 1999. p. 19–50.

[44] Francis D, Kaufman R, Bevan Y, et al. Air bag induced orbital blowout fractures. Laryngoscope 2006;116(11):1966–72.

ELSEVIER
SAUNDERS

Emerg Med Clin N Am
26 (2008) 125–136

EMERGENCY
MEDICINE
CLINICS OF
NORTH AMERICA

Chemical, Thermal, and Biological Ocular Exposures

Jordan Spector, MD[a,b],
William G. Fernandez, MD, MPH[a,*]

[a]Boston Medical Center, Department of Emergency Medicine, Boston University School
of Medicine, One BMC Place, Dowling 1 South, Boston, MA 02118, USA
[b]Department of Emergency Medicine, Albert Einstein Medical Center, 5501 Old York Road,
Philadelphia, PA, USA

Chemical or radiant energy injuries to the eyes are considered ocular burns. The majority of these injuries are occupation-related [1]. Chemical burns are by far more common and represent a true emergency. Thermal and UV injuries are associated with severe pain, but often result in less long-term sequelae than chemical injuries do. The term "biologic exposure" refers to an exposure to human blood or other body fluid. This article describes patterns of these injuries and exposures, with particular emphasis on emergent management and including acute diagnostic and treatment considerations.

Chemical burns

Chemical burns to the eye are common, particularly in industrial settings, and constitute an ocular emergency. In fact, chemical burns were the second leading cause of work-related eye injury treated in United States emergency departments in 1999 [2]. A burn may occur with exposure of the eye to any chemical, solid, liquid, or aerosol. Household cleaning supplies and cosmetics are common offenders. The potent alkaline or acidic substances contained within these products cause the burn injury. Accidents involving industrial materials in the workplace are a frequent cause of eye burns.

Chemical exposures to the eye can result in significant damage to the ocular surface epithelium, the cornea, and the anterior segment. Permanent unilateral or bilateral visual impairment may result. Alkaline substances can

---

* Corresponding author.
E-mail address: william.fernandez@bmc.org (W.G. Fernandez).

be particularly injurious. An alkali causes liquefactive necrosis of the surface epithelium, leading to rapid penetration of the substance to the deeper layers of the eye. There can be irreversible damage to the corneal stroma and endothelium, as well as to anterior segment structures. Most acidic substances cause coagulation necrosis when exposed to the cornea. The reaction precipitates surface proteins, which serve as a barrier to deeper damage, and acidic injury tends to be superficial [3].

Pathophysiology

The external portion of the eye is covered by the cornea centrally and the conjunctiva peripherally. The cornea is a multilayered structure atop a basement membrane, all covered by a thin film of tears. Both the cornea and the conjunctiva produce a nonkeratinized epithelium, and both have the ability to rapidly regenerate and renew surface epithelium during injury repair [3]. Within minutes of a small injury to the corneal epithelium, the regenerative process begins. However, after a larger injury, healing may take 4 to 5 hours to begin. Injuries that destroy the basement membrane may require up to 6 weeks to complete healing. After significant injuries, full restoration of the cornea may never occur [4].

Alkali injury

The severity of chemical burn injury is directly proportional to the surface area of contact on the cornea and the depth of penetration of the substance. Alkalis penetrate into the eye more readily than do acids. The hydroxyl ion of a base causes saponification of the fatty acids within the cornea, resulting in epithelial cell disruption and death. The associated cation then penetrates toward deeper structures. Depending on the degree of penetration, a number of structures may suffer injury, including the corneal and conjunctival epithelium, the basement membrane, stromal keratocytes, the lens, stromal nerve endings, the episclera, the iris, and the ciliary body (Figs. 1 and 2) [3].

A number of alkaline substances cause ocular injury. Some of the more common agents are listed in Table 1. The most serious alkali injuries are associated with exposures to ammonia (anterior segment injury in <1 minute) and to lye (deep injury within 3–5 minutes). Magnesium hydroxide, which is present in fireworks, may produce a severe injury because of the coexistent thermal burn [3]. Eye injuries secondary to methamphetamine production have been described as well [5].

On presentation, a patient with an alkaline eye burn demonstrates conjunctival hyperemia, chemosis, and corneal clouding. The stroma may have mild edema, and the anterior chamber may develop cells and flare. Severe alkali burns are characterized by corneal opacification and limbal ischemia [6].

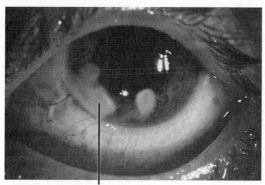

Corneal alkali burn

Fig. 1. Alkali burn demonstrating corneal burns and conjunctival injection on the day of the accident. (*From* Kaiser PK, Friedman NJ, Pineda II R. The Massachusetts Eye and Ear Infirmary illustrated manual of ophthalmology, second edition. China: Saunders; 2004. p. 122, 123 ; with permission.)

Acid injury

Acids cause less severe, more focal tissue injury. The corneal epithelium offers moderate protection against weaker acids. The hydrogen ion alters surface pH, while the associated anion reacts with epithelial and superficial stromal cells to precipitate and denature surface proteins [3]. The coagulated proteins function as a superficial barrier and prevent intraocular injury. Stronger acids may penetrate and produce an injury pattern comparable to that of an alkali burn, as deep tissue damage occurs when the exposed eye reaches a pH of 2.5 or less [6].

Some common acidic agents that cause ocular injury are listed in Table 2. Sulfuric acid is the most common cause of acid injury. It seldom produces

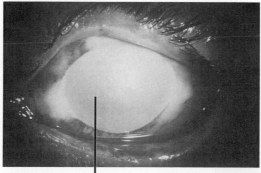

Corneal alkali burn

Fig. 2. Complete corneal tissue destruction 7 days after alkali burn. (*From* Kaiser PK, Friedman NJ, Pineda II R. The Massachusetts Eye and Ear Infirmary illustrated manual of ophthalmology, second edition. China: Saunders; 2004. p. 122, 123; with permission.)

Table 1
Common products containing alkali

Product	Chemical
Lime	Calcium carbonate or magnesium carbonate
Plaster and mortar	Calcium hydroxide
Oven and drain cleaner (lye)	Sodium hydroxide or potassium hydroxide
Fireworks and sparklers	Magnesium hydroxide
Ammonia (in cleaning agents and fertilizers)	Ammonium hydroxide
Dishwasher detergent	Sodium tripolyphosphate

Data from Xiang H, Stallones L, Chen G, et al. Work-related eye injuries treated in hospital emergency departments in the US. Am J Ind Med 2005;48(1):57–62; and Farjo AA, Soong HK. Corneal epithelium. In: Yanoff M, Duker JS, editors. Ophthalmology. 2nd edition. St. Louis (MO): Mosby; 2004.

serious injury unless there is additional damage from thermal injury or high-velocity penetration of a foreign body into the eye, as may occur in the explosion of an automobile battery [3]. Acids containing heavy metals may penetrate and produce injury patterns similar to those seen in alkali burns [6].

Hydrofluoric acid (HF) exposure can cause the most potentially serious ocular acid injury and deserves special consideration. HF is a low molecular-weight acid found in many industrial and commercial products. It can exist in gaseous or aqueous form. After exposure, HF penetrates deeply in tissues and causes liquefaction necrosis, much like an alkali. HF contamination may cause significant injury to multiple organ systems. In the eye, HF can rapidly penetrate to anterior chamber structures and cause devastating ocular injury [7,8].

In burns caused by strong acids, the cornea and conjunctiva rapidly become white and opaque. The epithelium may slough, leaving a relatively clear stroma. This may initially mask the severity of the injury. The cornea eventually becomes opacified. Very severe acid burns also cause complete corneal anesthesia, limbal pallor, and uveitis [6].

Table 2
Common products containing acid

Product	Chemical
Toilet cleaner	Sulfuric acid (80%)
Battery fluid	Sulfuric acid (30%)
Pool cleaners	Sodium hypochlorite or calcium hypochlorite (70%)
Bleaches	Sodium hypochlorite (3%)
Vinegar or essence of vinegar	Acetic acid
Glass polishers, silicone production agents, rust removal agents	Hydrofluoric acid
Food- and leather-processing compounds	Hydrochloric acid

Data from Xiang H, Stallones L, Chen G, et al. Work-related eye injuries treated in hospital emergency departments in the US. Am J Ind Med 2005;48(1):57–62; and Farjo AA, Soong HK. Corneal epithelium. In: Yanoff M, Duker JS, editors. Ophthalmology. 2nd edition. St. Louis (MO): Mosby; 2004.

Cyanoacrylate exposure

Cyanoacrylate is an adhesive that results in strong polymer bonds with a variety of materials and is used in both industrial and domestic settings [9]. It is a substance considered to have relatively little toxicity. It has also been used by ophthalmologists during surgical procedures to seal globe injuries without incident [10]. However, the emergency department clinician may encounter a patient who inadvertently instilled cyanoacrylate-containing adhesives into the eye. Alternatively, the clinician may accidentally spill skin adhesives into a patient's eye when repairing lacerations on the forehead or face. Such occurrence can result in adherence of the upper and lower eyelids. This may lead to local dermatitis of the eyelids, as well as to eyelash loss [10]. Occasionally, cyanoacrylate may collect over the cornea and irritate the eyes, resulting in mild to moderate corneal abrasions [11]. In such exposures, treatment as per the management for corneal abrasions in indicated. Attempting to pry the eyelids open should be done with caution, as this may result in further injury [12]. In the vast majority of cases, the adhesive separates from the eyelids within 1 week. As needed, irrigation with normal saline may remove particulate debris in and about the eye. Otherwise, no other specific interventions are indicated, and expectant management is appropriate [9–12].

Treatment

For the emergency physician, the management of chemical burns is contingent upon the time elapsed since injury. Eye injury due to chemical exposure occurs in phases. The immediate or acute phase occurs at the time of the injury and results in corneal and conjunctival epithelium necrosis and chemical invasion into the anterior chamber, the ciliary body, and the iris. The later phases of eye burns (intermediate and chronic) occur over the subsequent days to weeks and require management by ophthalmologic and plastic surgery specialists.

The goal of treatment after a chemical burn is to restore physiologic pH of the eye as rapidly as possible. If the external pH is restored to normal, the aqueous pH within the eye returns to normal within 30 minutes [3]. The most important initial intervention for all chemical exposures is irrigation. Delays in the initiation of irrigation by as little as 20 seconds have been demonstrated in animal models to result in a higher maximal pH and higher risk for more severe injury after alkaline exposure [13]. If possible, irrigation should begin immediately after injury, even before a patient presents to an emergency department. A number of studies have looked for the best agent for irrigation, and certain solutions containing buffering agents have been proposed as ideal [14]. However, even tap water is an appropriate irrigating solution [15,16], and any nontoxic solution, such as normal saline or lactated Ringer's solution, is effective. If the nature of the chemical injury is unknown, one may apply a piece of pH paper to the inferior fornix to determine if the offending substance was basic or acidic, but this should not delay the start of irrigation.

To permit appropriate irrigation of the chemically exposed and inflamed eye, topical anesthesia with 0.5% proparacaine may be necessary. Lid retractors or a lid speculum may be helpful. Prolonged irrigation can be accomplished with the use of a polymethylmethacrylate scleral lens with an attached perfusion tube. If such a lens is not available, an angiocath may be inserted percutaneously across the upper lid, though this should be reserved for rare instances and after discussion with consultants [6].

Chemical burns can be quite painful. Topical anesthesia may help. Additionally, the clinician should be prepared to provide the patient with systemic analgesics. For rapid pain relief and for ease of administration during irrigation, parenteral nonsteroidal anti-inflammatories or narcotic analgesics should be strongly considered.

Classically, ophthalmologists have suggested irrigation for 30 minutes or until 2 L of irrigant has been applied [6]. However, most now advocate continued irrigation until the eye is restored to normal pH (checked at 30-minute intervals). In animal models, greater than 2 hours of irrigation were necessary to achieve normal pH in the aqueous humor after a severe alkali burn [17]. Many ophthalmologists recommend reassessing pH approximately 30 minutes after the eye is restored to normal pH, especially after alkali burns, as particulate matter lodged in the conjunctiva can dissolve slowly and cause persistently increased pH, requiring further irrigation [6].

Emergent referral to an ophthalmologist is indicated in all but the most minor of injuries. Considering that injury severity can be difficult to ascertain upon emergent presentation, urgent follow-up is recommended for all chemical burns that cannot be evaluated by the ophthalmologist in the emergency department.

In a patient that reports an eye splash of rust remover, leather-tanning fluid, high-octane gasoline or glass or enamel etching materials, the clinician should be suspicious for an HF exposure. This is significant because, even though irrigation with water or saline should be instituted immediately, some reports suggest prolonged or repetitive irrigation can increase corneal ulceration and worsen outcome following HF exposure [8,18]. As topical calcium gels are indicated for dermal exposures to HF, some have suggested that application of 1% calcium gluconate drops to affected eyes may be protective after an HF burn [18,19]. However calcium salts can be quite irritating to the eye, and most would advise use of calcium gluconate drops only after discussion with an ophthalmologist [7,8].

Once irrigation is complete, a thorough evaluation for any particulate matter should be performed. This must include eversion of both upper and lower lids, and retraction of redundant conjunctival tissue. Topical anesthetic may be helpful. Any particles can be removed with a moistened cotton-tip applicator. Larger particles can be removed with smooth forceps.

As with all patients who present to an emergency department with eye complaints, an assessment of visual acuity must be performed. For patients who do not arrive in the emergency department with their corrective lenses, pinhole refraction can aid in the evaluation. A comprehensive slit-lamp examination is indicated for all patients. All but the mildest of burns develop a significant uveitis. In such cases, a clinician should appreciate cells and flare in the anterior chamber. For pain relief and prevention of synechiae (adhesion of the iris to the cornea or lens), cycloplegic eye drops (eg, cyclopentolate 0.5%) are indicated. Phenylephrine is contraindicated because it can exacerbate ischemic injury to deeper structures. Intraocular pressure should be assessed after a burn and, if elevated, systemic treatment with carbonic anhydrase inhibitors is indicated [6].

As with all patients presenting with superficial injury to the eye, a flourescein exam is indicated. Flourescein uptake occurs in all areas where the chemical exposure produced injury. An ophthalmologist will follow the observed injury pattern over time.

The goal of treatment is to promote epithelial cell growth as rapidly as possible. Topical antibiotic ointment, such as erythromycin or tetracycline, should be applied. Some investigators suggest topical corticosteroid to reduce the inflammatory response to chemical injury (ie, prednisolone or dexamethasone) [6]. However, this should be used in close collaboration with an ophthalmologist [20]. Although a semipressure patch can be applied to relieve pain [4,6], this has been shown to provide no benefit in the emergent treatment of traumatic corneal abrasions [21–23]. Rapid follow-up with an ophthalmologic specialist to manage care is vital.

Thermal injuries

Thermal injuries to the eye generally occur as a result of exposure to scalding liquid, direct flame, or such items as cigarettes and curling irons. Although a direct thermal injury to the eye is a rare event, burns to the surrounding adnexal structures (ie, eyebrow, eyelid, eyelashes) are not uncommon [6,20]. Due to the rapidity of the lid reflex, the eyelid provides protection for the eye itself, and long-term visual acuity is preserved. However, the eyelid takes on the majority of insult in a thermal injury, which leads to an inordinately high rate of postinjury lid contractures [24]. Much like chemical burns, the severity of thermal eye burns is related to the duration of exposure and the nature of the causative agent. Compared to water-based liquids, hot oils and greases are more adherent and subsequently result in deeper thermal injury [25,26]. The grading system for thermal burns to the eyelid is similar to that for burns in other areas of skin [27]. First-degree or superficial partial-thickness burns to the eyelid affect only the epidermal layer of skin. This type of burn pattern is characterized by pain, erythema, and edema. Second-degree or deep partial-thickness burns affect both the epidermal and dermal layers of skin, and also exhibit pain and erythema. However, second-degree burns blister. Third-degree or full-thickness burns of the eye-lid affect the entire dermal layer and may extend into the subcutaneous tissue. Patients present with a black or white eschar over the adnexal structures of the eye, which may lead to contractures. Full-thickness burns damage nerve endings and are less painful or even painless.

Radiation injuries

UV radiation (wavelengths 295–400 nm) is primarily absorbed by the corneal surface [28,29]. Prolonged unprotected exposure to sunlight, particularly at high elevation or with highly reflective surfaces, result in damage to the corneal surface (eg, snow blindness) [6,30]. UV damage to the corneal epithelium results in an inflammatory keratitis known as superficial punctuate keratitis. The pinpoint corneal defects characteristic of superficial punctuate keratitis can readily be found on flourescein staining. Additionally, there is often a varying degree of conjunctival injection and eyelid edema. The onset of pain and decreased visual acuity is delayed and occurs approximately 6 to 12 hours after prolonged UV light exposure. Overall, the epithelial layer heals within 72 hours of the injury, and the long-term prognosis for UV burns is excellent.

Artificial sources of UV radiation include welding arcs, sun-tanning beds, electric sparks, and halogen desk lamps. In contrast, prolonged exposure to infrared radiation (wavelengths of > 700 nm) damages the anterior lens and may lead to cataract formation (eg, glassblowers cataracts) [6,30]. This occupational injury is rarely seen now that appropriate eye protection is used.

Prolonged exposure to visible solar light (wavelengths 400–700 nm) may rarely result in retinal injury and subsequent visual loss [6,30]. This delayed photochemical retinal injury most commonly occurs among beachgoers and persons engaged in maritime industries who are exposed for long periods in the sun without eye protection. Patients often present 1 to 2 days after exposure with complaints of pain and visual change. On examination, there are often minimal findings apart from a reduction in visual acuity. Although no immediate management is necessary, outpatient ophthalmology follow-up is necessary, as the visual loss may take several months to improve.

Treatment

The treatment for thermal injuries is comparable to treatment for chemical burns. For all thermal injuries of the eye, the first priority is to remove the individual from the source and to cool the tissues as rapidly as possible. The eye should be irrigated with copious normal saline, lactated Ringer's solution, or tap water. Ideally, this should be instituted at the scene (eg, coworkers at the worksite) or before emergency department evaluation (eg, by pre–hospital-care providers), and should be continued in the emergency department. The removal of adherent debris or retained contact lenses is facilitated via copious irrigation. The initial use of topical anesthetic (eg, proparacaine 0.5%) is suggested in the emergency department, but long-term application of these agents delays epithelial healing. Cold compresses should be applied to the affected areas to decrease thermal injury and to relieve discomfort. Both thermal and UV injuries are quite painful, so oral and parenteral nonsteroidal and narcotic analgesics should be prescribed. Topical analgesics have not been shown to be superior to oral agents [31,32]. Once pain control is addressed, visual acuity testing should be performed to identify any baseline visual deficits. Pinhole refraction may optimize visual acuity assessment among selected patients who arrive in the emergency department without their corrective lenses. While evaluating the eye, the eyelids should be everted so that a complete inspection of the stromal structures can be performed. Frequent application of artificial tears or ointment should be instituted in the event that tear production has been affected. This also helps to prevent long-term adhesion formation between the eyelid and the globe itself. The patient's tetanus status should be updated. Systemic antibiotics are unnecessary unless the source of infection has been identified.

In addition to the above actions, the specific treatment for first- and second-degree thermal eye burns includes an antibiotic ointment (erythromycin 0.5%) or eye drops. Cycloplegic agents (eg, cyclopentolate 0.5%) are commonly administered. However, a recent systematic review found no compelling evidence to support this practice [33]. For third-degree burns, a nonocclusive dressing should be applied to prevent infection, and urgent ophthalmologic consultation is warranted.

The traditional therapy for UV keratitis is cycloplegic drops (eg, cylcopentolate 0.5%) to reduce reflex ciliary muscle spasm and to potentially reduce pain. However, as noted above, no studies have proven the efficacy of this treatment [33]. Topical antibiotic drops or ointment (eg, erythromycin 0.5%) should be prescribed. Although some ophthalmologists continue to recommend eye patching, this is viewed as controversial and should be done with caution [21–23].

Biologic exposures

In practical terms, a "biologic" exposure refers to contact with human blood or body fluids (eg, saliva, semen, urine). The key issue that the emergency physician must confront is that such an exposure may result in an infection with blood-borne pathogen. The most serious of these pathogens include hepatitis B virus (HBV), hepatitis C virus, and HIV [34,35]. The infectious risk increases if the biologic exposure (ie, blood, body fluid) comes into direct contact with the exposed person's bloodstream (eg, needle-stick incident). However, exposure to the mucous membranes of the eye can potentially result in infection. The risk of infection via exposure through mucous membranes or injured skin is considerably less than that via a percutaneous needle-stick event. Although the true risk is lower with mucous membrane exposures, the risk is not zero [34]. The risk of infection is related to the amount (ie, volume) and concentration (ie, viral load) of the biologic exposure.

Treatment

The most important action that the emergency physician can make in the treatment of biologic exposures to the eye is to irrigate the eye with water or normal saline. For those who wear contact lenses, recommendations call for the lenses to be kept on during irrigation because the lens itself serves as a protective barrier for the eye. The use of soap or other agents may irritate and compromise the mucosal barrier of the eye. Lenses may be removed after irrigation and either discarded or cleaned as per the usual manner. Soap and water may be used, however, for biologic exposures to nonintact skin of the orbital adnexal structures [34].

Of the three viral agents discussed, the risk of hepatitis B infection is greatest. Fortunately, in the health care environment, most hospital personnel are vaccinated against HBV. Among unvaccinated persons, the emergency department clinician should consider initiating treatment with HBV vaccination in ocular exposures with blood from source individuals where the HBV status is unknown. The first dose should be given at the time of exposure; a follow-up vaccination is given at 1 month and 6 months postexposure. If the blood is known to be from an HBV-positive source, then hepatitis-B immune globulin, which contains antibodies to HBV, is recommended [34,35].

The Centers for Disease Control and Prevention recommends postexposure prophylaxis to reduce HIV infection if the exposure is discovered within 72 hours and one or more of the following bodily fluids was involved: blood, semen, vaginal secretions, rectal secretions, breast milk, or any body fluid that is visibly contaminated with blood [35]. However, given that mucous membranes of the eye are an extremely unlikely route of HIV transmission, it is recommended that each situation be considered on an individual basis [34,35].

Unfortunately, for biologic exposure to hepatitis C virus, there is no known effective preventive measure apart from copious irrigation with water or saline.

In cases of occupational biologic exposures to the eye, health care workers may be referred to the hospital's occupational health clinic for same-day or next-day baseline serum testing, as well as follow care. All others should be referred to a primary care provider for further management.

Disposition

Most first-degree thermal burns and radiation injuries may be discharged from the emergency department with outpatient ophthalmology follow-up in 24 to 48 hours. Second-degree burns of the eye merit at least a phone call to the on-call ophthalmologist, or referral for urgent ophthalmology consultation. Third-degree eye burns require ophthalmologic consultation and either hospital admission or early burn-center transfer. All those with biologic exposures should be referred for baseline and follow-up testing and management.

References

[1] Schrage NF, Langefeld S, Zschocke J, et al. Eye burns: an emergency and continuing problem. Burns 2000;26(8):689–99.
[2] Xiang H, Stallones L, Chen G, et al. Work-related eye injuries treated in hospital emergency departments in the US. Am J Ind Med 2005;48(1):57–62.
[3] Wagoner MD. Chemical injuries of the eye: current concepts in pathophysiology and therapy. Surv Ophthalmol 1997;41(4):275–313.
[4] Farjo AA, Soong HK. Corneal epithelium. In: Yanoff M, Duker JS, editors. Ophthalmology. 2nd edition. St. Louis (MO): Mosby; 2004. p. 413–20.
[5] Charukamnoetkanok P, Wagoner M. Facial and ocular injuries associated with methamphetamine production accidents. Am J Ophthalmol 2004;138(5):875–6.
[6] Belin MW, Catalano RA, Scott JL. Burns of the eye. In: Catalano RA, Belin MW, editors. Ocular emergencies. Philadelphia: WB Saunders; 1992. p. 179–96.
[7] Salzman M, O'Malley RN. Updates on the evaluation and management of caustic exposures. Emerg Med Clin North Am 2007;25(2):459–76.
[8] Su M. Hydrofluoric acid and fluorides. In: Flomenbaum NE, Goldfrank LR, Hoffman RS, et al, editors. Goldfrank's toxicologic emergencies. 8th edition. New York: McGraw-Hill Medical Publishing Division; 2002. p. 1417–23.
[9] Fisher AA. Reactions to cyanoacrylate adhesives: instant glue. Cutis 1985;35:18–24.
[10] Patel KC, Hussain U, Zia R. Cyanoacrylate injuries in the eye: a review of management. 2007. Available at: http://www.karnesh.com/downloads/documents/articles/cyanoacrylate.pdf. Accessed October 8, 2007.
[11] Derespinis PA. Cyanoacrylate nail glue mistaken for eye drops. JAMA 1990;263(17):2301.
[12] McClean CJ. Ocular superglue injury. J Accid Emerg Med 1997;14(1):40–1.
[13] Rihawi S, Frentz M, Becker J, et al. The consequences of delayed intervention when treating chemical eye burns. Graefes Arch Clin Exp Ophthalmol 2007;245(10):1507–13.
[14] Rihawi S, Frentz M, Schrage NF. Emergency treatment of eye burns: Which rinsing solution should we choose. Graefes Arch Clin Exp Ophthalmol 2006;244(7):845–54.
[15] Ikeda N, Hayasaka S, Hayasaka Y, et al. Alkali burns of the eye: effect of immediate copious irrigation with tap water on their severity. Ophthalmologica 2006;220(4):225–8.
[16] Hall AH, Maibach HI. Water decontamination of chemical skin/eye splashes: a critical review. Cutan Ocul Toxicol 2006;25(2):67–83.
[17] Grant WM, Schuman JS. Treatment of chemical burns of the eye. In: Grant WM, Schulman JS, editors. Toxicology of the eye. 4th edition. Springfield (MA): Thomas Books; 1993.
[18] Bertolini JC. Hydrofluoric acid: a review of toxicity. J Emerg Med 1992;10(2):163–8.
[19] Bentur Y, Tannenbaum S, Yaffe Y, et al. The role of calcium gluconate in the treatment of hydrofluoric acid eye burn. Ann Emerg Med 1993;22(9):1488–90.
[20] Chen AI, Reenstra-Buras WR, Rosen C, et al. Burns, ocular. Emedicine 2006. Available at: http://www.emedicine.com/emerg/topic736.htm. Accessed August 9, 2007.
[21] Kaiser PK. A comparison of pressure patching versus no patching for corneal abrasions due to trauma or foreign body removal. Corneal Abrasion Patching Study Group. Ophthalmology 1995;102(12):1936–42.
[22] Flynn CA, D'Amico F, Smith G. Should we patch corneal abrasions? A meta-analysis. J Fam Pract 1998;47(4):264–70.

[23] Le Sage N, Verreault R, Rochette L. Efficacy of eye patching for traumatic corneal abrasions: a controlled clinical trial. Ann Emerg Med 2001;38(2):129–34.

[24] Stern JD, Goldfarb IW, Slater H. Ophthalmological complications as a manifestation of burn injury. Burns 1996;22(2):135–6.

[25] Schubert W, Ahrenholz DH, Solem LD. Burns from hot oil and grease: a public health hazard. J Burn Care Rehabil 1990;11(6):558–62.

[26] Allen SR, Kagan RJ. Grease fryers: a significant danger to children. J Burn Care Rehabil 2004;25(5):456–60.

[27] Pham TN, Gibran NS. Thermal and electrical injuries. Surg Clin North Am 2007;87(1):185–206.

[28] Taylor HR. The biological effects of UV-B on the eye. Photochem Photobiol 1989;50(4):489–92.

[29] Roberts JE. Ocular phototoxicity. J Photochem Photobiol B 2001;64(2–3):136–43.

[30] Brozen R, Fromm C. Ultraviolet keratitis. Emedicine 2006. Available at: http://www.emedicine.com/EMERG/topic759.htm. Accessed August 9, 2007.

[31] Szucs PA, Nashed AH, Allegra JR, et al. Safety and efficacy of diclofenac ophthalmic solution in the treatment of corneal abrasions. Ann Emerg Med 2000;35(2):131–7.

[32] Weaver CS, Terrell KM. Evidence-based emergency medicine. Update: Do ophthalmic non-steroidal anti-inflammatory drugs reduce the pain associated with simple corneal abrasions without delayed healing? Ann Emerg Med 2003;41(1):134–40.

[33] Carley F, Carley S. Towards evidence based emergency medicine: best BETs from the Manchester Royal Infirmary. Mydriatics in corneal abrasion. Emerg Med J 2001;18(4):273.

[34] Zaleznik D. Patient information: blood and body fluid exposure. 2007. Available at: http://patients.uptodate.com/topic.asp?file=inf_immu/8025. Accessed October 18, 2007.

[35] CDC. Exposure to blood: what healthcare personnel need to know. 2003. Available at: http://www.cdc.gov/ncidod/dhqp/pdf/bbp/Exp_to_Blood.pdf. Accessed October 18, 2007.

ELSEVIER
SAUNDERS

Emerg Med Clin N Am
26 (2008) 137–180

EMERGENCY
MEDICINE
CLINICS OF
NORTH AMERICA

Neuro-Ophthalmology

David K. Duong, MD, MS[a], Megan M. Leo, MD[a],
Elizabeth L. Mitchell, MD[b],*

[a]Emergency Medicine Residency, Boston Medical Center, 1 Boston
Medical Center Place, Boston, MA 02118, USA
[b]Department of Emergency Medicine, Boston University School of Medicine, Boston
Medical Center, 1 Boston Medical Center Place, Dowling 1, Boston, MA 02118, USA

Neuroanatomy and neuro-ophthalmologic examination

Neuro-ophthalmologic disorders arise from all areas of the neuro-ophthalmologic tract. They may be expressed simply as loss of vision or double vision, or as complex syndromes or systemic illnesses, depending on the location and type of lesion. Problems may occur anywhere along the visual pathway, including the brainstem, cavernous sinus, subarachnoid space, and orbital apex, and may affect adjacent structures also. A firm understanding of the neuroanatomy and neurophysiology of the eye is essential to correct diagnosis [1–3].

The visual pathway

Functionality of the visual pathway requires the afferent innervation of the optic nerve, cranial nerve (CN) II. A lesion can occur anywhere along the pathway and is manifested according to distinct location and fiber involvement. An adequate understanding of the visual pathway from the retina, through the optic nerve and chiasm, with projection dorsally to the occipital lobe, allows for localization of the insult (Fig. 1). The fibers from the temporal retina (capturing the images from the nasal visual field) and nasal retina (capturing images from the temporal visual field) converge at the optic disc and proceed dorsally to form the optic nerve. The ophthalmic artery supplies the retina and optic nerve. It is the first intracranial division off the internal carotid artery. The optic nerve is subject to ischemic, compressive, infiltrative, or inflammatory damage because of its vulnerability to increased

* Corresponding author.
E-mail address: emitchel@bu.edu (E.L. Mitchell).

0733-8627/08/$ - see front matter © 2008 Elsevier Inc. All rights reserved.
doi:10.1016/j.emc.2007.11.004
emed.theclinics.com

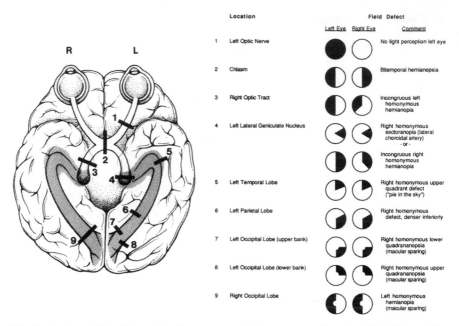

Fig. 1. Lesions of the afferent visual pathway and their corresponding visual field defects. The term hemianopsia (or hemianopia) refers to a visual field defect that respects the vertical meridian. Homonymous indicates that the defect involves the same side of the visual field in both eyes. An incongruous defect is that for which the extent of visual field loss is asymmetric between the two eyes. (*Adapted from* Mason C, Kandel ER. Central visual pathways. In: Kandel ER, Schwartz JH, Jessell T, editors. Principles of neural science. 3rd edition. Norwalk (CT): Appleton & Lange; 1991. p. 437; with permission.)

intraocular pressure or papilledema. An optic nerve deficit may result in unilateral, complete vision loss, without macular sparing.

As the fibers approach the optic chiasm intracranially, the temporal fibers remain ipsilateral and the nasal fibers cross within the chiasm to join the contralateral optic tracts. The optic chiasm is located directly above the pituitary fossa, anterior to the pituitary stalk, and inferior to the hypothalamus and third ventricle. Infarction of the optic chiasm is extremely rare because of its collateral blood supply. The superior hypophyseal arteries perfuse the chiasm inferiorly, which are fed by the internal carotid, posterior communicating, and posterior cerebral arteries. Superiorly the optic chiasm is perfused by the branches of the anterior cerebral arteries. A lesion in the chiasm classically presents as bitemporal hemianopsia, although this can vary depending on the specific area of the chiasm that is affected (see Fig. 1).

Posterior to the chiasm, the optic fibers course superiorly and around the infundibulum, below the third ventricle. They contain fibers from the ipsilateral temporal retina and the contralateral nasal retina. Most of the blood supply is from the thalamic perforators of the posterior cerebral artery and branches of the anterior choroidal artery. Most of the fibers synapse in the lateral geniculate nucleus (LGN), whereas those axons that are responsible for the pupillary light reflex branch off before the LGN and synapse in the pretectal nuclei of the midbrain.

The optic radiations that emerge from the LGN are called the geniculo-calcarine fibers. These separate into superior and inferior bundles, containing the afferent signal from the contralateral inferior visual fields and the contralateral superior visual fields, respectively. The superior bundles that pass through the parietal lobe project back to the upper bank of the calcarine cortex of the occipital lobe, thus receiving the image from the contralateral inferior visual field. The inferior bundles pass through the temporal lobe to form the Meyer loop and project back to the lower bank of the calcarine cortex of the occipital lobe, thus receiving the image from the contralateral superior visual field. The optic radiations receive blood supply from the middle cerebral arteries and anterior choroidal arteries. The macular area of the visual cortex, which represents the central 30° of vision, is processed by one half of the visual cortex. The fovea, or very center of the visual field, is represented within the tips of the occipital poles and has a dual blood supply, including branches of the posterior and middle cerebral arteries, providing the basis for macular sparing in the setting of occipital lobe infarct.

Efferent and afferent pupillary innervation

The efferent innervation of the pupil, which is responsible for pupillary constriction and dilation, involves parasympathetic and sympathetic fibers. Afferent pupillary innervation involves the retina, optic nerve, chiasm, optic tract and optic radiations.

The parasympathetic preganglionic fibers originate in the Edinger-Westphal subnucleus, adjacent to the oculomotor nucleus in the periaqueductal midbrain. The fibers travel on the superficial aspect of the oculomotor nerve (CN III) until it synapses in the ciliary ganglion in the orbit. The superficial location of the parasympathetic fibers explains why a blown pupil is an early sign of a compression lesion, including aneurysm or uncal herniation. From the ciliary ganglion, the postganglionic nerve fibers travel to the ciliary muscle and the iris sphincter and provide the tone for pupillary constriction. The pupillary light reflex pathway, allowing the pupil to constrict when exposed to light, consists of four neurons (Fig. 2). The image obtained from the retinal ganglionic cells travels through the optic nerve and follows the nasal retinal fibers across the chiasm, where they synapse in both of the pretectal nuclei of the dorsal midbrain. Each pretectal nucleus sends axons bilaterally to the two Edinger-Westphal nuclei, which contain the parasympathetic preganglionic fibers. These fibers travel with the third nerve to the ciliary ganglion within the orbit, which then sends parasympathetic postganglionic fibers to the pupillary sphincter muscle and ciliary muscle for lens accommodation. The projections to bilateral pretectal and Edinger-Westphal nuclei explain consensual pupillary constriction to light. Near inputs, such as

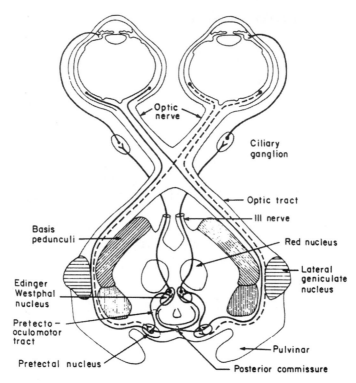

Fig. 2. The pupillary light reflex pathway. (*Adapted from* Walsh FB, Hoyt WF. The autonomic nervous system. In: Clinical neuro-ophthalmology. 3rd edition. Baltimore (MD): Williams & Wilkins; 1969. p. 473; with permission.)

an object placed directly in front of a patient being examined, project directly to both Edinger-Westphal nuclei, bypassing the pretectal area, which can serve to distinguish some forms of light-near dissociation in which the dorsal midbrain is involved. Adie syndrome, or Adie tonic pupil, is an example of light-near dissociation.

The sympathetic pathway originates in the posterolateral hypothalamus and descends along the lateral brainstem to synapse at the ciliospinal center of Budge-Waller, at the level of C8-T2 (Fig. 3). The preganglionic fibers exit the spinal cord with the ventral rootlets at this level and travel across the apex of the lung before ascending the neck to synapse in the superior cervical ganglion. The postsympathetic fibers form a plexus around the cervical internal carotid artery and reenter the skull. The oculosympathetic fibers leave the carotid artery in the cavernous sinus and enter the orbit with the ophthalmic division of the trigeminal nerve. The sympathetic fibers continue with the long ciliary nerves to the radial iris muscle, causing pupillary dilatation. There are also fibers that innervate the smooth muscle in the upper and lower eyelids (Mueller muscle) and the blood vessels in the skin and conjunctiva. Classic symptoms of sympathetic dysfunction, Horner

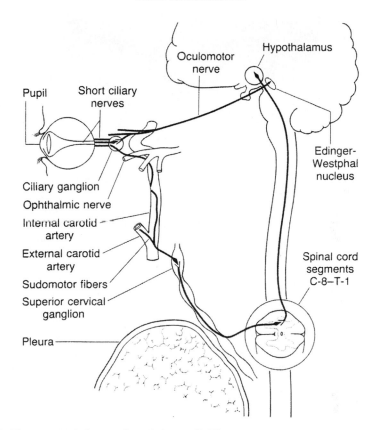

Fig. 3. The autonomic innervation of the pupil. The two-neuron parasympathetic pathway begins in the Edinger-Westphal nucleus of the midbrain and synapses in the ciliary ganglion in the orbit. Short ciliary nerves innervate the iris sphincter. The three-neuron sympathetic pathway begins in the hypothalamus, synapses in the lower cervical cord, ascends the neck on the carotid artery, and synapses again in the superior cervical ganglion to innervate the pupillodilator. (*From* Selhorst J. The pupil and its disorders. Neurol Clin 1983;1:861; with permission.)

syndrome, occur ipsilateral to the side of the lesion and include mild ptosis, papillary miosis, and inconsistently anhidrosis (Fig. 4). There is a small area of sweat glands above the eyebrows innervated by branches directly from the superior cervical ganglion, which explains why some third-order neuron Horner syndromes do not involve anhidrosis.

The cranial nerves

The five cranial nerves that innervate the eye are the optic nerve (CN II), the oculomotor nerve (CN III), the trochlear nerve (CN IV), the abducens nerve (CN VI), and the first division of the trigeminal nerve (CN V$_1$). A review of the course of these cranial nerves is important for understanding ocular pathology.

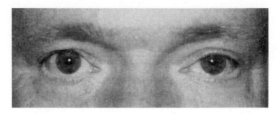

Fig. 4. A patient who had a left Horner syndrome secondary to an apical lung tumor. (*From* Balcer LJ, Galetta SL. Pancoast's syndrome. N Engl J Med 1997;337:359; with permission. Copyright © 1997, Massachusetts Medical Society.)

Ocular motility

Eye movement is controlled by a group of muscles innervated by the oculomotor nerve (CN III), the trochlear nerve (CN IV), and the abducens nerve (CN VI). The coordinated action of these muscles is accomplished by supranuclear control and is what allows for conjugate gaze of both eyes (Fig. 5).

Cranial nerve III. The oculomotor nerve (CN III) innervates the superior rectus muscle, inferior rectus muscle, medial rectus muscle, inferior oblique, levator palpebrae, and ciliary ganglion, providing motor and parasympathetic innervation to the eye. Partial dysfunction is common but a classic dysfunction of the entire nerve results in ptosis (attributable to loss of levator palpebrae function), papillary dilation (with loss of parasympathetic tone of ciliary ganglion), and the eye deviated down and out (attributable to the sole action of superior oblique and lateral rectus muscles) (Fig. 6). The origin

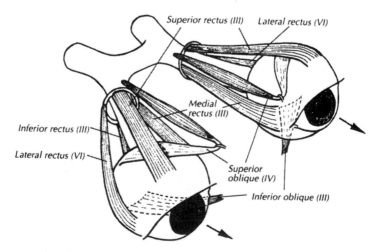

Fig. 5. The extraocular muscles. The medial rectus, superior rectus, inferior rectus, and inferior oblique are innervated by the third nerve (III); the superior oblique is innervated by the fourth nerve (IV); the lateral rectus is innervated by the sixth nerve (VI). (*From* Patten J. Vision, the visual fields, and the olfactory nerve. In: Patten J, editor. Neurological differential diagnosis. 2nd edition. New York: Springer-Verlag; 1996; with permission.)

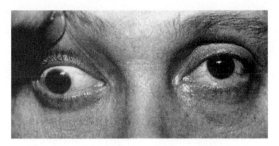

Fig. 6. Complete right third nerve palsy resulting in hypotropia, exotropia, and pupillary mydriasis. The ptotic eyelid is elevated manually. (*From* Bennett JL, Pelak VS. Palsies of the third, fourth, and sixth cranial nerves. Ophthalmol Clin North Am 2001;14(1):169–85; with permission.)

of the oculomotor nerve is in the periaqueductal midbrain, from a paired nuclear complex (Fig. 7). Within the complex are several paired subnuclei that send projections ipsilaterally to its target organ. The two exceptions to this are the axons originating from the unpaired midline central caudal nucleus, which innervate the levator palpebrae muscles, and the axons innervating the superior rectus muscles, which travel from the contralateral subnucleus. The parasympathetic preganglionic axons originate from the Edinger-Westphal nuclei, then travel to innervate the ciliary ganglion.

The fascicles that form from the oculomotor nuclei project anteriorly through the midbrain, passing through the red nucleus, then run adjacent to the substantia nigra and cerebral peduncle. The oculomotor nerve emerges from the ventral surface of the midbrain, where it passes between the superior cerebellar artery and the posterior cerebral artery. It is at this point that it is vulnerable to aneurysmal compression. Within the subarachnoid space, the nerve travels adjacent to the posterior communicating artery and the tip of the basilar artery, making a CN III deficit one of the ominous signs of aneurysm in this area. The oculomotor nerve continues to track anteriorly and enters the cavernous sinus and runs along the wall where it lies superior to CN IV. As the nerve exits the cavernous sinus, it passes through the superior orbital fissure and divides into superior and inferior branches. The superior branch provides motor function to the superior rectus and levator palpebrae, whereas the inferior branch provides motor function to the inferior rectus, medial rectus, inferior oblique, and the parasympathetic fibers for the ciliary ganglion.

Cranial nerve IV. The trochlear nerve (CN IV) innervates the superior oblique muscle (see Fig. 5). The dysfunction of this muscle is the most common cause of vertical strabismus. The superior oblique muscle depresses the eye in adduction and intorts the eye in abduction, making the deficit more apparent and exaggerating symptoms when the gaze is deviated downward and inward toward the affected side (Fig. 8). The nucleus is dorsal to the medial longitudinal fasciculus and inferior to the oculomotor nuclear

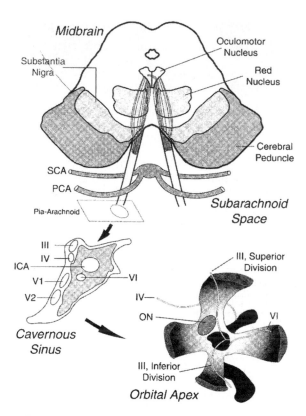

Fig. 7. Anatomy of the oculomotor nerve. The dotted lines depict the crossed fibers emanating from the superior rectus subnucleus. ICA, internal carotid artery; III, oculomotor nerve; IV, trochlear nerve; ON, optic nerve; PCA, posterior cerebral artery; SCA, superior cerebellar artery; VI, abducens nerve; V1, trigeminal nerve, ophthalmic division; V2, trigeminal nerve, maxillary division. (*From* Bennett JL, Pelak VS. Palsies of the third, fourth, and sixth cranial nerves. Ophthalmol Clin North Am 2001;14(1):169–85; with permission.)

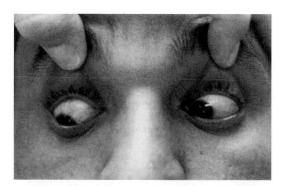

Fig. 8. Left fourth nerve palsy in a patient who had head trauma. There is a significant left hypertropia in down and right gaze. (*From* Bennett JL, Pelak VS. Palsies of the third, fourth, and sixth cranial nerves. Ophthalmol Clin North Am 2001;14(1):169–85; with permission.)

complex within the midbrain (Fig. 9). As the fascicles leave the nucleus, they course posteriorly and inferiorly, where they decussate in the superior medullary velum of the dorsal midbrain. It emerges at this point at the level of the inferior colliculus and runs within the subarachnoid space anteriorly, between the lateral midbrain and the tentorium cerebelli, between the superior cerebellar and posterior cerebral arteries. The trochlear nerve has the longest course outside of the midbrain. It courses around the cerebral peduncle as it enters the cavernous sinus, which makes it the most vulnerable cranial nerve to injury. Within the cavernous sinus, the trochlear nerve holds a position that is inferior to the oculomotor nerve and superior to the first division of the trigeminal nerve. The trochlear nerve then passes through the superior orbital fissure to enter the orbit and innervate the superior oblique muscle.

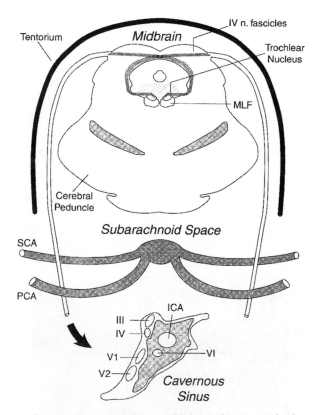

Fig. 9. Anatomy of the trochlear nerve. The speckled area demarcates the descending preganglionic sympathetic fibers. ICA, internal carotid artery; III, oculomotor nerve; IV, trochlear nerve; MLF, medial longitudinal fasciculus; PCA, posterior cerebral artery; SCA, superior cerebellar artery; VI, abducens nerve; V1, trigeminal nerve, ophthalmic division; V2, trigeminal nerve, maxillary division. (*From* Bennett JL, Pelak VS. Palsies of the third, fourth, and sixth cranial nerves. Ophthalmol Clin North Am 2001;14(1):169–85; with permission.)

Cranial nerve VI. The abducens nerve (CN VI) innervates the lateral rectus muscle (see Fig. 5). Paresis of this muscle results in binocular, horizontal diplopia that is worse in the direction of the affected side. Examination reveals an inability to abduct the affected eye on lateral gaze (Fig. 10). The abducens nerve fascicles originate in the dorsal pons, on the floor of the fourth ventricle, adjacent to the medial longitudinal fasciculus (MLF), paramedian pontine reticular formation (PPRF), and the fascicles of the facial nerve (CN VII). These fascicles are grouped to innervate the ipsilateral lateral rectus muscle and another group to innervate the contralateral medial rectus subnucleus by way of the MLF. The fascicles that course to the lateral rectus muscle project ventrally from the abducens nucleus and course through the tegmentum of the pons, where it emerges caudally. The nerve courses superiorly along the clivus to the level of the petroclinoid (Gruber) ligament, where it leaves the subarachnoid space and enters the Dorello canal and into the cavernous sinus. Within the cavernous sinus, the abducens nerve courses freely along with the carotid artery ventrally until it leaves the cavernous sinus and enters the orbit through the superior orbital fissure (Fig. 11). The abducens nerve is often the first deficit to be seen with cavernous sinus pathology because of its vulnerable position within the space.

Corneal reflex. The corneal reflex is accomplished by the afferent action of the ophthalmic branch of the trigeminal nerve (CN V_1) and the efferent action of the facial nerve (CN VII). When the cornea is touched, an impulse is sent by way of CN V_1 to the chief sensory nucleus of CN V, which is located in the rostral pons. Axons then project bilaterally to motor nucleus of CN VII, leading to coordinated eye closure with touch stimulation of CN V_1.

Conjugate eye movements. The coordination of eye movements in a determined direction is orchestrated by a supranuclear and internuclear pathway between the frontal eye fields and the contralateral side of the body. The

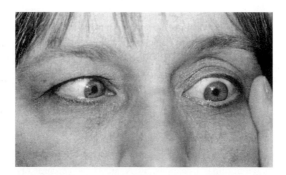

Fig. 10. Left abducens palsy caused by vasculopathic injury. There is a large angle esotropia in left lateral gaze. (*Data from* Bennett JL, Pelak VS. Palsies of the third, fourth, and sixth cranial nerves. Ophthalmol Clin North Am 2001;14(1):169–85.)

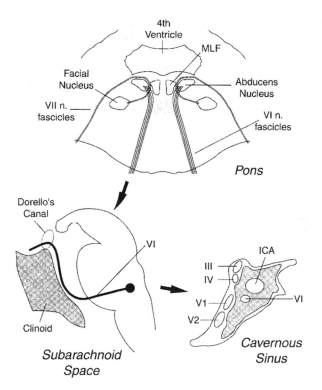

Fig. 11. Anatomy of the abducens nerve. The speckled area demarcates the paramedian pontine reticular formation. ICA, internal carotid artery; III, oculomotor nerve; IV, trochlear nerve; MLF, medial longitudinal fasciculus; VI, abducens nerve; V1, trigeminal nerve, ophthalmic division; V2, trigeminal nerve, maxillary division. (*Data from* Bennett JL, Pelak VS. Palsies of the third, fourth, and sixth cranial nerves. Ophthalmol Clin North Am 2001;14(1):169–85.)

frontal eye fields send a signal to the superior colliculus, the contralateral PPRF, and the rostral interstitial nucleus of the MLF (Fig. 12). Axons from the cell bodies in the PPRF project to the ipsilateral sixth nerve nucleus and synapse. Axons of the abducens motor nucleus travel to the ipsilateral lateral rectus muscle and axons from the abducens internuclear neurons cross over and ascend the contralateral MLF to the medial rectus subnucleus of the third cranial nerve. This internuclear connection between the PPRF of CN VI and the contralateral third nerve nucleus by way of the MLF allows for horizontal conjugate gaze. Distinction between sixth nerve palsies and lesions of the PPRF, or internuclear ophthalmoplegia (INO), can be distinguished by performing the oculocephalic (doll's eyes) maneuver or caloric testing. One of these maneuvers will overcome the ipsilateral horizontal gaze palsy if the sixth nerve is intact, whereas a PPRF lesion prevents the voluntary movement of the eye past midline.

The vestibulo-ocular system allows for stabilization of conjugate vertical and horizontal gaze. Inputs from each vestibular nucleus produce conjugate horizontal gaze by sending signals to the contralateral sixth nerve nucleus, serving the lateral rectus muscle. Interneurons then cross back by way of the MLF ipsilateral to the vestibular nucleus to allow for horizontal gaze toward the contralateral size of the body (Fig. 13). Vertical gaze holding occurs through the contralateral fourth nerve nucleus, third nerve nucleus, INO, and MLF. Vertical alignment is maintained by coordination through the fourth nerve nucleus (contralateral superior oblique muscle) and the third nerve subnuclei (contralateral superior rectus muscle, ipsilateral inferior oblique muscle, and inferior rectus muscle).

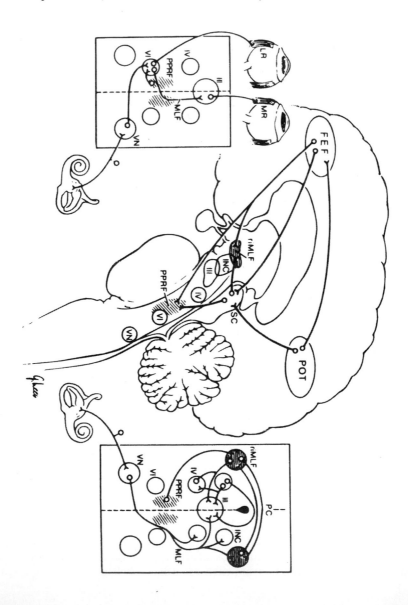

Neuro-ophthalmologic examination

Visual acuity

Visual acuity is a vital part of the neuro-ophthalmologic examination. Any change in visual acuity should be noted. Please refer to the article by Robinett and Kahn elsewhere in this issue.

Visual fields

Testing the visual field is essential for the neuro-ophthalmology evaluation. The visual field of each eye should be assessed individually. The patient begins by covering one eye and fixating on the nose of the examiner. The patient should note any obvious differences in upper and lower face. Hemianopic defects can be detected in this manner. If the nose is not clear to the patient, he or she likely has a central scotoma. The patient should then count fingers in the four quadrants. Simultaneous presentations of fingers in two separate quadrants can increase the sensitivity of finding a visual field defect. If a defect is found, the hand should be moved from the defected field to the normal one to establish the boundaries of the defect. Recordings of the visual fields are taken from the patient's perspective. If the cap held off midline is a clearer red, a central scotoma is suggested. By mapping out the visual field defect, the location of the lesion can be isolated using the anatomy of the neuro-ophthalmic pathways (see Fig. 1).

Visual field defects may be associated with higher cortical functioning, such as neglect (parietal lesion) or visual agnosia. Neglect is present if a patient can perceive a single stimulus (such as a finger), but on introduction of a second stimulus, one stimulus is neglected. An example of visual agnosia is prosopagnosia, which is a condition in which the patient cannot recognize familiar faces. These defects should be distinguished from pure visual field defects.

◄───

Fig. 12. Summary of eye movement control. The center shows the supranuclear connections from the frontal eye fields (FEF) and the parieto-occipital-temporal junction region (POT) to the superior colliculus (SC), rostral interstitial nucleus of the medial longitudinal fasciculus (riMLF), and the paramedian pontine reticular formation (PPRF). The FEF and SC are involved in the production of saccades, whereas the POT is believed to be important in the production of pursuit. The left shows the brainstem pathways for horizontal gaze. Axons from the cell bodies located in the PPRF travel to the ipsilateral sixth nerve (abducens) nucleus (VI) where they synapse with abducens motoneurons whose axons travel to the ipsilateral lateral rectus muscle (LR) and with abducens internuclear neurons whose axons cross the midline and travel in the medial longitudinal fasciculus (MLF) to the portions of the third nerve (oculomotor) nucleus (III) concerned with medial rectus (MR) function (in the contralateral eye). The right shows the brainstem pathways for vertical gaze. Important structures include the riMLF, PPRF, the interstitial nucleus of Cajal (INC), and the posterior commissure (PC). Note that axons from cell bodies located in the vestibular nuclei (VN) travel directly to the sixth nerve nuclei and, mostly by way of the MLF, to the third (III) and fourth (IV) nerve nuclei. (*From* Miller NR. Neural control of eye movements. In: Miller RN, editor. Walsh and Hoyt's Clinical Neuro-Ophthalmology. 4th edition. Baltimore (MD): Williams & Wilkins; 1985. p. 627; with permission.)

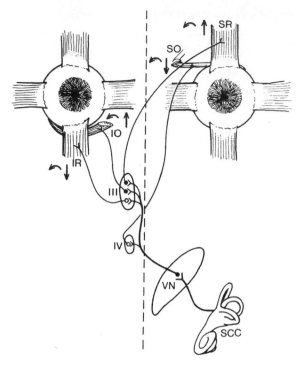

Fig. 13. The main excitatory vestibulo-ocular connections from the vertical semicircular canals. Dashed line, midline of the brainstem; arrows, directions of eye movement when individual extraocular muscles are stimulated; solid circles, receivers of the anterior canal projection; open circles, receivers of the posterior canal projection. Lesions occurring within these vestibulo-ocular pathways result in skew deviation. III, third nerve (oculomotor) subnuclei; IV, fourth nerve (trochlear) nucleus; IO, inferior oblique muscle; IR, inferior rectus muscle; SCC, semicircular canals; SO, superior oblique muscle; SR, superior rectus muscle; VN, vestibular nuclei. (*Adapted from* Zee DS. The organization of the brainstem ocular motor subnuclei. Ann Neurol 1978;14:384; with permission. Copyright © 1978. Reprinted with permission of John Wiley & Sons, Inc.)

Funduscopic examination

Evaluation of the visual pathway is not complete without a funduscopic examination. A swollen and elevated optic disc may be present in a patient who has papilledema. In other conditions, the optic disc may be pale and atrophic. The presence of spontaneous venous pulsations should be noted, which suggests that the intracranial pressure is not elevated. Getting a general sense of the condition of the retina can help guide a differential diagnosis for visual complaints (see the article by Robinette and Kahn elsewhere in this issue for a more complete discussion of the funduscopic examination).

Testing efferent and afferent pupillary innervation

Pupillary size is determined by the efferent dilating tone of the sympathetic nervous system and the efferent constricting tone of the parasympathetic nervous system. The pupils should be assessed for size and reactivity to light with the patient's vision fixated on an object in the distance. The pupils should be round and equal in diameter, although 1 mm of inequality may be a normal variation. Direct response to light is assessed one eye at a time by bringing the light source from below to avoid triggering near reaction.

Near response is tested by having the patient look at an object, such as a pen, starting at 14 in away. The examiner should note the pupillary change as the object is drawn closer. Pupillary constriction indicates a response to convergence. An absent response to light with normal response to convergence suggests the presence of light-near dissociation. Argyll Robertson pupil is an example of this and is often seen in patients who have untreated syphilis or encephalitis that has damaged the pretectal area of the dorsal midbrain. These pupils also dilate with anticholinergic eye drops but do not constrict with light because of the damaged pretectal area.

Afferent pupillary defects (APD) are examined using the swinging flashlight test. Marcus Gunn pupil is an example of an APD in which the pupils do not react equally to light, indicating a disturbance in the anterior afferent visual pathway, including retina, optic nerve, chiasm, or optic tract. Ask the patient to fixate on an object at a distance. A light is directed in the pupil for 1 to 2 seconds and the light is moved rapidly across the bridge of the nose to the other eye and moved back in a rhythmic fashion to equally stimulate both eyes (Fig. 14). The pupillary size should be compared bilaterally. In the presence of an afferent pupillary defect, there is a paradoxic dilation in the affected eye as light is directed into it, despite a normal consensual response (Fig. 15). Afferent pupillary defects can also be uncovered indirectly in the setting of a third nerve palsy with a dilated pupil by shining a light in the affected eye and observing the response in the opposite eye. Adequate constriction in the opposite eye indicates an intact optic nerve in the interrogated eye, despite its lack of direct response. Another example of a tonically dilated pupil with intact optic nerve is Adie tonic pupil, a lesion of the ciliary ganglion, which holds the cell bodies for the postsynaptic parasympathetic fibers that allow pupillary constriction. The lesion is often unilateral and in the setting of a traumatic or postviral injury. At about 8 weeks past the initial insult, the accommodating fibers can regenerate and the pupil begins to act like a light-near dissociation with improvement in the patient's near vision.

The corneal reflex can be tested by touching the cornea lightly with the edge of a sterile piece of gauze. A lack of response indicates a deficit in the afferent fibers of CN V_1 or the efferent fibers of CN VII. Testing both corneas is important to reveal direct and consensual reflexes.

Testing ocular motility

The motility examination assesses the integrity of the supranuclear pathways, ocular motor nuclei and nerves, and the muscles they innervate. The examination should begin with eyelid examination, observing for asymmetry and lid retraction, which could suggest CN III palsy or thyroid disease,

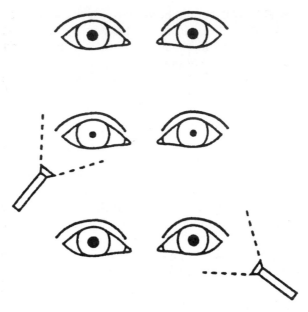

Fig. 14. The swinging flashlight test is used to test the integrity of the afferent visual pathway. In this example, the left optic nerve is not functioning properly, and there is a paradoxic dilation of the left pupil as the light is directed into it (left relative afferent pupillary defect). (*From* Wilhelm H. Neuro-ophthalmology of pupilary function–practical guidelines. J Neurol 1998;245:573–83; with permission.)

respectively. Myasthenia gravis is suggested when fatigable ptosis or Cogan lid twitch sign (transient improvement of lid function after sustained down gaze) is present. Ocular deviation is assessed from the neutral position and is classified as esotropia with inward displacement, exotropia with outward displacement, or hypertropia with vertical displacement. Corneal light reflex, in which a penlight is held directly in front of the patient, can be used to compare position as the light reflects off the cornea. Deviation is suggestive of strabismus, extraocular muscle dysfunction, or oculomotor nerve dysfunction.

Diplopia is often binocular, although monocular diplopia can be caused by early cataract formation or astigmatism and can be relieved by viewing through a pinhole device. Palsies of the third, fourth, or sixth cranial nerves or the muscles they innervate result in binocular diplopia, typical of paretic strabismus. In assessing a patient who has complaints of diplopia, it is important to establish whether the double vision is vertical, horizontal, or oblique, and determine in which direction the two images are most widely separated. The patient is then taken through the six cardinal fields of gaze to localize any involved nerve or muscle. This examination is usually done by asking the patient to follow an object, usually the examiner's finger, to the patient's upper right, upper left, lower left, lower right, right, and left,

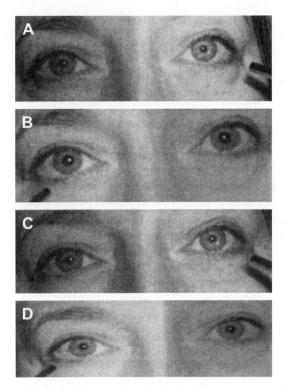

Fig. 15. The alternating light test in a patient who had a right optic neuropathy. (*A*) Patient is fixating a distant target while in dim room light. Light stimulation of the good left eye produces brisk, strong pupilloconstriction in both eyes. Clinically, the observer watches only the reaction of the illuminated pupil. (*B* and *C*) Light stimulation of the right eye produces lesser pupilloconstriction compared with light stimulation of the good left eye. (*D*) Rapid alternation of the light stimulus back to the bad right eye results in pupillodilation because that eye "sees" a relative decrement in light intensity. There is thus a relative afferent pupillary defect in the right eye. (*From* Kawasaki A, Kardon R. Disorders of the pupil. Ophthalmol Clin North Am 2001;14(1):149–68; with permission.)

returning to midline between each field. Any paralysis or weakness of the extraocular muscles can be isolated in this manner. Nystagmus is also observed if present in any of these six cardinal positions. Horizontal nystagmus usually indicates a lesion in the cerebellar or vestibular pathways, whereas downbeat nystagmus localizes to the cervicomedullary junction.

Saccades or fast eye movements are assessed by having the patient fixate on two targets, usually the examiner's nose and an eccentrically placed finger. Have the patient follow a swinging reflex hammer from side to side to test pursuit. Pursuit can also be assessed vertically by moving the reflex hammer up and down in a constant manner. Lastly, the vestibular ocular reflex (VOR) can be tested by having the patient fixate on the examiner's finger while rotating the head from side to side. A defective VOR results in catch-up saccadic eye movements.

Finally, a complete neurologic examination should be done on any patient in whom a neuro-ophthalmologic problem is suspected. Most lesions involving the optic tract, cranial nerves, or occipital lobe affect adjacent structures. These are manifest in physical examination findings consistent with pathology in those areas.

Pupillary disorders

Neurologic dysfunction of the pupils may be classified as an afferent or efferent defect based on the neuroanatomic site of the lesion. An afferent pupillary lesion refers to the retina, the optic nerve, chiasm, and tract, and the optic radiations. An efferent pupillary lesion refers to lesions of parasympathetic and sympathetic innervation, controlling constriction and dilation, respectively (see Fig. 3). Disorders of the pupils may also be defined by a clinical presentation, such as asymmetry of pupils, bilaterally abnormal pupil size, abnormal light reactivity, or deficits with other associated neurologic abnormalities. For the purposes of this article, we describe pupillary disorders by the defect and clinical presentation.

Pupil size and reactivity

Anisocoria

Anisocoria is defined as asymmetry of pupillary size. Physiologic, or simple, anisocoria occurs in about 20% of people [4,5]. The asymmetry is more prominent in dim light and rarely more than 1 mm. On examination, there is symmetric, rapid papillary constriction and dilatation. There has been no clear physiologic explanation, but it is believed to be attributable to an asymmetric supranuclear inhibition of the Edinger-Westphal parasympathetic nuclei in the pupilloconstrictor pathway [5].

Horner syndrome

Horner syndrome is classically described as ptosis, miosis, and anhidrosis. Ptosis and anhidrosis may be present to varying degrees, however, and may be clinically subtle (Fig. 16). When anisocoria is present and there is sluggish dilation of the miotic pupil, one should suspect Horner syndrome. The pupillary lag in dilation takes about 15 to 20 seconds, with the most prominent asymmetry at 4 to 5 seconds [5,6]. Normally, or in the case of physiologic anisocoria, there is no such lag and the pupils dilate with equal speed. Pupillary lag is present in about 50% of those who have Horner syndrome [5]. Ptosis is attributable to denervation of the tarsal muscles. The degree of ptosis is usually mild, partly because of compensation of the levator palpebrae and frontalis muscles. Anhidrosis is not always present, although its presence can be helpful diagnostically and usually implies an acute cause, because there is reinnervation of sweat glands in chronic cases. If Horner syndrome is present, localization of the lesion is the next step because the

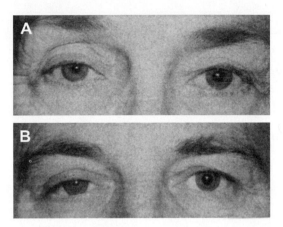

Fig. 16. (*A*) Right upper lid ptosis and ipsilateral miosis in a patient who had pseudo-Horner syndrome (levator dehiscence and simple anisocoria). (*B*) Right upper and lower lid ptosis and ipsilateral miosis in a patient who had true Horner syndrome (oculosympathetic defect). (*From* Kawasaki A, Kardon R. Disorders of the pupil. Ophthalmol Clin North Am 2001;14(1):149–68; with permission.)

differential is broad and ranges from benign to serious (Box 1). There should be a search for associated signs and symptoms to help localize the lesion. For instance, if anhidrosis is present over the entire body, this indicates a central lesion. If anhidrosis affects the face, neck, and arm only, there is a cervical lesion. Consultation with neurology or ophthalmology for pharmacologic tests (cocaine or hydroxyamphetamine provocation) may be necessary. For further localization, imaging is usually indicated.

Tonic (Adie) pupil

Another cause of a unilateral sluggishly reactive pupil is Adie, or tonic, pupil. Adie pupil is caused by degeneration of the ciliary ganglion, followed by aberrant reinnervation of the pupilloconstrictor muscles. On slit-lamp examination, segmental pupillary sphincter palsies may be appreciated. Most cases are idiopathic, with a minority of cases caused by ocular trauma or surgery, infections such as zoster, neoplasm, or ischemia from temporal arteritis. In general, a finding of a tonic pupil requires no further evaluation. In the elderly, however, giant cell arteritis should be considered because prompt therapy can slow visual loss, reduce the risk for contralateral eye involvement, and may restore vision [7]. Although corticosteroids have been the mainstay of treatment, a small, randomized, double-blinded trial showed that combination oral methotrexate and oral prednisone significantly reduces disease relapse compared with prednisone alone (Fig. 17) [8].

Pharmacotherapy and pupils

The sympathetic and parasympathetic innervation of the pupil (see Fig. 3) makes the response to certain pharmacologic agents predictable.

Box 1. Etiologies of Horner's Syndrome

Central
Hypothalamus/brainstem
   Ischemia
   Hemorrhage
   Demyelination
Cervical Cord
   Trauma
   Tumor
   Syrinx
Arteriovenous malformation

Preganglionic
Cervicothoracic Cord
   Trauma
   Intramedullary paravertebral tumor
   Syrinx
   Cord arteriovenous malformation
   Cervical spondylosis
   Epidural anesthesia
Lower brachial plexus
   Birth trauma
   Acquired trauma
Pulmonary apex/mediastinum
   Vascular anomalies of ascending aorta or subclavian artery
   Apical lung tumor (Pancoast)
   Mediastinal tumors
   Cervical rib
   Iatrogenic (eg, chest tube, cardiothoracic surgery)
   Infection (eg, apical tuberculosis)
Anterior neck
   Iatrogenic (eg, neck surgery, internal jugular/subclavian
     catheter)
   Trauma
   Tumor (eg, thyroid, lymphoma)

Postganglionic
Superior cervical ganglion
   Trauma
   Jugular venous ectasia
   Iatrogenic (eg, ganglionectomy, tonsillectomy)
Internal carotid artery
   Dissection
   Trauma

Thrombosis
Tumor
Migraine/cluster
Skull base/carotid canal
    Trauma
    Tumor (eg, nasopharyngeal carcinoma)
Cavernous sinus
    Tumor (eg, meningioma, pituitary adenoma)
    Inflammation
    Carotid aneurysm
    Carotid-cavernous fistula
    Thrombosis

Data from Kawasaki A, Kardon R. Disorders of the pupil. Ophthalmol Clin North Am 2001;14(1):158.

Pharmacologic dilation can result with sympathomimetics and with parasympatholytics. Mydriasis by way of sympathomimetics occurs through alpha-adrenergic stimulation with agents, such as phenylephrine, ephedrine, and naphazoline, found in over-the-counter and prescription eye drops. Parasympatholytics, mainly anticholinergic agents, such as scopolamine, tropicamide, cyclopentolate, and bronchodilating inhalers, also cause pharmacologic mydriasis. These give anisocoria that is most pronounced in bright light in the case of ophthalmic application. There may still be

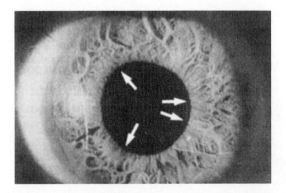

Fig. 17. A slit-lamp view of a 33-year-old man who had Adie tonic pupil. The white arrows are pointing to sectors of the sphincter that are contracting well, and the dark arrows indicate areas in which the iris sphincter is weak. Notice that the curvature of the pupillary margin is usually tighter in the sections that are functional and flatter in the palsied parts. (*From* Kardon RH, Thompson HS. The pupil. In: Rosen ES, Eustace P, Thompson HS, et al, editors. Neuro-ophthalmology. London: Mosby International Limited; 1998. p. 13.1–9; with permission.)

constriction to bright light with these agents. Pharmacologic constriction mainly occurs through cholinergic drugs, such as pilocarpine. Glaucoma ophthalmic drops, such as brimonidine, also cause pupillary constriction. There is more pronounced anisocoria in dim light in these instances.

Relative afferent pupillary defect

Any unilateral or asymmetric decreased afference of the optic nerve may manifest as a relative afferent pupillary defect (RAPD). An RAPD should not be assumed to be caused by a media disturbance (ie, cataracts) because light flashed directly into the pupil is still scattered onto the macula [6]. One exception may be a dense intraocular hemorrhage, which is generally not diagnostically elusive. Optic nerve disease also presents as a deficit in visual sensory function and possibly a change in the appearance of the optic disc. Optic neuropathies are caused by a myriad of processes and differentiating these causes is difficult (Table 1). The history may be the most helpful tool in narrowing the differential.

Preservation of visual acuity or preventing further visual loss is the goal of management. Determining which patients need emergent intervention may require further testing and consultation with an ophthalmologist, depending on the history and physical examination findings.

Traumatic optic neuropathy

Patients who present with an RAPD after trauma must be presumed to have optic nerve injury. Penetrating trauma requires prompt ophthalmologic evaluation and consultation for possible surgical intervention and

Table 1
Conditions producing relative afferent pupillary defect

Condition	Site
Intraocular hemorrhage	Anterior chamber or vitreous (dense or diffuse)
Intraocular hemorrhage	Preretinal
Central serous retinopathy	Retina (fovea)
Cystoid macular edema	Retina (fovea)
Central or branch retinal vein occlusion	Inner retina
Central or branch retinal artery occlusion	Inner retina
Retinal detachment	Outer retina
Anterior ischemic optic neuropathy	Optic nerve head
Optic neuritis—acute	Optic nerve
Optic neuritis—recovered	Optic nerve
Compressive optic neuropathy	Optic nerve
Chiasmal compression	Optic chiasm
Optic tract lesion	Optic tract
Postgeniculate damage	Visual radiations, visual cortex
Midbrain tectal damage	Olivary pretectal area of pupil, midbrain

Data from Kawasaki A, Kardon RH. Disorders of the pupil. Ophthalmol Clin North Am 2001;14(1):166.

a search for foreign bodies. In addition to careful examination, these patients should undergo CT scanning and tetanus prophylaxis, and be placed on systemic antibiotics [9,10]. Indirect trauma, from concussive forces, can result in shearing forces that result in mechanical and ischemic damage to the optic nerve. This type of traumatic optic nerve injury is much more common. The treatment of this type of injury is less well studied. In the International Optic Nerve Trauma Study, there was no clear benefit on visual acuity for treatment with corticosteroids, decompression surgery, or observation alone [11]. This conclusion should be taken in the context of the study design, however. This study was non-randomized, uncontrolled, unblinded, and retrospective, making the conclusions weakly generalizable.

Optic neuritis

Optic neuritis refers to inflammatory optic neuropathies, but more specifically to those neuropathies in which demyelination is predominant (idiopathic or secondary to multiple sclerosis [MS]). Optic neuritis is mainly a clinical diagnosis. Patients generally present with monocular visual deficits associated with periorbital or ocular pain. The pain may precede or present concurrently with the vision loss. Eye pain is present in 92% of patients and is almost universally worsened by eye movement [12–14]. There may also be decreased color perception or central scotoma. The optic disc has a normal presentation in about 70% of patients initially, because the inflammatory process is usually posterior to the optic disc [4,13]. Optic disc swelling and, less commonly, flame-shaped hemorrhages at or near the disc may be present, however. RAPD is usually seen, but may be subtle, requiring advanced ophthalmologic evaluation. MRI imaging of the brain is helpful diagnostically and prognostically but is not always needed emergently. In those who have monocular optic neuritis, there is a 50% incidence of MS if the initial MRI shows at least three typical white matter lesions. Conversely, the 5-year incidence of MS drops to 15% if the MRI is normal [14]. Consultation with an ophthalmologist is important. If the examination shows a macular star figure, this represents an infectious cause. In general, further investigation with chest radiograph, anti-nuclear antibody, or testing for syphilis are generally noncontributory in the emergency department setting and not recommended for evaluation in the patient who has typical optic neuritis [12,14]. Emergency physicians should be aware of more recent treatment recommendations based on the Optic Neuritis Treat Trial data [14–16]. Oral prednisone was associated with an increased incidence of recurrent optic neuritis in a 5-year follow-up period and was no better than placebo in improvement of visual outcomes. Intravenous methylprednisolone (over 3 days followed by a prednisone taper) was associated with faster recovery in visual function if given within 8 days of symptom onset. The difference in benefit seems to wash away after about 6 months. There is no current convincing data on the use of immunoglobulin or plasma exchange therapy in optic neuritis [13].

Oculomotor nerve palsy

Pupillary disorders may occur in the context of a third nerve lesion as discussed in the next section.

Extraocular movement disorders

Cranial nerve palsies and binocular diplopia

There are three cranial nerves involved in controlling the six extraocular muscles, the oculomotor nerve (III), the trochlear nerve (IV), and the abducens nerve (VI). The eyes have equal and opposed actions of the muscles of extraocular movement, which are in turn coordinated by supranuclear control to produce conjugate and divergent gaze. These supranuclear controls consist of brainstem gaze centers and cortical input. When there is a disruption of extraocular muscle function, the eye is unable to move in the direction of the action of the affected muscle (ie, ophthalmoplegia). Palsies of the extraocular muscles commonly present as binocular diplopia because the images fall on a different region of each retina. It is important to identify associated signs and symptoms and establish in which gazes double vision occurs to determine which cranial nerves are affected. During the examination, all six cardinal positions of gaze should be tested, not only for muscle palsies but also to see if diplopia is elicited. The examiner may use a light source to see if the light falls on the same spot on both corneas in each position of gaze, which determines which cranial nerves are affected. The most common palsy is a sixth nerve palsy, followed by third nerve and fourth nerve palsies. Involvement of multiple cranial nerves is the least common presentation [17,18].

In this section, we divide the causes of binocular diplopia by each cranial nerve, and then neuroanatomically for each cranial nerve. When presented with diplopia, the emergency physician should determine which cranial nerves are affected. This determination may help in formulating a differential diagnosis and the urgency of such a presentation.

Cranial nerve III

The oculomotor nerve innervates the medial, superior, and inferior rectus, the inferior oblique, the levator palpebrae, and the parasympathetic pupillary constrictors. There is ptosis, pupillary dilation, and lateral deviation from unopposed action of the lateral rectus in a complete CN III lesion (see Fig. 6). The patient reports diplopia in all directions of gaze except on lateral gaze to the affected side. This discussion focuses on lesions according to their location: brainstem (nuclear and fascicular), subarachnoid, cavernous sinus, orbital apex, and neuromuscular lesions. Despite the wide differential, urgent evaluation is generally warranted for a patient presenting with new third nerve palsy, because this may herald serious diseases, such as brainstem infarction, aneurysm, and neoplasm. Vascular causes are the most common known causes of oculomotor nerve palsy, whereas aneurysms are the second most common. Usually, the cause is never determined (Table 2) [17].

Brain stem lesions. Brainstem oculomotor lesions classically present with bilateral ptosis and contralateral superior rectus and ipsilateral oculomotor paresis. This presentation occurs because the levator palpebrae are innervated by an unpaired central nucleus and the superior recti are innervated by contralateral subnuclei. The most common cause is ischemia [19]. The patient should thus undergo a stroke evaluation with appropriate accompanying management. Besides mass lesions, compression, and inflammation, other causes for higher-order third nerve palsies are Wernicke encephalopathy and progressive supranuclear palsy. In Wernicke encephalopathy, the third nerve ophthalmoplegia is usually bilateral and is associated with a history of chronic alcohol use or malnutrition, ataxia, nystagmus, and altered mentation. There may be ophthalmoplegia because of involvement of CN

Table 2
Lesions of the oculomotor nerve

Anatomic location	Cause	Associated symptoms
Nuclear	Infarction, mass, infection, inflammation, compression	Bilateral ptosis and paresis of the contralateral superior rectus; lid function may be spared
	Wernicke-Korsakoff syndrome	Ataxia, abducens palsy, nystagmus, altered mentation
Fascicular	Infarction, mass, infection, inflammation, compression	Contralateral hemiparesis or tremor; pupil may be spared
	Demyelination	
Subarachnoid space	Aneurysm	Headache, stiff neck, pupil-involved
	Vasculopathic	Pupil generally spared
	Meningitis	Headache, CN involvement, meningismus, fever
	Miller-Fisher syndrome	Areflexia, ataxia, previous viral illness
	Migraine	Headache, family history
	Uncal herniation	Early pupil involvement, altered mentation, ipsilateral hemiparesis
Cavernous sinus	Neoplasm	Cavernous sinus syndrome, pain, sensory changes, ± sympathetic involvement
	Fistula	Exophthalmos, bruit, chemosis
	Thrombosis	Previous infection/trauma, pain, exophthalmos, chemosis
Superior orbital fissure	Neoplasm	Superior division involvement
Neuromuscular junction	Myasthenia gravis	No pupil involvement, frequent fluctuation, ptosis, ophthalmoparesis, orbicularis oculi weakness, dysarthria

Data from Bennett JL, Pelak VS. Palsies of the third, fourth, and sixth cranial nerves. Ophthalmol Clin North Am 2001;14(1):173.

IV and VI also. Progressive supranuclear palsy is an idiopathic degenerative disease that mainly affects the subcortical gray matter regions of the brain in older men. The ocular manifestations are ophthalmoplegia in all directions, although initially more severe with voluntary vertical gaze. This disease is also associated with dementia, decreased facial expression, pseudobulbar palsy, and axial dystonia. These patients should have routine follow-up with a neurologist. Although prognosis is poor, quality of life may be improved with multidisciplinary symptom management [20].

Subarachnoid lesions. The subarachnoid segment of CN III is that section after the nerve leaves the midbrain and before it enters the cavernous sinus (Fig. 18). Lesions generally present as unilateral ptosis and third nerve paresis, with or without pupillary dilation. A search for associated signs and symptoms is helpful because there are many causes of lesions of this portion of the oculomotor nerve, including meningitis, migraines, Miller-Fisher variant of Guillian-Barre, vasculopathy, uncal herniation, and aneurysm. The nerve travels near the junction of the internal carotid and posterior communicating artery and between the posterior cerebral and the superior cerebellar arteries, and is thus susceptible to compression from aneurysms. In fact, about 30% of oculomotor palsies are from aneurysms, most

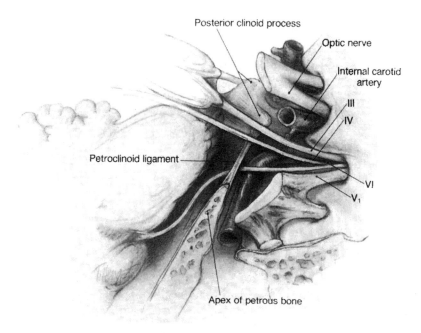

Fig. 18. Subarachnoid and intracavernous courses of the third, fourth, and sixth cranial nerves. (*From* Porter JD, Baker RS. Anatomy and embryology of the ocular motor system. In: Miller NR, Newman NJ, editors. Walsh and Hoyt's clinical neuro-ophthalmology. 5th edition. Baltimore (MD): Williams & Wilkins; 1998. p. 1066; with permission.)

commonly from the posterior communicating artery [21]. A third nerve palsy may also result from aneurysms of the basilar, superior cerebellar, and posterior cerebral arteries. The aneurysm causes oculomotor paresis by compression of the nerve. Parasympathetic fibers travel in the periphery of the subarachnoid portion of the nerve, with the motor fibers centrally located. Oculomotor involvement from an aneurysm commonly causes pupillary dilation. Aneurysm is extremely unusual if there is not pupillary involvement in the presence of a complete palsy [21]. CT angiography is the study of choice for noninvasive diagnosis of unruptured aneurysms, with sensitivities ranging from 85% to 90% for aneurysms larger than 5 mm and 79% for aneurysms smaller than 5 mm [22]. MR angiography is an alternative, able to detect aneurysms as small as 3 mm. It is not as sensitive, however, especially for aneurysms smaller than 5 mm [19,21,22]. CT scan with or without lumbar puncture should be undertaken if aneurysmal rupture with subarachnoid bleed is suspected. Definitive treatment includes surgical clipping or endovascular coil placement.

Migraine headache variants, such as cranial neuralgias and ophthalmoplegic migraine, present with ocular and pupillary dysfunction. This diagnosis usually requires the exclusion of other, more serious disease processes. Presentations supportive of a migraine diagnosis are a previous history of migraines, especially with childhood onset, aura, typical positive and negative visual phenomena (scotoma, transient visual distortions), and migraine-like headache. The International Headache Society requires at least two attacks of a migrainelike headache accompanied or followed by oculomotor paresis within 4 hours, not attributed to other disorders, for diagnosis of ophthalmoplegic migraine [23]. This condition is rare and usually presents in the pediatric population [24]. The ophthalmoplegia is usually transient but rarely may become permanent. Consultation with a neurologist is important because acute treatment with corticosteroids has been shown to provide relief and may prevent a permanent deficit [23,25].

Cavernous sinus lesions. Diplopia may be the presenting symptom of a cavernous sinus fistula, seen in about 60% to 70% of cases [21]. These fistulas are abnormal communications between the cavernous sinus and the carotid artery, usually the result of trauma, but also occur as a complication of surgery or after rupture of a cavernous carotid artery aneurysm. They typically present days to weeks after traumatic head injury with conjunctival chemosis, proptosis, and a cranial bruit, either subjective or objective. Conjunctival chemosis occurs from the arterialization of the conjunctival veins. Proptosis occurs from the arterialization of the orbital veins and edema of the orbital tissue. Pulsating exophthalmos may be visually or palpably appreciated on examination, and occurs in about 95% of cases [21]. Diplopia occurs through compression or ischemia of the ocular nerves by the fistula itself. Most commonly CN VI is involved, although ophthalmoplegia may be attributable to any combination of ocular nerve involvement. Definitive diagnosis requires arteriography with selective injection of the internal and external carotid arteries, although CT and MR imaging may be suggestive of a fistula and can help exclude other disease processes. Visual loss may be delayed or immediate and is the main morbidity associated with this condition, occurring in up to 90% of cases. Other complications include intracranial or subarachnoid hemorrhage, venous infarction, and epistaxis, although life-threatening sequelae are rare [21]. Addressing these high-flow carotid-cavernous fistulas usually requires urgent treatment.

Superior orbital fissure lesions. The most common cause of a third nerve palsy from a superior orbital fissure lesion is a neoplasm. When vision is affected, the lesion is almost always in the orbital apex [19]. Other associated signs include conjunctival injection and chemosis, proptosis, and lid swelling. CN IV, CN VI, and also CN V_1 may be involved because of their proximity to one another. MR imaging is the modality of choice, keeping in mind that the most common cause is a neoplasm. CT may have a role, but early in the growth of a tumor the neoplasm may be isodense with normal brain tissue.

Neuromuscular disease. Neuromuscular disease, such as myasthenic syndromes, may mimic isolated nerve palsies. There is a separate discussion later in this article.

Cranial nerve IV

Trochlear nerve palsy presents with paresis of the superior oblique muscle. The function of this muscle is tested in isolation with downward gaze with the eye adducted, which is the position of gaze that elicits the most pronounced diplopia. The involved eye is elevated in neutral position and the degree of elevation is increased with adduction and decreased with abduction (see Fig. 8).

A lesion causing a fourth nerve palsy can also occur anywhere along the path of the nerve, from the nucleus to the superior oblique muscle. Determining where the lesion lies may be difficult, requiring a search for associated, or absent, symptoms and signs along with neurologic consultation and imaging. For instance, association with an oculomotor palsy strongly suggests a cavernous sinus lesion. Most fourth nerve palsies have no known cause, but of the known causes, most are attributable to head trauma. Vasculopathies are the next most common cause (Table 3) [17,26].

Brain stem lesions. Nuclear and fascicular lesions of the fourth cranial nerve present as a contralateral superior oblique palsy because of the crossing of the fascicles in the brainstem. They may be caused by ischemia, trauma, inflammation, a mass, or in the case of a fascicular lesion, MS. There are usually other associated neurologic findings attributable to involvement of nearby structures. The periaqueductal gray matter carries sympathetic

Table 3
Lesions of the trochlear nerve

Anatomic location	Cause	Associated symptoms
Nuclear	Infarction	Internuclear ophthalmoplegia, Horner syndrome, relative afferent pupillary defect
	Trauma, tumor, infection, inflammation	As above
Fascicular	Infarction	As above
	Trauma, tumor, infection, inflammation	As above
	Demyelination	Isolated or with midbrain signs above
Subarachnoid space	Trauma, hydrocephalus	May be bilateral
	Vasculopathic	Usually isolated
	Mass lesion	Contralateral hemiparesis or ipsilateral ataxia
Cavernous sinus	As with third nerve palsy	Cavernous sinus syndrome
	Herpes zoster ophthalmic	Rash, trigeminal sensory loss V1 or V2 distribution
Orbit	Inflammation, trauma, tumor	Oculomotor, abducens, optic nerve dysfunction, proptosis

Data from Bennett JL, Pelak VS. Palsies of the third, fourth, and sixth cranial nerves. Ophthalmol Clin North Am 2001;14(1):180.

fibers. There may thus be a preganglionic Horner syndrome. The medial longitudinal fasciculus is just anterior to the nucleus and a lesion affecting this causes an internuclear ophthalmoplegia. Evaluation for a nuclear trochlear nerve lesion should include MR imaging and a stroke workup [5].

Subarachnoid lesions. The trochlear nerve has a relatively long subarachnoid course after it leaves the brainstem posteriorly, which makes it susceptible to trauma, the most common cause of a fourth nerve palsy [17,26]. The trauma may cause unilateral or bilateral isolated trochlear nerve palsy. Other causes of fourth nerve palsies in the subarachnoid space are meningitis, aneurysm of the superior cerebellar artery, schwannoma, and small vessel infarction [17,19,26]. Work-up includes MR imaging to rule out a mass lesion, detect the extent of trauma, and direct any possible neurosurgical intervention.

Distal nerve lesions. Just as with third nerve palsies, orbital fissure lesions and neuromuscular lesions may produce a fourth nerve palsy. A nonneurologic entity that may mimic isolated trochlear nerve palsy is Brown superior oblique tendon syndrome, likely caused by a tenosynovitis or scarring of the superior oblique tendon. The superior oblique tendon is prohibited from free movement through the trochlear pulley. There is inhibition with a forced duction test where the entrapped muscles resist forced movement, indicating mechanical trapping of the superior oblique muscle. Referral to an ophthalmologist is required because surgery may be the best option for the patient.

Cranial nerve VI

Of the three cranial nerves involved in extraocular movement, the abducens nerve is the most commonly affected [17]. A unilateral sixth nerve lesion results in diplopia on lateral gaze, attributable to paresis of the lateral rectus muscle. In neutral position, the affected eye is adducted and fails to abduct with examination (see Fig. 10). Similar to the third and fourth cranial nerve, lesions of the sixth cranial nerve can be subdivided anatomically with some distinguishing features associated with each lesion. The most commonly determined cause for a sixth nerve palsy is a neoplasm, most often metastatic disease or a meningioma, followed by head trauma and vascular disease (Table 4) [17].

Brainstem lesion. A nuclear sixth nerve lesion produces conjugate, horizontal gaze palsy toward the side of the lesion. Nuclear lesions of the abducens nucleus rarely present with an isolated ophthalmoplegia, however. These lesions are associated with damage to the surrounding brainstem structures, such as the facial nerve nucleus, the pontine lateral gaze centers, and the reticular activating system. There may thus be facial weakness, impaired conjugate gaze, and depressed level of consciousness, respectively. The sixth cranial nerve has two projections, one to the ipsilateral lateral rectus and the other to the contralateral CN III nucleus by way of the MLF (see Fig. 12). A pontine lesion involving the adjacent MLF and the pontine lateral gaze centers produces a one-and-a-half syndrome, seen as a complete gaze palsy

Table 4
Lesions of the abducens nerve

Anatomic location	Cause	Associated symptoms
Nuclear	Infarction	Ipsilateral facial paralysis, INO
	Infiltration, trauma, inflammation	
	Wernicke-Korsakoff	Ataxia, nystagmus, altered mentation
Fascicular	Infarction, tumor, inflammation, MS	Ipsilateral facial nerve paralysis and contralateral hemiplegia
	Anterior inferior cerebellar artery infarction	Ipsilateral facial paralysis, loss of taste, ipsilateral Horner, ipsilateral trigeminal dysfunction, and ipsilateral deafness
Subarachnoid	Mass	Contralateral hemiparesis
	Ischemia	Usually isolated
	Trauma	Papilledema, headache
	Intracranial hypertension or hypotension	Headache
Petrous apex	Mastoiditis, skull fracture, lateral sinus thrombosis, neoplasms, tumor	Ipsilateral facial paralysis, severe facial pain
Cavernous sinus	As with third nerve palsy	Cavernous sinus syndrome

Data from Bennett JL, Pelak VS. Palsies of the third, fourth, and sixth cranial nerves. Ophthalmol Clin North Am 2001;14(1):180.

in one direction and a unilateral (half) gaze palsy in the other direction. The lesion to the MLF causes an internuclear ophthalmoplegia and the lesion to the pontine lateral gaze center causes a conjugate gaze palsy to the side of the lesion. Attempted gaze away from the lesion activates the unaffected contralateral lateral gaze center and abducens nucleus but with paresis of ipsilateral adduction. On gaze toward the lesion, neither eye can effectively move laterally, because the pontine lateral gaze center cannot be activated. The most common causes of a one-and-a-half syndrome include pontine infarct, pontine hemorrhage, and multiple sclerosis. Wernicke encephalopathy may present with a nuclear sixth nerve palsy. If a nuclear abducens nerve lesion is suspected, the patient should undergo MR imaging and a stroke workup, because infarction may be the cause of such a lesion.

Subarachnoid lesions. The sixth cranial nerve has a unique course in the subarachnoid space. It emerges from the brainstem just between the pons and the medulla and courses just lateral to the basilar artery and just posterior to the clivus in the prepontine cistern before entering the cavernous sinus. This course makes it susceptible to injury from trauma and changes in intracranial pressure (ICP). The nerve may be compressed between the pons and the basilar artery or the clivus. In addition to MR imaging, the patient may require evaluation for elevated or diminished ICP.

Aneurysms of the basilar artery, and less commonly of the anterior and posterior inferior cerebellar arteries, and the vertebral arteries can produce a sixth nerve palsy. Sixth nerve palsy from an aneurysm is less common than a third nerve palsy [21]. Diagnosis and management have been mentioned previously.

Cavernous sinus lesions. Ophthalmoplegia may be the presenting symptom of a cavernous sinus thrombosis, usually affecting all the extraocular muscles. These occur from trauma, but more commonly from infection. CN VI is usually affected first, however, because it lies freely within the sinus and not within the lateral walls of the sinus as CN III and CN IV do [19,27]. Besides headache, which is present in about 90% of cases, the most common accompanying signs are fever, ptosis, proptosis, and chemosis, occurring in 80% to 100% of infectious cases [19,27,28]. Periorbital swelling and papilledema only occur in 50% to 80% of cases [27]. MRI with MR angiography is the most sensitive noninvasive modality, approaching 100% sensitivity for all types of sinus thromboses in small studies [28,29]. Another promising diagnostic option is CT venography, but more study is required [27]. The gold standard is angiography, although its diagnostic use has dramatically declined. Therapeutically, cavernous sinus thromboses may be treated with anticoagulation and antibiotics, in addition to supportive measures and management of elevated intracranial pressures. There are no rigorous, large trials on the use of anticoagulation in venous sinus thrombosis. A recent prospective observational study showed that more than 80% of the

624 patients received anticoagulation with a good safety profile [30]. The outcomes were fairly encouraging in this subgroup, with only 5% rated as severely handicapped and 8% having died. In cases of septic cavernous sinus thrombosis, broad-spectrum antibiotics should be given. The most common offending organism is *Staphylococcus aureus*, and less commonly streptococcus, gram-negative bacilli, and anaerobes [27]. Surgical drainage of the sinus thrombosis is rarely performed, although decompression of a hemorrhagic infarction may be indicated.

Nystagmus

Nystagmus is rhythmic oscillation of the eyes. To detect nystagmus, the eyes should be observed in primary position and each of the six positions of gaze. Nystagmus is described by the position in which it occurs, precipitating factors, such as head position, and the direction of the fast phase. It is useful to classify nystagmus as physiologic or pathologic, and subdivide the pathologic causes as peripheral or central.

Physiologic nystagmus occurs normally at the extremes of gaze. In this instance a clear image is preserved as reflexes reset the position of the eyes and prevent the image from slipping on the retina [31]. These reflexes are collectively known as the slow eye movement system. Their function is to maintain clear vision with a quick corrective saccade, resulting in nystagmus. Pathologic nystagmus is usually accompanied by vertigo, oscillopsia, nausea, gait disturbance, and other symptoms depending on the cause. The patient may complain of oscillopsia, a sensation of oscillation of the environment in the direction of the fast phase.

Peripheral nystagmus

In general, pathologic peripheral vestibular causes of nystagmus and vertigo are less worrisome and less emergent than central causes. The nystagmus from vestibular causes usually has a combined horizontal and torsional component, which can be inhibited by visual fixation onto an object. The horizontal component does not change direction with gaze (unidirectional). Nausea, vomiting, auditory symptoms, and vertigo are significant components of the presentation. Vertical nystagmus may be present in addition to horizontal nystagmus, but is far less common in peripheral causes. Vertical nystagmus has been shown to be about 80% sensitive for central causes of vertigo in a small prospective trial (Table 5) [32].

A common emergency department presentation of horizontal nystagmus is benign paroxysmal positional vertigo (BPPV). BPPV presents with a combined horizontal and torsional nystagmus and vertigo on provocation with the Dix-Hallpike maneuver. The nystagmus lasts for less than 1 minute, and fatigues on repeated testing. It has a positive predictive value of 83% and negative predictive value of 52% for BPPV. If the induced nystagmus is vertical, and not preceded by a latency, or does not fatigue with repeated

Table 5
Peripheral versus central nystagmus

Feature	Peripheral	Central
Direction of nystagmus	Horizontal/torsional	Pure vertical, pure torsional, or mixed
Visual fixation	Inhibits nystagmus	No inhibition
Severity of vertigo symptoms	May be severe	Usually mild
Associated eye movements	None	May have pursuit or saccadic defects
Other findings	Hearing loss	May have other CN or long tract signs

Data from Moster, ML. Nystagmus. Ophthalmol Clin North Am 2001;14(1):205.

provocation, then a central cause cannot be excluded [33]. If BPPV is diagnosed, the treatment of choice is canalith repositioning, such as the Epley maneuver. In a meta-analysis of nine studies, canalith repositioning was 4.6 times more likely to have symptom resolution at the time of first follow-up, compared with those who did not have repositioning [34]. Although commonly used, vestibular suppressant (anticholinergic and benzodiazepine) pharmacotherapy has not been well studied or shown to improve symptoms in those who have BPPV. Its use is discouraged because it does not seem to reduce the frequency of attacks and may even worsen a patient's imbalance [35].

Drug intoxication from alcohol, anticonvulsants, and sedative-hypnotics is the most common cause of nystagmus. The nystagmus is usually in the horizontal plane, but can occasionally appear in the vertical plane. Antiepileptic medications, including the newer agents, may cause a gaze-evoked nystagmus and even diplopia. Other types of nystagmus are rare with anticonvulsants, so other causes for the nystagmus should be sought if they are not gaze-evoked [36]. Other peripheral causes of nystagmus and vertigo include BPPV, Ménière disease, labyrinthitis, perilymphatic fistula, and Ramsey-Hunt syndrome.

Central nystagmus

In contrast to peripheral causes of nystagmus, central causes (from the brainstem or cerebellum) generally produce a purely vertical, horizontal, or torsional nystagmus that is not inhibited by visual fixation, and the fast phase may change direction with gaze (bidirectional). Vertical nystagmus should not be considered as arising from a vestibular cause. Downbeat nystagmus, which is always of central origin, is characteristic of lesions in the medullary–cervical region, Chiari malformation, and demyelinative plaques. Upbeat nystagmus has less localizing value [31]. Rarely are there auditory symptoms with central nystagmus [37]. Instead, there are other neurologic symptoms, including dysarthria, weakness, and diplopia. These differences between peripheral and central nystagmus are only guidelines and not absolute rules. Brainstem and cerebellar lesions causing central nystagmus include cerebellopontine angle tumors, cerebellar disease, cerebrovascular disease, seizures, migraine, and MS.

Cerebellopontine angle tumors, including vestibular schwannomas, ependymomas, brainstem gliomas, medulloblastomas, and neurofibromatosis can cause vertigo and nystagmus. The nystagmus is usually coarse and bidirectional. Hearing loss of insidious onset is usually the initial symptom, and then gait ataxia, facial pain, tinnitus, a sensation of fullness in the ear, or facial weakness may ensue.

Cerebellar mass lesions or ischemia may cause nystagmus that is gaze-evoked, bidirectional, downbeat, or even pendular [38]. Pendular nystagmus is nystagmus with no fast component. Rather, the eyes move back and forth with slow velocity; this is also seen in MS. Cerebellar lesions usually have associated dysfunction in coordination, equilibrium, and gait.

Arnold-Chiari malformations are congenital abnormalities at the base of the brain that cause extensions of a tongue of cerebellar tissue into the cervical canal with displacement of the medulla into the cervical canal, along with the inferior part of the fourth ventricle. The herniated tissue blocks the circulation of cerebrospinal fluid in the brain and can lead to the formation of a cavity (syrinx) within the spinal cord. Without the meningomyelocele, it is classified as a type I malformation, and with a meningomyelocele, a type II malformation. The nystagmus is generally downbeating. Other associated symptoms are occipital headache (from increased intracranial pressure), ataxia, quadriparesis, and sensory loss (from cervical syringomyelia) [37].

MS may cause various types of nystagmus [13,39]. The most common is the nystagmus exhibited by INO, discussed in more detail later. The nystagmus in INO is seen during abduction of the unaffected eye, and the affected eye is unable to adduct. Demyelinating lesions of the cerebellum may cause a downbeat nystagmus, whereas bilateral internuclear ophthalmoplegia can cause an upbeat nystagmus. Multiple sclerosis is the most common cause of pendular nystagmus, in any direction [13,31].

The extraocular movement disorders of Alzheimer disease and Parkinson disease are usually delays of saccades and impairment of smooth pursuit, but not nystagmus [40].

Myasthenia gravis

Half of all patients who have myasthenia gravis (MG) present with pure ocular findings. Of these, 70% eventually develop generalized myasthenia [41]. Ptosis and diplopia are the presenting complaint in 75% of patients and develop eventually in 90% of patients who have MG [41–43].

The clinical hallmarks of myasthenia gravis are variable muscular weakness and fatigability, with amelioration after rest. Normally, there are more than enough acetylcholine receptors to ensure a muscle action potential after repeated ligand and receptor interactions. In MG, however, the number of available receptors quickly diminishes with each muscle contraction, resulting in variability and fatigability. Variability is caused by the decreased probability that acetylcholine will trigger an action potential given the reduced number of acetylcholine receptors. Fatigability results from depletion of acetylcholine after repeated action potentials.

Propensity for the muscles of extraocular movement is not well understood [41]. Ptosis is a common manifestation, which may be unilateral or asymmetric, and is exacerbated with prolonged upward gaze. Diplopia results from weakness of one or more of the extraocular muscles. There may be strabismus evident on examination, or loss of conjugate gaze on prolonged eccentric gaze. There are no sensory changes, loss of muscle bulk, or reflex changes. In general, the pupils are not affected, although there is disagreement if this is universal [41,42]. On examination there may be weakness of the orbicularis oculi muscles. The examiner may find weakness in forced eyelid closure, whereas normally it is very difficult to retract the eyelids against forced eye closure.

The differential may be fairly limited in more advanced disease or with generalized myasthenia, but can be broader in the earlier stages because there are fewer stigmata of MG. MG can mimic a single nerve palsy and other peripheral or central neuropathic diseases described previously. There are also other neuromuscular junction diseases, although they are less common. Lambert-Eaton myasthenic syndrome, like MG, is an autoimmune disease affecting the neuromuscular junction. It affects the presynaptic nerve terminal, however. With repeated stimulation, the nerve terminal eventually releases adequate acetylcholine. This process is clinically evident with improvement of power as a contraction is maintained, most prominently affecting the proximal muscles. Lambert-Eaton rarely affects the extraocular muscles [4,41]. Treatment of Lambert-Eaton syndrome is similar to treatment of MG as described later. Botulism may cause a myasthenic-like syndrome. The *Clostridium botulinum* toxin prevents the release of acetylcholine at the neuromuscular junction and autonomic synapses. Weakness begins 2 to 36 hours after toxin ingestion and fulminating weakness begins 12 to 72 hours after ingestion with a distinctive pattern of development [4,44]. There is descending flaccid paralysis, with virtually all cases starting with cranial nerve palsies, including extraocular nerve palsies. Unlike MG, there are also autonomic symptoms in botulism, such as dry mouth, ileus, postural hypotension, and blurring of vision. There may be similar symptoms in clusters of people, strongly indicating botulism. It is also important to consider botulism in intravenous drug users who have cranial nerve palsies, including diplopia. Treatment includes hospitalization because respiratory compromise may develop quickly. Elective intubation should be considered because there seems to be a mortality benefit over those who suffer a respiratory arrest before intubation [44]. Antitoxin should be administered, although this only binds circulating toxins and does not reverse established paralysis. All cases are public health emergencies and must be reported to public health officials. Organophosphate poisoning may also present with a combination of neuromuscular and autonomic symptoms and signs, classically as a cholinergic crisis. Treatment is supportive, along with atropine or pralidoxime. Finally, medications may produce myasthenic syndromes or exacerbate the symptoms of those who have MG (Table 6).

Table 6
Drugs that exacerbate myasthenia gravis

Antibiotics	Aminoglycosides
	Polymyxin
	Clindamycin
	Lincomycin
	Tetracycline
	Ciprofloxacin
	Chloroquine
	Pyrantel
Antiarrhythmics	Quinidine
	Procainamide
	Lidocaine
	Propafenone
Beta blockers	
Calcium channel blockers	
Anticonvulsants	Phenytoin
	Trimethadione
Psychiatric drugs	Lithium
	Chlorpromazine
	Phenelzine
Other	Cocaine
	Steroids
	Magnesium
	Iodinated contrast

Data from Barton JJS, Fouladvand M. Ocular aspects of myasthenia gravis. Semin Neurol 2000;20(1):17.

Diagnosis of MG and differentiation from other neuromuscular disorders is generally confirmed with clinical response to acetylcholinesterase inhibitors, EMG, and antibody/toxin assays. Treatment of ocular MG is generally not emergent, but timely referral or consultation with a neurologist is important. These patients may be offered symptomatic treatment, immunosuppressive therapies, and thymectomy if there is a demonstrated thymoma. Those in a myasthenic crisis (ie, weakness of respiration requiring mechanical ventilation) temporarily benefit from plasmapheresis or intravenous immunoglobulins [4,43].

Multiple sclerosis

In addition to optic neuropathy, MS may cause ocular motility dysfunction, mimicking cranial nerve lesions at any neuroanatomic level. It is clinically defined by neurologic disturbances separated by time and space. In other words, deficits involve different areas of the central nervous system at different times. After the initial symptoms resolve in days to weeks, there may be an interval of months to years before other neurologic deficits appear.

The most common oculomotor nerve palsy in multiple sclerosis is CN VI palsy, which may be the initial presentation of MS [39]. After trauma and mass lesions, it is one of the most common causes of an abducens palsy. Trochlear nerve palsies are rare in MS because of the limited myelination of the trochlear nerve [39].

INO is a distinctive feature of MS, caused by a demyelinating lesion of the MLF (see Fig. 12). The MLF carries ascending projections from the CN VI nucleus to the contralateral CN III nucleus to coordinate horizontal gaze. It is characterized by lost or limited adduction of one eye and a horizontal nystagmus, during abduction, of the contralateral eye. Many cases of INO are subtle because the deficit is partial and no diplopia with lateral gaze is reported [39]. It is present in 17% to 41% of patients who have MS [13]. Other common causes of INO include vascular disease and infection, whereas less common causes include trauma, tumor, hemorrhage, and vasculitis [13]. Isolated INO without other accompanying symptoms or signs is uncommon, but work-up should still include neurologic consultation and MRI.

Stroke syndromes and gaze palsies

Stroke syndromes and the visual system

Stroke should be considered in any evaluation of visual or ocular disturbance. Visual field defects are a common consequence of a large vessel cerebrovascular accident (CVA). The type of visual field defect depends on the location of the lesion, which can range anywhere from the retina to the occipital lobe (Fig. 19). These lesions lead to predictable patterns of visual field deficits. The simplest and most appropriate emergency method of testing visual fields is the confrontation technique described previously. Oculomotor dysfunction in the setting of CVA is more indicative of brainstem and posterior circulation ischemia. Ischemia of the brain has been mentioned in virtually all sections thus far, but we dedicate a section to the effects of stroke on the visual and oculomotor system, organized by the affected artery. A full discussion of stroke and its diagnosis and management is outside the scope of this article.

Anterior cerebral artery

The anterior cerebral artery supplies the parasagittal cerebral cortex. A CVA involving the anterior cerebral artery does not typically result in a visual or oculomotor defect.

Internal carotid artery

The internal carotid artery (ICA) feeds into the circle of Willis, and because of collateral circulation, no part of the brain is completely dependent on it. In fact, 30% to 40% of occlusions are asymptomatic [37]. The ICA gives rise to two branches of interest to the visual system: the ophthalmic artery and the anterior choroidal artery. A lesion of these branches may cause monocular blindness and homonymous hemianopia, respectively. An

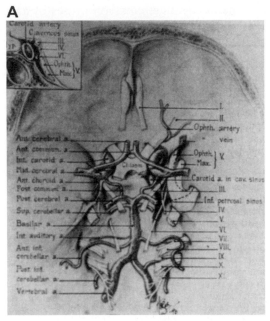

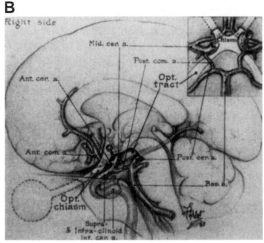

Fig. 19. (*A*) The regional anatomy of the base of the skull, cranial nerves, and circle of Willis. (*B*) The section through the brain showing the relationship between arteries of the circle of Willis and adjacent component parts of the visual pathways. (*From* Walsh FB. Visual field defects due to aneurysms at the circle of Willis. Arch Ophthalmol 1964:71:49; with permission.)

ICA lesion must be considered in these presentations. Vascular studies of the carotid system should be performed as part of the stroke work-up to determine if carotid endarterectomy is indicated.

The ophthalmic artery supplies the retina. Ischemia from ICA occlusion may initially manifest as transient monocular blindness attributable to retinal artery ischemia, whereas infarction leads to more persistent monocular blindness. Because the ICA is connected to the middle and anterior cerebral arteries by the circle of Willis, other symptoms, such as hemiplegia and hemisensory deficits, may accompany the ocular blindness.

The anterior choroidal artery comes off the ICA near the posterior communicating artery. It supplies parts of the globus pallidus, internal capsule, and various contiguous structures, including the optic tract. In addition to the motor and sensory deficits in an anterior choroidal artery infarct, there is also a homonymous hemianopia contralateral to the side of the lesion. In general, there is preservation of language and cognition. Anterior choroidal artery strokes have not been well studied or documented and there is debate as to whether there is a distinct syndrome [37].

Middle cerebral artery

The middle cerebral artery (MCA) supplies the lateral convexity of the cerebral hemisphere, including the frontal eye field, the lateral geniculate nucleus, and the optic radiations, the region of the cortex related to macular vision. Deep branches supply the basal ganglia and the internal capsule. It is the most commonly involved vessel in strokes. MCA strokes are anatomically separated into a superior division and an inferior division depending on which branch is affected after the MCA bifurcates, although a more proximal lesion can occur that includes the superior and inferior divisions.

The superior division of the MCA does not supply the optic tract or the radiations, but it does supply the frontal eye field and the cortical region responsible for voluntary lateral conjugate gaze. Superior division strokes thus do not result in a visual field defect, but may cause a conjugate gaze deviation [4,37]. This phenomenon is discussed further in the section on gaze palsies. Inferior division strokes may cause a homonymous quadrantanopia or hemianopia depending on how extensively the optic radiation is affected.

Posterior cerebral artery

The posterior cerebral artery (PCA) supplies the occipital visual cerebral cortex, the medial temporal lobes, thalamus, and rostral midbrain. Ischemia in the PCA distribution is most commonly attributable to embolic PCA infarcts that affect the visual cortex causing a homonymous hemianopia because of unilateral ischemia of the occipital lobe. There may be macular sparing (central visual field) because of the collateral blood supply to the section of cortex involved in macular vision from the MCA.

Involvement of the extraocular muscles occurs through ischemia of cranial nerve nuclei, resulting in nerve palsies, vertical gaze palsies, and internuclear ophthalmoplegia. When deep branches of the posterior cerebral artery in the midbrain are affected, there can be involvement of the third cranial nerve nucleus, causing an oculomotor palsy. These arterial branches also supply other nearby structures and, in addition to the third nerve palsy, can cause an accompanying contralateral hemiplegia (Weber syndrome) if the corticospinal tracts are involved, or a contralateral ataxia and tremor (Claude syndrome), if the red nucleus is involved [37].

Cortical blindness may result from bilateral occlusion of the PCA, which is a rare event, and more commonly cortical blindness is the result of trauma to the occipital lobe, or global ischemia, such as in cardiac arrest. The hallmark of cortical blindness or cortical visual impairment is normally functioning pupils and a normal funduscopic examination with no perceptible vision. The occipital lobe is particularly vulnerable to insult from global ischemia because of its location in the border zone between the middle and posterior cerebral arteries. Cortical blindness from global ischemia is usually transient, but may be permanent [4].

Basilar artery

The basilar artery supplies deep structures of the cerebrum and the entire brainstem and cerebellum. Occlusion of the basilar artery is usually incompatible with life [4]. If the proximal basilar artery is affected there may be unilateral or bilateral abducens nerve palsy, usually with associated neurologic findings, such as paresis.

"Top of the basilar" syndrome occurs when there is an embolism small enough to lodge at the basilar artery bifurcation into the posterior cerebral arteries. Unilateral or bilateral third nerve palsies are characteristic in this syndrome. The basilar artery supplies a large number of structures and is associated with numerous other defects, however. There is generally coma because of involvement of the reticular activating system and multiple motor-sensory deficits.

Vertebal arteries

The vertebral arteries supply the medulla and their branches supply the cerebellum. Occlusion of the vertebral artery and its branch, the posterior inferior cerebellar artery, may cause lateral medullary (Wallenberg) syndrome because of infarction of a lateral wedge of the medulla. This is the most common ischemic lesion involving the vertebral arteries. The complete syndrome involves the vestibular nuclei (vertigo, nystagmus, vomiting); spinothalamic tract (impairment of pain and thermal sense over half the body); descending sympathetic tract (ipsilateral Horner syndrome); the ninth and tenth cranial nerves (hoarseness, dysphagia, diminished gag reflex); otolithic nucleus (vertical diplopia and illusion of tilting of vision); olivocerebellar or spinocerebellar tracts (ipsilateral ataxia of limbs, falling or toppling to the ipsilateral side, or lateropulsion); the fifth cranial nerve (pain, burning, and impaired sensation over half of the face); and nucleus and tractus solitarius (loss of taste) [37]. The most common findings are vertigo, nystagmus, lateropulsion, and limb ataxia. This syndrome does not characteristically involve the motor system.

Gaze palsies/conjugate gaze deviation

The decision to move one's eyes laterally begins in the cerebral hemisphere. Cortical fibers then travel down to the CN VI nucleus and the contralateral CN III nucleus through the MLF as described previously for conjugate horizontal gaze (see Fig. 12). A gaze palsy, or impairment of conjugate eye movement, mainly results from lesions above the level of the cranial nerve nuclei. In this case, an impairment of one hemisphere results in an imbalance in neural tone between the two hemispheres. The result is a conjugate gaze deviation. In this section we discuss gaze palsies and their causes by their location in the cerebral cortex, midbrain, or pons.

Hemispheric lesions

The most common cause of gaze palsy is a hemispheric lesion. In destructive lesions of the frontal eye field (Brodmann area 8) of the cerebral cortex, there is gaze palsy toward the side of the lesion in the area of the anterior circulation. Hemispheric ischemia or infarction can result in a conjugate gaze deviation. Seizure activity to the frontal eye field causes a gaze deviation away from the affected hemisphere because of uninhibited neural stimulation.

The incidence of gaze palsy in stroke has been documented to be approximately 20% to 32% and its presence has been associated with poorer functional outcomes [45]. In an acute stroke or transient ischemic attack, the eye is deviated away from the side of the hemiparesis and toward the side of the lesion. At times this physical examination finding is subtle if the patient's gaze is fixated during examination. The eyes are still yoked, so there is usually no diplopia. Visualization of the conjugate eye deviation on CT scanning has been offered as a sign supporting acute stroke. Patients usually close their eyes, removing gaze fixation and revealing underlying tonic eye deviation [46,47]. This phenomenon has not been prospectively studied, however.

Midbrain lesions

The dorsal midbrain has centers responsible for voluntary upward gaze. This area may be damaged by trauma, hydrocephalus, compressive masses such as pineal tumors, demyelinating disorders, infection, ischemia, or hemorrhage, resulting in features of Parinaud syndrome [46,48]. The syndrome is characterized by up-gaze paresis. There is preservation of vertical eye movements with the doll's eye maneuver and with voluntary downward gaze, and nystagmus mainly on downward gaze, eyelid retraction, midposition pupils, and loss of accommodation. These patients require MRI for further delineation of the cause and confirmation of a midbrain lesion. Although most case reports describe clinically stable patients [46,48], patients who are suspected to have Parinaud syndrome should have prompt neurologic consultation and admission given the potentially life-threatening causes and location of the lesion.

Pontine lesions

The paramedian pontine reticular formation, mentioned previously, is involved in conjugate horizontal gaze. Unlike lesions of the cerebral hemisphere, the gaze deviation is away from the side of the lesion and toward the side of the hemiparesis, as in the case of unilateral ischemia to the pons, because of the level of the lesion in relation to the decussation of the motor pathways. Also in contrast to hemispheric or midbrain lesions, gaze paresis from pontine lesions is more resistant to attempts to move by doll's eye maneuver or caloric stimulation [4]. It is rare to have isolated gaze palsy from a pontine lesion, except in MS. Evaluation is similar to other gaze palsies and usually requires neurologic consultation, neuroimaging, and treatment of the underlying cause.

Summary

Neuro-ophthalmology is a complex, broad-ranging area of ophthalmology. Appropriate work-ups, correct diagnosis, treatment, and referral all depend on a thorough understanding of the neuroanatomy and neuro-ophthalmologic examination. Recognizing subtle physical findings, such as cranial nerve abnormalities or visual field cuts, may be the key to finding significant pathology in emergency department patients.

References

[1] Balcer LJ. Anatomic review and topographic diagnosis. Ophthalmol Clin North Am 2001; 14(1):1–21.
[2] Liu GT, Galetta SL. The neuro-ophthalmologic examination (including coma). Ophthalmol Clin North Am 2001;14(1):23–39.
[3] Bradford CA, et al, editors. Basic ophthalmology for medical students and primary care residents. 7th edition. American Academy of Ophthalmology. Library of Congress Cataloging-in-Publication Data; 1999.
[4] Simon RP, Aminoff MJ, Greenberg DA. Clinical neurology. 4th edition. Appleton and Lange; 1999.
[5] Kawasaki A, Kardon R. Disorders of the pupil. Ophthalmol Clin North Am 2001;14(1): 149–68.
[6] Wilhelm H. Neuro-ophthalmology of pupillary function—practical guidelines. J Neurol 1998;245:573–83.
[7] Balcer LJ. Evidence-based neuro-ophthalmology: advances in treatment. Curr Opin Ophthalmol 2001;12:387–92.
[8] Jover JA, Hernandez-Garcia C, Morado IC, et al. Combined treatment of giant-cell arteritis with methotrexate and prednisone: a randomized, double-blind, placebo-controlled trial. Ann Intern Med 2001;134:106–14.
[9] Kaiser PK, Friedman NJ. The Massachusetts eye and ear infirmary illustrated manual of ophthalmology. 2nd edition. Elsevier Sciences; 2004.
[10] Van Stavern GP, Newman NJ. Optic neuropathies: an overview. Ophthalmol Clin North Am 2001;14(1):61–72.
[11] Levin LA, Beck RW, Joseph MP, et al. The treatment of traumatic optic neuropathy: the International Optic Nerve Trauma Study. Ophthalmology 1999;106(7):1268–77.

[12] Eggenberger ER. Inflammatory optic neuropathies. Ophthalmol Clin North Am 2001;14(1): 73–82.

[13] Chen L, Gordon LK. Ocular manifestations of multiple sclerosis. Curr Opin Ophthalmol 2005;16:315–20.

[14] Optic Neuritis Study Group. The clinical profile of optic neuritis: experience of the Optic Neuritis Treatment Trial. Arch Ophthalmol 1991;109:1673–8.

[15] Optic Neuritis Study Group. Visual function more than 10 years after optic neuritis: experience of the Optic Neuritis Treatment Trial. Am J Ophthalmol 2004;137(1):77–83.

[16] Beck RW, Cleary PA, Anderson MM, et al. A randomized, controlled trial of corticosteroids in the treatment of acute optic neuritis. The Optic Neuritis Study Group. N Engl J Med 1992; 326(9):581–8.

[17] Richards BW, Jones FR, Younge BR. Causes and prognosis in 43,278 cases of paralysis of the oculomotor, trochlear, and abducens cranial nerves. Am J Ophthalmol 1992;113(5): 489–96.

[18] Sobel J. Botulism. Clin Infect Dis 2005;41:1167–73.

[19] Bennett JL, Pelak VS. Palsies of the third, fourth, and sixth cranial nerves. 2001,14(1). 169–85.

[20] Warren NM, Burn DJ. Progressive supranuclear palsy. Pract Neurol 2007;7(1):16–23.

[21] Biousse V, Newman NJ. Intracranial vascular abnormalities. 2001;14(1):243–65.

[22] Vaphiades MS. Imaging the neurovisual system. Ophthalmol Clin North Am 2004;465–80.

[23] Friedman DI. The eye and headache. Ophthalmol Clin North Am 2004;357–69.

[24] Manzouri B, Sainani A, Plant GT, et al. The aetiology and management of long-lasting sixth nerve palsy in ophthalmoplegic migraine. Cephalalgia 2007;27(3):275–8.

[25] Crevits L, Verschelde H, Casselman J. Ophthalmoplegic migraine: an unresolved problem. Cephalalgia 2006;26(10):1255–9.

[26] Keane JR. Fourth nerve palsy: historical review and study of 215 inpatients. Neurology 1993;43(12):2439–43.

[27] John R, Ebright MD, Mitchell T, et al. Septic thrombosis of the cavernous sinuses. Arch Intern Med 2001;161(22).

[28] Stam J. Thrombosis of the cerebral veins and sinuses. N Engl J Med 2005;352:1791.

[29] Lafitte F, Boukobza M, Guichard JP, et al. MRI and MRA for diagnosis and follow-up of cerebral venous thrombosis (CVT). Clin Radiol 1997;52:672–9.

[30] Ferro JM, Canhao P, Stam J, et al. Prognosis of cerebral vein and dural sinus thrombosis: results of the International Study on Cerebral Vein and Dural Sinus Thrombosis (ISCVT). Stroke 2004;35:664–70.

[31] Moster ML. Nystagmus. Ophthalmol Clin North Am 2001;14(1):205–15.

[32] Kroenke K, Lucas CA, Rosenberg ML, et al. Causes of persistent dizziness. A prospective study of 100 patients in ambulatory care. Ann Intern Med 1992;117(83)):163–77.

[33] Labuguen RH. Initial evaluation of vertigo. Am Fam Physician 2006;(2):244–54.

[34] Woodworth BA, Gillespie MB, Lambert PR. The canalith repositioning procedure for benign positional vertigo: A meta-analysis. Laryngoscope 2004;114:1143–6.

[35] Koeliker P, Summers RL, Hawkins B. Benign paroxysmal positional vertigo: diagnosis and treatment in the emergency department—A review of the literature and discussion of canalith-repositioning maneuvers. Ann Emerg Med 2001;(4):392–8.

[36] Hadjikoutis S, Morgan JE, Wild JM, et al. Ocular complications of neurologic therapy. Eur J Neurol 2005;12:499–507.

[37] Ropper AH, Brown RH. Adams and Victor's principles of neurology. 8th edition. McGraw-Hill; 2005.

[38] Abadi RV. Mechanisms underlying nystagmus. J R Soc Med 2002;95:231–4.

[39] Jacobs DA, Galetta SL. Multiple sclerosis and the visual system. Ophthalmol Clin North Am 2004;17:265–73.

[40] Pelak VS, Hall DA. Neuro-ophthalmic manifestations of neurodegenerative disease. Ophthalmol Clin North Am 2004;17:311–20.

[41] Barton JJS, Fouladvand M. Ocular aspects of myasthenia gravis. Semin Neurol 2000;20(1): 7–20.
[42] Elrod RD, Weinberg DA. Ocular myasthenia gravis. Ophthalmol Clin North Am 2004;17: 275–309.
[43] Drachman DB. Myasthenia gravis. N Engl J Med 1994;330(25):1797–810.
[44] Cherington M. Botulism: update and review. Semin Neurol 2004;24(2):155–63.
[45] Singer OC, Humpich MC, Laufs H, et al. Conjugate eye deviation in acute stroke: incidence, hemispheric asymmetry, and lesion pattern. Stroke 2006;37(11):2726–32.
[46] Simon JE, Morgan SC, Pexman JH, et al. CT assessment of conjugate eye deviation in acute stroke. Neurology 2003;60:135–7.
[47] Bhola R, Olson RJ. Dorsal midbrain syndrome with bilateral superior oblique palsy following brainstem hemorrhage. Arch Ophthalmol 2006;124(12):1786–8.
[48] Baloh RW, Furman JM, Yee RD. Dorsal midbrain syndrome: clinical and oculographic findings. Neurology 1985;35:54–60.

ELSEVIER
SAUNDERS

Emerg Med Clin N Am
26 (2008) 181–198

EMERGENCY
MEDICINE
CLINICS OF
NORTH AMERICA

Pediatric Ophthalmology in the Emergency Department

Kimball A. Prentiss, MD, David H. Dorfman, MD*

*Boston University School of Medicine, Boston Medical Center,
1 Boston Medical Center Place, Boston, MA 02118, USA*

Examining the young child with a visual or ocular complaint can be a daunting challenge. Understanding the basic concepts of visual and behavioral development will facilitate the examination of the child who presents to the emergency department with eye complaints. Ocular complaints may include pain and visual impairment which may lead to anxiety and interfere with the examination of the child. Keeping the child calm and taking the time to engage the child in a manner he or she is comfortable with will allow a more accurate examination.

Visual development

Vision development is a complex system that requires the development of neuro-ocular pathways and depends on proper visual stimulation of both eyes. The first 3 to 4 months of life are most critical for this development. If significant disruption of a child's vision occurs during this period and is not quickly corrected, lifelong visual deficit is the likely result despite later treatment. The rate of vision development remains steep until about 2 years of life, at which time three-dimensional binocular depth perception develops. It is not until 9 years of age that the brain's development of vision is complete.

Full-term newborns do not generally respond well to visual targets. Visual acuity at birth is approximately 20/400. In newborns, the presence of vision may be demonstrated by pupil responses or by aversive behavior to bright lights. Eye position at birth varies greatly. Outward deviation may be normal eye alignment in the newborn period. After birth, the eyes tend

---

* Corresponding author.
E-mail address: david.dorfman@bmc.org (D.H. Dorfman).

0733-8627/08/$ - see front matter © 2008 Elsevier Inc. All rights reserved.
doi:10.1016/j.emc.2007.11.001 *emed.theclinics.com*

to move to a more convergent position and should be well aligned and stable by 4 months of age [1]. The pupils of newborns are often constricted.

Although fixation is generally present at birth in the full-term newborn, the ability to follow targets is not developed until about 3 months of age. Accommodation, the ability to focus, develops by 4 months [2,3]. Vision improves dramatically during infancy. By 1 year of age, children's vision is 20/50 and by 2 years of age 20/20.

The eye examination in a child

Assessing vision in a child can be difficult but should be evaluated in every child with an eye complaint. To accomplish this it is necessary to adjust the examination to the age and cognitive ability of the child. There are many aspects of the eye examination, but in the emergency department, the practitioner may focus on the skin and the surrounding tissues, light responses, fixation responses, and visual acuity. The discussion herein focuses on those parts of the eye examination which differ in children and adults and describes the examination appropriate for children of different ages [4].

Testing of visual acuity varies markedly depending on the age, verbal skills, and cooperation of the child. Eye alignment is an important part of the evaluation in children. In infants, misalignment or strabismus can lead to severe visual deficits. Misalignment may also be associated with a range of acute processes including orbital cellulitis.

Examination of the newborn and young infant

The first part of any eye examination is to observe the child. In children of all ages, it is best to leave the most invasive part of the examination that will cause the most distress to the child until the end. One should evaluate the lids and the periorbital area for swelling, redness, drainage. One should observe how the child moves their eyes and note the color of the conjunctiva and sclera. The macula in young infants is not fully developed; therefore, the eyes do not fixate well centrally and do not follow objects until about 3 to 4 months of age. To examine infants in this age group some recommend having the parent hold the child in the feeding position and then move the child's head from side to side. The baby should follow this movement with his or her eyes or head and should also blink when a light is shone into their eyes. Another method of evaluating an infant for fixing is to cradle him or her in one arm upright and facing the examiner while gently rocking the infant side to side. If an infant has the eyes closed, he or she will generally open them when rocked in this manner, allowing for examination.

Of note, young infants may have intermittent downward deviation of the eyes. This finding usually lasts only a few weeks. If this sunsetting is constant or associated with poor feeding, lethargy, a large head size or bulging fontanelle, or occurs in a child in whom it had not been present, it may be caused by increased intracranial pressure. Downward eye deviation that persists pasts a few weeks may be a sign of neurologic conditions, and the child should be evaluated by neurology and ophthalmology.

The retina is indirectly evaluated by examining the red reflex. Fundoscopic examination of a young child who is awake and has not had his or her pupils dilated can be extremely difficult. The red reflex allows the examiner to assess light that enters the child's eye and is reflected off the retina. The examiner should dim the lights in the room and calm the baby by giving the child a pacifier or bottle or by gentle side-to-side rocking. With the child's eyes open, the direct ophthalmoscope can be used to look at the red reflex. The key to evaluating the red reflex is symmetry and uniformity in the child's eyes. In light skinned infants, the red reflex appears orange-red. In dark skinned infants, the reflex looks dull orange or whitish orange. This finding should not be confused with leukokoria (Fig. 1), which is a whitish appearance of the pupil that, if present, is not generally found in both eyes. Leukokoria indicates a problem with reflection of light from the retina and may be caused by an array of pathologic entities including cataracts and tumor.

Older infants and preverbal children

One should start with the least invasive, least painful parts of the examination in older infants and preverbal children. Some young children are afraid of physicians because stranger anxiety is most pronounced around 10 months of age. One should begin the examination by observing the child from a distance to determine whether there is any swelling or redness to the eyes and surrounding tissues and how the child uses and moves their eyes. Children in this age group usually fix on and follow a toy or other object of interest. With some children, it may be necessary to seat the child in the guardian's lap and have him or her hold the child's head still while the examiner moves the object from side to side and up and down.

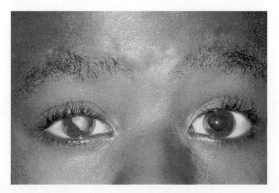

Fig. 1. Right eye leukokoria from a traumatic cataract. (*From* Levine LM. Pediatric ocular trauma and shaken baby. Pediatr Clin North Am 2003;50:145; with permission).

In preverbal children visual acuity can be difficult to assess. A child who consistently protests to having one eye covered as opposed to the other likely has better visual acuity in the favored eye. To check for such a preference, the examiner should cover one eye of the child and observe whether the child fixes and follows with the uncovered eye. If the child objects to having the eyes covered by the physician, sometimes enlisting the aid of a guardian to hold a hand in front of the child's eye can be helpful. Again, the child who consistently favors viewing with a particular eye likely has better vision on that side, and more detailed testing is indicated.

A similar technique can be used to evaluate for eye movement and strabismus (Fig. 2). Using a thumb to cover one eye of the child (a patch or parent's hand can be used as well), the examiner holds a toy or penlight and checks that the child fixes on the object with the uncovered eye and follows the object as it is moved. The examiner then moves the thumb to the other eye to check for strabismus. If the child has been focused on the light or object, in the absence of strabismus, the newly uncovered eye should not move. Strabismus should also be suspected if the light reflex does not fall on the center of both pupils. If one is concerned about the presence of esotropia (eye turning in), a light or lighted toy can be held in front of the child and then brought closer. In some cases esotropia is only revealed with focusing on near objects.

A third test is needed to check for intermittent exotropia (eye turning out). Intermittent exotropia often occurs only with viewing objects from a distance. This condition is brought out by presenting the child with a toy or object at a distance and looking at the corneal light reflex. This reflex can be difficult to assess; if a history of an intermittent out turning of an eye is obtained, the child should be referred to a pediatric ophthalmologist.

In practice, certain parts of the examination may be reasonably omitted in the emergency department setting, because a young child who has eye

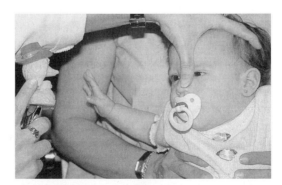

Fig. 2. Fixation examination in children 4 months and older. Use of a toy will often help with the examination. Use the thumb to cover each eye in turn to check for fixation. Move the thumb from one eye to the other to check for strabismus (cover testing). (*From* Drack AV. Pediatric ophthalmology. In: Palay DA, Krachmer JH, editors. Primary care ophthalmology. 2nd edition. Philadelphia: Mosby; 2005. p. 234; with permission).

pain or discomfort may not be cooperative with some or all of the examination. As long as the child is opening both eyes for any length of time, fixation and corneal light reflex can be assessed.

If the child has pain and the history suggests a corneal abrasion or foreign body (and not a ruptured globe), instilling a topical anesthetic may decrease eye pain and allow for an easier examination. The intervention may also be diagnostic as the relief of symptoms isolates the pathology to disruption of the conjunctiva or corneal surface.

In children with a large amount of swelling around the eye, it may be necessary to retract the eyelids to perform the examination. If the history suggests significant trauma and globe rupture is a possibility, it is important to avoid putting pressure directly on the eye by placing the examiner's thumbs on the infraorbital and supraorbital rims and separating the lids. In some instances, lid retractors may be needed to examine the eye. If only one retractor is being used, it is most helpful to apply it to the upper lid. Cotton swabs can also be used to open the eyes. In this method, one swab is placed on the upper eyelid and one on the lower. The swabs are then rotated toward the eyeball, the upper swab rotated down, and the lower swab rotated up. Simultaneous with rotation, the swabs are moved toward the orbital margins [5]. This method should not be used if trauma is suspected because it places pressure on the eyeball.

Verbal children

The examination becomes much easier in children who can talk and allow for objective testing of visual acuity. In young children who do not yet know numbers or letters, the Allen card or other calibrated picture tests may be used (Fig. 3). Before testing, one should have the child identify the objects up close. The Tumbling E chart is also commonly used. With this test, one should make the instructions clear to the child. Some recommend telling the child that the E is a table, sometimes right side up, sometimes on its side, and sometimes upside down [4]. The examiner should have the child point the direction legs of the table are pointing. As in adults, each eye should be tested individually; however, in children, special attention should be paid to whether they are using the covered eye to see. Children tend to look around the hand-held eye covers, and it may be necessary to patch the child. Vision should be 20/50 or better at a distance in children aged less than 5 years but 20/30 or better at near distance in all ages. In the absence of nystagmus, there should be no significant improvement in acuity viewing with both eyes open. One should remember children have short attention spans. There is no need to start on the line with the largest figures or to have the child read every figure in a given line.

With patience, an understanding of children's development, and a few techniques, it is possible to perform an eye examination on children in the emergency department. The following sections discuss an array of disease

A   B

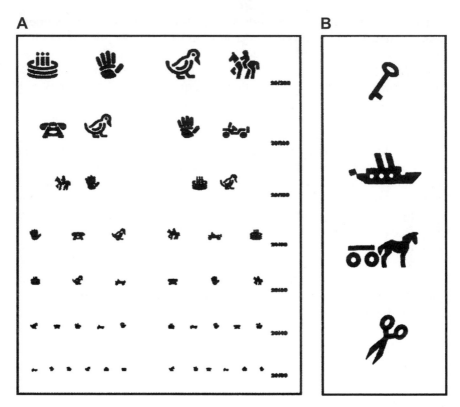

Fig. 3. Allen chart (*A*) and Osterberg chart (*B*) used to assess vision in verbal children who do not know the alphabet. (*From* Kniestedt C, Stamper RL. Assessing visual function in clinical practice. Ophthalmol Clin North Am 2003;16:166; with permission).

processes that are particular to, or more common in, the pediatric age group.

Conjunctivitis

Ophthalmia neonatorum (neonatal conjunctivitis)

Ophthalmia neonatorum is defined as conjunctivitis within the first month of life. There are three main types of neonatal conjunctivitis: chemical, bacterial, and viral. Although these entities may present with similar symptoms, the timing of the development of symptoms can often be a useful diagnostic clue. Chemical conjunctivitis secondary to perinatal ocular prophylaxis generally presents within the first 24 to 48 hours of life [6]. Erythromycin ointment is the agent most commonly used today and only rarely causes chemical conjunctivitis. Silver nitrate was used in the past and has been more frequently associated with chemical conjunctivitis. Infants with chemical conjunctivitis typically present with bilaterally inflamed lids and watery discharge. Gram stain reveals white cells without bacteria. Treatment initially is supportive and involves the discontinuation of any ophthalmic medications and observation, with an expected resolution of symptoms within 48 hours. If no improvement is seen, a culture should be obtained and topical antibiotic therapy initiated, with care to avoid whatever agent was used for initial prophylactic therapy.

The epidemiology of neonatal infections is related to the transmission of organisms at the time of delivery; therefore, pathogens found in the genital tract and enteric system should be suspected. *Chlamydia trachomatis* is more commonly acquired from the birth canal than are *Neisseria gonorrhoeae* and herpes viruses (herpes simplex virus [HSV]) [7]. In addition, gram-negative enteric organisms and several staphylococcus and streptococcus species may also be acquired peri- and postnatally. Gonorrheal infections typically occur 2 to 5 days after birth but can be delayed if neonatal prophylactic therapy provides partial suppression. Chlamydial infections present slightly later, often between 5 and 14 days of life [6].

Physical examination findings can be helpful with diagnosis, but there is tremendous overlap of symptoms from different pathogens. Accurate diagnosis on the basis of physical examination alone is challenging and often requires supplementary laboratory data. Gonorrheal infections are classically characterized by a hyperacute mucopurulent discharge with lid edema, bulbar conjunctivitis, and chemosis. Chlamydial infections can also present with copious discharge but more commonly are characterized by palpebral conjunctival injection and inflammation with less associated lid edema and thick discharge [6,8]. A statim Gram stain and culture, including chocolate agar, should be obtained to aid in the diagnosis but should not delay the initiation of therapy when a high clinical suspicion for disease is present. In addition to Gram stain and culture, Giemsa stain, direct fluorescent antibody, ELISA, and polymerase chain reaction can be used to diagnose chlamydial infections, and laboratory investigation should be guided based on method availability [9]. Intracellular gram-negative diplococci are consistent with gonorrheal infection and constitute an ocular emergency because this organism can penetrate through and ulcerate the cornea, rapidly causing blindness [8]. An ophthalmology consult should be obtained immediately without delay in therapy. Current recommendations for treatment are a single dose of intravenous or intramuscular ceftriaxone with admission and hourly saline eye lavage. The infant should simultaneously be covered for chlamydial disease until cultures are negative using oral erythromycin therapy to treat ophthalmic disease and prevent the late onset of chlamydial pneumonitis [7,8].

Staphylococcus aureus, Streptococcus epidermis, Haemophilus influenzae, Escherichia coli, and *Pseudomonas* are other causes of neonatal conjunctivitis and typically present from 5 to 7 days of life. Clinical findings are often indistinguishable from that of other pathogens. Diagnosis is by Gram stain and culture, and polymyxin/bacitracin/neomycin topical ointment is generally accepted as standard treatment. Diagnosis of typeable *Haemophilus influenzae* conjunctivitis is an exception and should be treated with systemic antibiotics, with consideration given to a full septic evaluation before parenteral antibiotic administration.

Neonatal conjunctivitis caused by HSV, typically, although not exclusively, HSV-2, may also be acquired through the birth canal, and ocular manifestations may be the only presenting symptoms of neonatal herpetic infections [6]. Clinical suspicion should be elevated with a maternal history of infection, vesicular blepharitis, or the presence of ocular dendritic ulcers with fluorescein staining. Diagnosis is made by immunofluorescence, smear, or culture. Treatment involves both topical and systemic parenteral acyclovir and the avoidance of steroids. Full septic evaluation should be performed in the neonate with HSV infection [10].

Childhood conjunctivitis

Acute conjunctivitis is the most common eye disorder in young children and is the most frequent ophthalmologic complaint seen in the pediatric emergency department [11]. To date, there are no evidence-based guidelines for the diagnosis and empirical treatment of conjunctivitis [12]. Bacterial infections are predominant and are chiefly caused by one of three pathogens— non-typeable *Haemophilus influenzae, Streptococcus pneumoniae,* and *Staphylococcus aureus* [7,11]. The clinical course of bacterial conjunctivitis generally has an abrupt uniocular onset, with spread to the opposite eye within 48 hours [13]. Tearing and irritation are the initial symptoms, followed by mucopurulent discharge, typically with a history of crusting or gluing of the eyelashes. Diffuse erythema of the bulbar and palpebral conjunctivae is generally present, whereas preauricular lymphadenopathy is not [14].

Laboratory studies to determine the causative organism are usually reserved for severe cases and those unresponsive to initial treatment. Empiric treatment is commonplace, particularly when a history of sticky eyelids is obtained in conjunction with a physical finding of purulent discharge [12]. Treatment typically involves erythromycin ointment, bacitracin-polymyxin B ointment, or topical fluoroquinolones [7]. Several clinical associations can also help guide diagnosis and subsequent treatment. Conjunctivitis-otitis syndrome is common, occurring about 25% of the time, and is most often associated with non-typeable *Haemophilus influenzae* infections [11,15]. In this scenario, monotherapy with systemic antibiotics is indicated, and a topical agent is not needed [16,17]. Several studies suggest that if *Haemophilus influenzae* is recovered from a culture, or if the patient has a history of recurrent otitis media, systemic treatment should be initiated even in the absence of acute otitis media in the hope of preventing its development [17].

Another common cause of pediatric conjunctivitis is viral illness. The overall frequency of pediatric viral illness is extremely high, but the presence of conjunctivitis in systemic pediatric viral disease varies. The most common type of viral conjunctivitis in children is adenoviral conjunctivitis, which can present as an isolated condition or as part of a viral syndrome [7]. Adenovirus can cause a nonspecific acute conjunctivitis characterized by red profusely watery eyes, or more severely, epidemic keratoconjunctivitis if corneal involvement is present. Pharyngoconjunctival fever caused by adenovirus is common in children and presents with the triad of pharyngitis, fever, and conjunctivitis, as the name implies. The typical course lasts 2 weeks and often begins with unilateral involvement, becoming bilateral within several days, with preauricular lymphadenopathy [18]. Although the typical course of pharyngoconjunctival fever is self-limited with an excellent prognosis, the same adenovirus types can also cause the rarer but more serious disseminated adenoviral disease which results in multisystem organ failure and death [18,19]. Upper respiratory tract infections caused by rhinovirus, enterovirus, and influenza virus are accompanied by a self-limited conjunctivitis less than 50% of the time, and less than one third of respiratory syncytial virus infections are accompanied by conjunctivitis. Conjunctivitis is also commonly associated with measles, although this pathogen is now rare in the United States [19].

The diagnosis of adenoviral conjunctivitis remains primarily clinical. Conjunctival hemorrhage can occur with adenoviral infection, as can punctate corneal epithelial defects; therefore, the slit lamp examination is an important part of the diagnostic evaluation, although it is often difficult to perform on a young patient. An ideal laboratory study does not yet exist. Viral cultures are epidemiologically useful, but delayed results have little use in the emergency department setting. Enzyme immunoassay and polymerase chain reaction tests are rapid, but the sensitivity varies considerably. Treatment options are also limited and are largely supportive because there is no proven effective treatment for adenoviral conjunctivitis [20,21]; however, topical antibiotics are often prescribed to prevent bacterial superinfection. Corticosteroids should be avoided in treating most cases of pediatric adenoviral conjunctivitis and should only be administered under the care of an ophthalmologist. In fact, the prescription of ophthalmic steroids in general in the emergency department should be limited, because steroids can be devastating in the presence of herpetic infections, which must always be considered and effectively ruled out.

Herpetic ocular infections outside of the neonatal period are typically from HSV-1 [6]. Herpetic keratitis with its classic dendritic pattern with fluorescein staining may be present, is most often unilateral, and is sometimes associated with vesicles in the distribution of the ophthalmic branch of the trigeminal nerve, involving the forehead, periorbital area, and tip of the nose [22]. More commonly, the clinical presentation of HSV conjunctivitis is nonspecific, although always painful, and very similar to other etiologies of conjunctivitis previously discussed. Treatment of HSV ocular infection, most often with a topical antiviral agent, should involve an ophthalmologist.

Orbital and periorbital cellulitis

Orbital and ocular adnexal infections are more common in children than adults and must be accurately distinguished from periorbital infections, because the pathogenesis, treatment, and potential severity of sequelae vary considerably. Knowledge of the region's anatomy helps one to clinically distinguish orbital from periorbital infections and aids in understanding the pathophysiology and the potential for spread of infection of each of these two entities. Orbital infections are defined by their location relative to the orbital septum, which is a thin membrane that extends from the periosteum and reflects into the upper and lower eyelids [23]. The septum separates the periorbital soft tissues (preseptal region) from the orbital space (septal) and provides a barrier to the spread of infection between the two regions. Preseptal processes do not directly progress into the septal space, nor do septal infections directly spread into the preseptal space [23,24]; however, infection can also travel through the valveless venous drainage system of the midfacial region involving the eye cavity and the ethmoid and maxillary sinuses, thereby allowing for the indirect spread of infection in an anterograde and retrograde fashion [25].

Another important anatomic consideration is the relationship between the sinus cavities and the orbit. The eye is surrounded by paranasal sinuses on three of its four walls. The floor of the frontal sinus is the roof of the orbit, and the roof of the maxillary sinus is the floor of the orbit. The medial border of the eye is formed primarily from the extremely thin lamina papyracea of the ethmoid bone. Infection can spread from the paranasal sinuses to the bone, forming osteitis or subperiosteal abscesses, and into the orbital space, producing an orbital abscess or orbital cellulitis (Fig. 4) [24,26]. These anatomic considerations help to explain the typical pathogens found in orbital cellulitis. The periorbital area is protected from the paranasal sinuses by the orbital septum; therefore, it is far less susceptible to infection by sinus pathogens. Infections in the periorbital area are usually secondary to skin pathogens and are often associated with soft tissue injuries such as insect

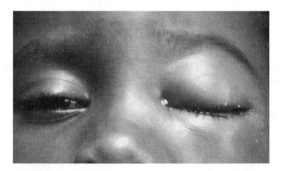

Fig. 4. Orbital cellulitis. (*From* Greenberg MF, Pollard ZF. The red eye in childhood. Pediatr Clin North Am 2003;50:106; with permission).

bites or the spread of local infection (impetigo, hordeolum, chalazion, dacryocystitis) [27].

Periorbital cellulitis is much more common than orbital cellulitis [25]. It presents clinically with erythema, induration, tenderness, or warmth of the periorbital tissues. Signs of systemic illness are often absent, although fever may be present, particularly if bacteremia served as the origin of the cellulitis. Extraocular motion is not affected and should be full. In fact, decreased movement of the eye is one of the cardinal features of orbital cellulitis, along with proptosis, decreased visual acuity, chemosis, and papilledema [8,23]. Orbital cellulitis is also associated with erythema, pain, and swollen eyelids, but the eyelid swelling of orbital cellulitis can be differentiated from that of periorbital cellulitis in that it will not extend beyond the superior orbital rim onto the brow [27]. This limitation of upper eyelid swelling is due to the extension of the orbital septum onto the periosteum of the inferior margin of the superior orbital rim, which effectively provides a structural barrier limiting the degree of upper eyelid swelling in orbital cellulitis.

Distinguishing between these two clinical entities is paramount. If one is unable to do so clinically, a CT scan should be obtained, as should ophthalmology consultation [25]. If CT scanning demonstrates sinus disease as a likely etiology of orbital cellulitis, otorhinolaryngology should also be consulted because surgical drainage may be necessary. Any child with orbital cellulitis must be admitted for parenteral antibiotics and close observation among a multidisciplinary team, with or without surgical intervention. The antibiotic choice should be aimed at the most likely pathogens, typically, respiratory pathogens and anaerobes originating from the paranasal sinuses. Ampicillin/sulbactam or cefuroxime with clindamycin or metronidazole are reasonable choices because they appropriately target the most common organisms, such as *Streptococcus pneumoniae,* non-typeable *Haemophilus influenzae*, group A streptococcus, *Staphylococcus aureus*, and anaerobic organisms [23].

For children with periorbital cellulitis, skin trauma is the most likely etiology. Antibiotics targeted at gram-positive organisms should be administered, because staphylococcus and streptococcus species are the most likely cause of post-traumatic periorbital cellulitis [23]. These patients should be followed up closely for any progression of symptoms. Primary bacteremia is another etiology of periorbital cellulitis but is rare due to effective vaccination against *Streptococcus pneumoniae* and *Haemophilus influenzae* [27]. If bacteremia is suspected as a source for infection, particularly in a child aged less than 3 months or in an unvaccinated or newly immigrated patient, *Streptococcus pneumoniae* and *Haemophilus influenzae* should be suspected. Any child aged less than 2 years or who has signs of systemic illness should be admitted for parenteral antibiotics and close observation. A full septic evaluation, including lumbar puncture, should be strongly considered before antibiotic administration in any toxic appearing child, or in the presence of any signs or symptoms suggestive of meningitis.

Another special consideration involves immunocompromised children, including children with diabetes. These children should immediately be referred to an ophthalmologist for evaluation because mucormycosis presents with eyelid erythema and is a diagnosis that generally requires surgical debridement [25].

Lacrimal system infections

Infections of the lacrimal system are named according to the location of infection. Infection of the nasal lacrimal duct, located between the medial canthus of the eye and the nasal bridge, is known as dacryocystitis and can occur in the setting of acute or chronic obstruction of the duct (Fig. 5). Often, a history of watery or even mucopurulent discharge from the eyes can be elicited, followed by the development of erythema, swelling, and tenderness over the lacrimal sac. The major complication of dacryocystitis is periorbital cellulitis [26] and, less commonly, orbital cellulitis [27] or cavernous sinus thrombosis [23]; meningitis, brain abscesses, and sepsis can also occur, although rarely. Diagnosis must be prompt, and treatment should include oral antibiotics. The most common pathogens in children with acute dacryocystitis are *Staphylococcus epidermidis* and *Staphylococcus aureus* [23]. Any child with dacryocystitis who appears ill or toxic should be admitted for parenteral antibiotic therapy [27].

Another infection of the lacrimal system is dacryoadenitis. This infection of the lacrimal gland is located in the supratemporal orbit. The gland is composed of two lobes. The palpebral lobe is easily visualized with eversion of the superior lid, but the orbital lobe cannot be directly visualized on physical examination. Dacryoadenitis may present as an acute or chronic problem. Acute disease is characterized by the abrupt onset of pain,

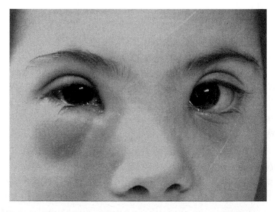

Fig. 5. Acute dacryocystitis. Maximal swelling nasally below the medial canthal ligament. (*From* Greenberg MF, Pollard ZF. The red eye in childhood. Pediatr Clin North Am 2003;50:108; with permission).

swelling, and erythema of the supraorbital region, often associated with chemosis, conjunctivitis, and mucopurulent discharge, and sometimes associated with limited ocular mobility, proptosis, fever, and malaise. More chronic infections typically present with swelling of the superior lid. Mild ptosis may be present secondary to the swelling, but pain, erythema, and fever are not present.

The treatment of dacryoadenitis is dependent on the acuity of the presentation and the most likely etiology. Imaging is often not necessary, although CT scanning can help to make the distinction between orbital cellulitis and dacryoadenitis if the orbital lobe of the gland is involved and clinical distinction is difficult. Acute dacryoadenitis is most commonly associated with viral infections, and treatment is supportive. Bacterial pathogens should be suspected if the discharge is mucopurulent. Cultures should be obtained while initiating treatment to cover the most common pathogens until culture data become available. A first-generation cephalosporin is generally recommended; however, an increasing prevalence of ocular methicillin-resistant *Staphylococcus aureus* (MRSA) has recently been reported. Choosing an oral antimicrobial agent to best fit the MRSA susceptibility profile within your institution is prudent [28,29].

Congenital

Nasal lacrimal duct obstruction

The most common congenital ophthalmologic finding in newborns is nasal lacrimal duct obstruction. Tears are produced in the lacrimal gland which rests within the temporal portion of the superior lid. They then circulate over the eye toward the punctum located in the nasal corner of the eye where the two lid margins unite. Typically, tears drain through the punctum and canalicular system into the nasolacrimal sac and then into the duct which drains intranasally through the valve of Hasner. When the drainage path is obstructed, most commonly at the level of the valve of Hasner, patients present with watery discharge from the eye, often bilaterally [21]. On further inspection, the tear lake in the inferior portion of the lid is often elevated. If bacterial superinfection exists, a chronic mucopurulent discharge is present, with parents commonly reporting lid adherence. If this adherence persists, symptoms may progress to include conjunctival injection with thickening of the periorbital skin. The examination of any newborn with these complaints should involve carefully applied pressure with a cotton tip to the region of the nasolacrimal sac. If nasal lacrimal duct obstruction is present, reflux of mucopurulent material from the punctum may occur. Careful examination of the skin that overlies the drainage system is also important, because identification of a bluish hued palpable mass is indicative of a mucocele, specifically, a cyst of the nasal lacrimal duct also known as a dacryocele [21]. Simple nasal lacrimal duct obstruction should not be associated with any photophobia, ocular cloudiness, or abnormal appearance of the red reflex. If any of these findings are present, the diagnosis of nasal lacrimal duct obstruction should be questioned, and congenital glaucoma or cataracts should be considered.

Treatment of nasal lacrimal duct obstruction in the newborn is simply supportive if no superinfection or dacryocele is suspected. Parents should be instructed to apply gentle massage over the nasal lacrimal duct with rapid downward motions three to four times daily to facilitate opening of the valve of Hasner. After the age of 6 months, the patient should be referred to an ophthalmologist, because obstructions rarely resolve on their own beyond the first several months of life and often require surgical probing [21]. If suspicion of a dacryocele exists, the patient should rapidly be referred to a pediatric ophthalmologist and otolaryngologist because obstructive intranasal cysts are often associated and require rapid intervention. The presence of mucopurulent discharge warrants the administration of topical antibiotics for 1 to 2 weeks in conjunction with daily massage as described previously. If this regimen does not clear the discharge, the patient should be referred to an ophthalmologist for further evaluation, independent of age. Continued infection in the lacrimal sac is associated with preseptal cellulitis, a more serious condition that often requires hospitalization in this age group.

Congenital cataracts

A cataract is an opacity of the lens of the eye requiring prompt diagnosis and treatment to prevent partial or complete blindness. Congenital cataracts can be present at birth and associated with certain congenital infections such as rubella, toxoplasmosis, HSV, or cytomegalovirus [30]. They can also develop in the first several months of life secondary to several metabolic conditions, such as galactosemia or peroxisomal disorders, or in genetic conditions such as trisomy 21 or Turner syndrome [21].

The clinical presentation of infants with cataracts is dependent on the density of the opacification and the presence in one or both eyes. Leukokoria is caused when the cataract is dense enough to prevent a significant amount of light from penetrating through the cornea to the retina (see Fig. 1). The red reflex is abnormal and may even be absent if the cataract is severe. Nystagmus or strabismus may also be noted if the cataract develops within the first several months of life. Vision may be mildly to severely decreased. In severe cases in which vision is absent, the infant may not even spontaneously open his or her eyes. In moderate cases, the infant may be noted to squint in bright sunlight in an effort to reduce the glare resulting from the reduced ability of the pupil to constrict [21].

Treatment of congenital cataracts should be initiated emergently through a pediatric ophthalmologist, because the first several months of life are critical to the development of the visual axis.

Congenital glaucoma

Pediatric glaucoma is divided into primary and secondary types depending on the presence of isolated angle malformations (primary) versus other underlying ocular abnormalities (secondary) [30]. Both types may be present at birth (congenital) or develop at any age (infantile or juvenile). The common finding with any form of glaucoma is increased intraocular pressure, which, if left undiagnosed and untreated, can lead to optic nerve damage and vision loss. Additional damage, such as large refractive errors, astigmatisms, strabismus, and amblyopia, may occur as a result of congenital or infantile glaucoma, because the visual system is undergoing crucial stages of development during infancy, and any disruption to the visual axis may have multiple sequelae [30].

Forty percent of cases are present at birth and 85% by age 1 year; however, the age of diagnosis varies from birth to late childhood. The most common finding in patients who have congenital glaucoma is excessive tearing, also known as epiphora, as well as photophobia and some degree of blepharospasm [30]. Corneal enlargement or asymmetry (when disease is unilateral) is often present, and a corneal diameter of greater than 12 mm in an infant younger than 1 year of age should prompt urgent referral to a pediatric ophthalmologist [30]. Other findings include corneal clouding, conjunctival injection, corneal edema, ocular enlargement, and ocular nerve cupping observed on fundoscopic examination [21].

Treatment of glaucoma in infants and children is almost always primarily surgical, complemented by medical therapy with topical or oral pressure-lowering agents. Prognosis is generally better the later the onset of symptoms, because the structural anomaly is typically less severe [30].

Misalignment

Ocular misalignment, generally referred to as strabismus, is not uncommon in newborns and young children and may be of enough concern to the parents to prompt an emergency room visit. It is important to distinguish normal misalignment from more worrisome clinical presentations. Newborns commonly have an ocular instability that is characterized by variable, intermittent ocular misalignment throughout their first several months of life. This misalignment is most commonly secondary to immaturity of the extraocular muscles and self-resolves by 3 to 4 months of life [21]. If the deviation is constant, or if it is bilateral, the patient should be referred to a pediatric ophthalmologist for further investigation, because these patterns may be more consistent with significant pathology such as primary neurologic or oncologic processes.

Patients with congenital strabismus typically have normal eye movements for the first several months of life and then develop the tendency for one or both eyes to deviate [21]. If this deviation is present without interruption of the visual axis, it is referred to as a "manifest strabismus." More specifically, it is termed *esotropia* if there is inward deviation of the eye or *exotropia* if the deviation is outward. The examination techniques for the evaluation of strabismus described earlier in this article, specifically the "cover uncover test," may elicit a latent strabismus also known as a "phoria" that is only present when fixation is interrupted by covering one eye [31]. Children who have either manifest or latent strabismus should be evaluated by an ophthalmologist because these conditions can lead to amblyopia, although much less commonly with phorias than tropias [31].

The emergency room physician should always rule out a sixth nerve palsy that could mimic congenital esotropia, particularly if accompanied by other signs of increased intracranial pressure such as nausea, vomiting, lethargy, and sunsetting of the eyes [8]. Similarly, third nerve palsies should be considered when evaluating a child with an exotropia [3,16]. In general, emergent presentations of cranial nerve palsies or mechanical restriction due to orbital fractures, cellulitis, masses, or other intracranial processes can effectively be ruled out by full extraocular muscle movements [8].

Oncology

Retinoblastoma is the most common primary intraocular malignancy of childhood and frequently presents with leukokoria, often detected by a parent who may seek medical evaluation in the emergency department. The white pupil is actually the tumor itself visualized through the pupil and vitreous [21]. The tumor may be unilateral, typically associated with a spontaneous mutation, or bilateral, almost always heritable. These children may also present with a unilateral fixed and dilated pupil, visual changes, a red and painful eye, proptosis, or different colored irises, also known as heterochromia iridis [21]. Any child with a white pupil or any other findings suspicious for retinoblastoma should be immediately referred to an ophthalmologist for a complete ocular examination, typically performed under anesthesia.

Other tumors that may present as orbital masses with proptosis include rhabdomyosarcoma, Langerhan's cell histiocytosis, acute myeloid leukemia, metastatic Ewing's sarcoma, Burkitt's lymphoma, or neuroblastoma [26]. Neuroblastoma can also present with the rare ocular finding of opsoclonus/myoclonus. This condition is often referred to as "dancing eyes," describing the simultaneous presence of rapid irregular eye movements and involuntary twitching of the eyelids, and is believed to be secondary to an autoimmune reaction. When present, opsoclonus/myoclonus should prompt an immediate evaluation for neuroblastoma, because this is the most commonly associated pediatric tumor.

References

[1] Weinacht S, Kind C, Mounting JS, et al. Visual development in preterm and full-term infants: a prospective masked study. Invest Ophthalmol Vis Sci 1999;40(2):346–53.

[2] Curry DC, Manny RE. The development of accommodation. Vision Res 1997;37(11): 1525–33.
[3] Hainline L, Riddell P, Grose-Fifer J, et al. Development of accommodation and convergence in infancy. Behav Brain Res 1992;49(1):33–50.
[4] Levin AV. Eye emergencies: acute management in the pediatric ambulatory setting. Pediatr Emerg Care 1991;7(6):367–77.
[5] Drack AV. Pediatric ophthalmology. In: Palay DA, Krachmer JH, editors. Primary care ophthalmology. 2nd edition. Philadelphia: Elsevier Mosby; 2005. p. 229–73.
[6] Erogul M, Shah B. Ophthalmology. In: Shah B, editor. Atlas of pediatric emergency medicine. New York: McGraw-Hill; 2006. p. 361–84.
[7] Morrow G, Abbott R. Conjunctivitis. Am Fam Physician 1998;57(4):735–48.
[8] Levin A. Ophthalmic emergencies. In: Fleisher G, Ludwig S, Henretig F, editors. Textbook of pediatric emergency medicine. Philadelphia: Lippincott Williams and Wilkins; 2006. p. 1653–62.
[9] American Academy of Pediatrics. *Chlamydia trachomatis*. In: Pickering LK, Baker CJ, Long SS, ct al, cditors. Rcd book: 2006 rcport of the committee on infectious diseases. 27th edition. Elk Grove Village (IL): American Academy of Pediatrics; 2006. p. 254–5.
[10] American Academy of Pediatrics. Herpes simplex. In: Pickering LK, Baker CJ, Long SS, et al, editors. Red book: 2006 report of the committee on infectious diseases. 27th edition. Elk Grove Village (IL): American Academy of Pediatrics; 2006. p. 364–5.
[11] Buznach N, Dagan R, Greenburg D. Clinical and bacterial characteristics of acute bacterial conjunctivitis in children in the antibiotic resistance era. Pediatr Infect Dis J 2005;24(9): 823–8.
[12] Patel P, Diaz M, Bennett J, et al. Clinical features of bacterial conjunctivitis in children. Acad Emerg Med 2007;14(1):1–5.
[13] Leibowitz H. The red eye. N Engl J Med 2000;343(5):345–51.
[14] Datner E, Tilman B. Pediatric ophthalmology. Emerg Med Clin North Am 1995;13(3): 669–79.
[15] Bingen E, Cohen R, Jourenkova N, et al. Epidemiologic study of conjunctivitis-otitis syndrome. Pediatr Infect Dis J 2005;24(8):731–2.
[16] Fischer P, Miles V, Stampfi D, et al. Route of antibiotic administration for conjunctivitis. Pediatr Infect Dis J 2002;21(10):989–90.
[17] Wald E. Conjunctivitis in infants and children. Pediatr Infect Dis J 1997;16(2):S17–20.
[18] Scott I. Pharyngoconjunctival fever. eMedicine. Available at: http://www.emedicine.com/ oph/topic501.htm. Updated February 27, 2007. Accessed February 27, 2007.
[19] R. Hered. Pediatric viral conjunctivitis. Northeast Florida Medical Journal 2002. Available at: http://www.dcmsonline.org/jaz-medicine/2002journals/augsept2002/conjunctivitis.htm. Accessed July 25, 2007.
[20] American Academy of Pediatrics. Adenovirus infections. In: Pickering LK, Baker CJ, Long SS, et al, editors. Red book: 2006 report of the committee on infectious diseases. 27th edition. Elk Grove Village (IL): American Academy of Pediatrics; 2006. p. 202–4.
[21] Drack AV. Pediatric ophthalmology. In: Palay D, Krachmer J, editors. Primary care ophthalmology. 2nd edition. New York: Elsevier/Mosby; 2005. p. 238–64.
[22] Baskin M. Ophthalmic and otolaryngologic emergencies. In: Fleisher G, Ludwig S, Baskin M, editors. Atlas of pediatric emergency medicine. Philadelphia: Lippincott Williams and Wilkins; 2004. p. 267–72.
[23] Wald E. Periorbital and orbital infections. Pediatr Rev 2004;25(9):312–9.
[24] Givner L. Periorbital versus orbital cellulitis. Pediatr Infect Dis J 2002;21(12):1157–8.
[25] Jain A, Rubin P. Orbital cellulitis in children. Int Ophthalmol Clin 2001;41:71–86.
[26] Greenburg M, Pollard Z. The red eye in childhood. Pediatr Clin North Am 2003;50: 105–24.
[27] Nield L, Kamat D. A 9-year-old girl who has fever, headache, and right eye pain. Pediatr Rev 2005;26(9):337–40.

[28] Asbell P, Sahm DF, Draghi DC, et al. Increasing prevalence of ocular methicillin-resistant Staphylococcus aureus [poster 62]. In: Programs and abstracts of the 2006 joint meeting of the American Academy of Ophthalmology and Asia Pacific Academy of Ophthalmology. Las Vegas (NV), 2006. Available at: http//:www.osnsupersite.com/view.asp?rID=19307. Accessed August 28, 2007.

[29] Johnson K. Overview of TORCH infections. UpToDate.com. Available at: http://www.utdol.com/utd/content/topic.do?topicKey=pedi_id/25219. Updated April 2007. Accessed July 16, 2007.

[30] Olitsky S, Reynolds J. Overview of glaucoma in infants and children. UpToDate.com. Available at: http://www.utdol.com/utd/content/topic.do?topicKey=pedi_opth/8856. Updated December 2006. Accessed April 3, 2007.

[31] Coats D, Paysse E. Evaluation and management of strabismus in children. UpToDate.com. Available at: http://www.utdol.com/utd/content/topic.do?topicKey=pedi_opth/7374. Updated December 2006. Accessed April 3, 2007.

ELSEVIER
SAUNDERS

Emerg Med Clin N Am
26 (2008) 199–216

EMERGENCY
MEDICINE
CLINICS OF
NORTH AMERICA

The Painful Eye

James M. Dargin, MD[a], Robert A. Lowenstein, MD[a,b,*]

[a]Department of Emergency Medicine, Boston University School of Medicine,
Boston Medical Center, 1 Boston Medical Center Place, Boston, MA 02118, USA
[b]Department of Emergency Medicine, Quincy Medical Center, 114 Whitwell Street,
Quincy, MA 02169, USA

Acute angle closure glaucoma

In 90% of cases, acute angle closure glaucoma (AACG) results from pupillary block in which pupillary dilation causes apposition of the lens and the iris, resulting in obstruction of aqueous outflow from the eye [1]. Accumulation of aqueous in the posterior chamber leads to a rapid elevation in intraocular pressure beyond the normal range of 10 to 21 mmHg, which causes pain and loss of vision [2]. Pupillary block often occurs in hyperopic (farsighted) eyes with a shallow anterior chamber angle [1]. AACG may be triggered by exposure to dim ambient lighting, topical mydriatics, anticholinergics, tricyclic antidepressants, selective serotonin reuptake inhibitors, or adrenergic agonists as a result of their dilating effect on the pupil [3]. There are case reports of intranasal phenylepherine [4], topiramate [5], and nebulized albuterol causing AACG [6]. Other etiologies of AACG may include peripheral anterior synechiae formed after uveits and previous ocular surgery. AACG is more common in Eskimo and Asian populations, women, patients with hyperopia, patients over 40 to 50 years of age, and in those with a family history of the disease [3,7]. In a British study, the overall incidence of AACG was found to be as high as 1 in 1000 people over the age of 40 [8], and the peak incidence occurs between ages 55 and 70 [1].

Patients with AACG complain of an acutely painful, red eye and blurred vision with halos around lights owing to corneal edema. Other commonly associated symptoms include frontal headache, nausea, vomiting, and abdominal pain. AACG is often misdiagnosed, particularly when systemic symptoms, such as abdominal pain, vomiting, and headache are more

---

* Corresponding author. Department of Emergency Medicine, Quincy Medical Center, 114 Whitwell Street, Quincy, MA 02169.
    E-mail address: robert.lowenstein@bmc.org (R.A. Lowenstein).

0733-8627/08/$ - see front matter © 2008 Elsevier Inc. All rights reserved.
doi:10.1016/j.emc.2007.10.001   emed.theclinics.com

prominent than ocular complaints [9,10]. Rarely, AACG may present as painless loss of vision [11]. In approximately 50% of cases, the patient will report similar past episodes. In these cases, the patient often describes evening headaches owing to pupillary constriction that are relieved with sleep [2]. Between attacks the patient is asymptomatic and the eye appears normal [8]. Most cases are unilateral, but AACG may be bilateral, particularly when medications are implicated [10].

Examination reveals circumcorneal conjunctival injection, a steamy cornea, impaired visual acuity, and a mid-dilated (4–6 mm) and fixed pupil (Fig. 1). The affected globe is tender and firm compared with the unaffected eye [2]. An intraocular pressure greater than 40 to 50 mmHg as measured by tonometry can cause rapid visual loss, and pressures greater than 70 mmHg can be seen in AACG [2]. A narrow anterior chamber angle, which predisposes to AACG, can be confirmed by the oblique flashlight test, during which a penlight is shone across the anterior chamber, parallel to the iris. The anterior chamber angle is considered wide if the entire iris is illuminated, and narrow if a shadow is cast across the nasal aspect of the iris [12]. This test, which has a specificity of 69% in AACG, can help confirm the diagnosis in the proper clinical setting [12].

AACG is an ocular emergency and prompt consultation with an ophthalmologist is imperative, as optic nerve atrophy and permanent loss of vision can occur within hours if the condition is not adequately treated [9]. Reduction of intraocular pressure and preservation of vision are the primary goals of treatment in AACG. Intraocular pressure is lowered by decreasing aqueous production with a topical beta blocker (timolol), alpha two agonist (apraclonidine), and a carbonic anhydrase inhibitor (acetazolamide) [7]. Topical timolol 0.5% can be expected to lower the intraocular pressure within 30 minutes to 1 hour. Topical beta blockers are systemically

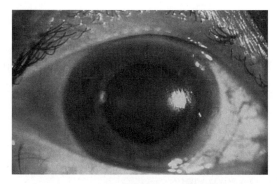

Fig. 1. Conjunctival injection, steamy cornea, and mid-dilated pupil caused by acute angle closure glaucoma. (*From* Bertolini J, Pelucio M. The red eye. Emerg Clin North Am 1995;13(3): 561–79; with permission.)

absorbed, and should be used cautiously if there is a history of reactive airway disease or cardiac conduction abnormality. Acetazolamide can be administered as an initial dose of 500 mg orally or intravenously, but is contraindicated in patients with a sulfa allergy. The intravenous osmotic agent mannitol can be used as an alternative to acetazolamide [7]. A topical corticosteroid may also be applied to reduce the inflammation associated with AACG. In addition to decreasing aqueous production with timolol and acetazolamide, aqueous outflow can be increased through pupillary constriction with pilocarpine [12,13]. Topical pilocarpine 2% can be administered every 15 minutes for the first 1 to 2 hours. The miotic effect of pilocarpine may not be observed until the intraocular pressure first has been reduced below 50 mmHg, at which point the ischemic paralysis of the iris is relieved [7]. The intraocular pressure should be repeated 1 hour after initial treatment to confirm that the pressure is dropping. Medical therapy should be continued if the intraocular pressure has not been reduced, and definitive surgical therapy with laser iridotomy or peripheral iridectomy may be necessary in refractory cases.

Scleritis

Scleritis, or inflammation of the sclera, is an uncommon disease, and many ophthalmologists see only a few cases per year. The emergency physician nevertheless should be familiar with this condition on account of its potential to cause visual loss and to threaten the integrity of the eye. Scleritis occurs more commonly in white females and the average age of onset is 49 years [14]. Most cases involve the anterior (visible) portion of the sclera. Posterior scleritis presents with a painless, red eye. Approximately 39% to 50% of patients with scleritis have an associated rheumatologic disease [14,15]. It is important to note that scleritis may be the first presentation of an underlying systemic disease. Infection causes scleritis in 8% of cases, with herpes zoster being the most common etiology [15]. Scleritis can be classified as diffuse, nodular, or necrotizing, and this distinction has implications for both treatment and prognosis.

Patients with scleritis complain of severe, boring pain that is worse with eye movement and often interferes with normal activity or sleep. The pain usually progresses insidiously over the course of weeks [14]. Headache may be the most prominent symptom, making the diagnosis more difficult. Tearing, blurred vision, and a red eye are also common symptoms. Examination reveals dilation of the deep episcleral vessels and thinning of the sclera, resulting in a bluish discoloration of the eye (Fig. 2). Visual acuity is impaired in 16% of patients [15] and, unlike in episcleritis, the globe is often tender to palpation. The condition is bilateral in 50% of all cases [15]. Diffuse anterior scleritis is characterized by the absence of nodules and a lack of scleral necrosis. In nodular scleritis, there are well-localized, tender areas of edema with dilation of the underlying vessels. In necrotizing

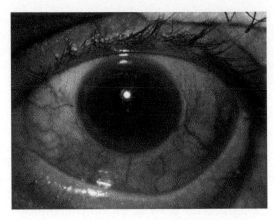

Fig. 2. Dilation of the deep episcleral vessels and a bluish discoloration of the eye in a patient with scleritis. (*Reprinted from* Lee AG, Beaver HA, Brazis PW. Painful ophthalmologic disorders and eye pain for the neurologist. Neurol Clin 2004;22(1):75–97. Plate 5; with permission.)

anterior scleritis, there is intense dilation of the deep vasculature and focal or generalized thinning of the sclera, exposing the underlying choroid. The eye is exquisitely tender to the touch in necrotizing scleritis, and this severe form of the disease represents a threat to the integrity of the eye. The bluish discoloration of the sclera helps differentiate scleritis from episcleritis. In addition, episcleritis tends to cause engorgement of only the more superficial vessels overlying the sclera, which are easily blanched with topical application of phenylepherine. In contrast, the deeper vessels involved in scleritis are unaffected by phenylepherine [14]. The distinction between scleritis and episcleritis has both therapeutic and prognostic implications, with the latter generally being a less malignant process, with fewer ocular complications [15]. Episcleritis is covered in more detail in an article about red eye that appears elsewhere in this issue.

Investigation of previously undiagnosed systemic disease, such as rheumatoid arthritis (RA), Wegener's granulomatosis, relapsing polychondritis, systemic lupus erythematosus, inflammatory bowel disease, and polyarteritis nodosa, becomes important in scleritis [14]. RA, the most commonly implicated systemic disease, accounts for up to 33% of all cases of scleritis referred to ophthalmologists [16]. Necrotizing scleritis often develops in the setting of peripheral ulcerative keratitis associated with vasculitis. Infectious etiologies include herpes zoster ophthalmicus, herpes simplex, Lyme disease, and HIV. Although the history and physical examination can help to focus testing in some cases, the painful, red eye of scleritis may be the only presenting symptom of an underlying systemic disease. In such cases, a complete blood count, blood urea nitrogen, creatinine, electrolyte panel, rheumatoid factor, antinuclear antibody, anticytoplasmic antibodies, and urinalysis may help to reveal an underlying systemic disease. The erythrocyte sedimentation rate and C-reactive protein are useful in assessing the severity of disease and evaluating response to treatment.

The treatment of scleritis is tailored based on the severity of disease and should involve consultation with an ophthalmologist. Mild cases of nodular or diffuse scleritis may respond to oral nonsteroidal anti-inflammatory drugs (NSAIDs) (oral indomethacin 50 mg 3 times/day), with symptoms generally resolving over the course of 1 month [15]. Oral corticosteroids (prednisone 1 mg/kg/day) may be required in refractory anterior scleritis and necrotizing scleritis. Other immunosuppressive drugs, such as cyclophosphamide and cyclosporine, can be added at the discretion of an ophthalmologist or rheumatologist when the condition does not respond to oral corticosteroids or with the goal of treating an underlying systemic disease [15]. Scleritis may be complicated by uveitis, keratitis, or glaucoma in up to 60% of cases [15], and these conditions require appropriate treatment when they arise. Topical corticosteroids are likely to be of little benefit in scleritis, but may be used to treat associated anterior uveitis. Patients with corneal or scleral perforation may require surgical intervention [14]. Most patients with mild scleritis will have little to no change in visual acuity. However, necrotizing scleritis is associated with a much higher incidence of visual loss and a 21% 8-year mortality [7], underscoring the importance of aggressive treatment and prompt referral for follow-up care.

Anterior uveitis (iritis)

The anterior uvea consists of the iris and ciliary body. Anterior uveitis refers to inflammation of one or both of these structures. The terms *iritis* (inflammation of the iris), *cyclitis* (inflammation of the ciliary body), and *iridocyclitis* (inflammation of both anterior uveal structures) are more specific anatomic descriptions of the involved structures in anterior uveitis. Anterior uveitis is typically associated with pain, redness, blurred vision, tearing, and photophobia. Anterior uveitis accounts for 50% to 92% of all cases of uveitis in Western countries [17]. In contrast, posterior uveitis, or inflammation of the choroid, is a less common type of uveitis and is typically painless [18]. The annual incidence of uveitis is 17 in 100,000 people [18]. Anterior uveitis occurs most commonly between the ages of 20 and 50 and rarely before the age of 10 or after the age of 70 [17].

Examination reveals conjunctival injection primarily involving the limbus. The presence of inflammatory cells and flare (protein extravasation from inflamed blood vessels) in the anterior chamber helps to confirm the diagnosis of anterior uveitis. A sterile hypopyon may develop in severe cases (Fig. 3). There may be miosis of the affected eye related to ciliary spasm. Photophobia is commonly present in the affected eye when a light is shone in either the affected or unaffected eye. The intraocular pressure should be measured as secondary glaucoma can result from blockage of the trabecular meshwork by inflammatory cells or from scarring.

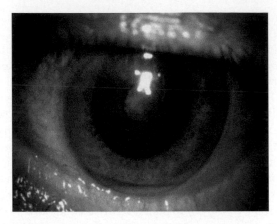

Fig. 3. Conjunctival injection due to anterior uveitis. Note the hypopyon in this patient with HLA-B27-associated disease. (*Reprinted from* Chang J, McCluskey PJ, Wakefield D. Acute anterior uveitis and HLA-B27. Surv Ophthalmol 2005;50(4):364–88. Fig. 1; with permission.)

HLA-B27-associated uveitis

Approximately 60% of all cases of uveitis are idiopathic [19]. Of the identifiable etiologies of anterior uveitis, HLA-B27-associated uveitis is the most common, accounting for 30% to 70% of cases. HLA-B27-associated anterior uveitis is characterized by acute (developing over hours to days), unilateral, alternating uveitis, with a high rate of recurrence [17]. The inflammation of HLA-B27-associated uveitis is often severe, but typically resolves within 2 to 4 months, leaving little to no visual impairment betweens episodes [7]. Only half of the HLA-B27-associated cases have an associated systemic disease, such as ankylosing spondylitis, Reiter syndrome, psoriatic arthritis, or inflammatory bowel disease [18]. The uveitis of Reiter syndrome and ankylosing spondylitis tend to be acute and unilateral, whereas those of psoriatic arthritis and inflammatory bowel disease are more insidious in onset and tend to be bilateral [7]. A small percentage of patients with HLA-B27-associated anterior uveitis develop synechiae (scarring), which can block the outflow of aqueous and result in AACG.

Other noninfectious etiologies

Other causes of anterior uveitis not typically associated with HLA-B27 include trauma, sarcoidosis, juvenile rheumatoid arthritis, Behçet's disease, and Kawasaki's disease. The history and physical examination can help to establish the etiology, particularly when there are signs and symptoms of systemic disease (Table 1). Uveitis associated with juvenile rheumatoid arthritis is unique in that it is often asymptomatic and can cause progressive visual loss if not detected on routine screening [18]. Other diseases may mimic anterior uveitis, including lymphoma and leukemia. These so-called

Table 1
Clinical features of uveitis associated with systemic disease

Disease	HLA-B27 positive (%)	Incidence of uveitis (%)	Clinical features of uveitis	Clinical features of systemic disease	Epidemiology
Ankylosing spondylitis	90	20–40	acute, unilateral, alternating	sacroiliitis, morning stiffness	male, young adult
Reiter syndrome	60	20–40	acute, unilateral	conjunctivitis, urethritis, arthritis, recent genitourinary or enteric infection	male, young adult, white
Psoriatic arthritis	40–50	7	insidious, bilateral	arthritis, rash, nail changes	male = female, ages 30–55, white
Inflammatory bowel disease	35–75	3–11	insidious, bilateral	diarrhea	female, bimodal peak in younger and older adults
Behçet's disease	—	80	acute, unilateral, hypopyon	oral and genital ulcers, skin lesions	male = female, ages 25–30, Asian, Mediterranean, Middle Eastern
Sarcoidosis	—	18	insidious, chronic, bilateral	respiratory symptoms, hilar adenopathy, skin lesions, fever, arthritis	female slightly more than male, young adult, African-American
Juvenile rheumatoid arthritis	—	5–20	asymptomatic, insidious, bilateral	fever, arthritis, rash	female, age younger than 16, white

Data from Refs. [16–20].

"masquerade syndromes," which are typically malignancies that mimic other causes of anterior uveitis, should be suspected when patients do not respond to treatment or when uveitis is diagnosed in the elderly.

In patients with unexplained anterior uveitis, performing serologic testing for syphilis and chest radiography to screen for sarcoidosis is a reasonable diagnostic approach. Knowing the HLA-B27 status may provide some prognostic information, as patients with a positive result tend to have a more severe uveitis [7]. Idiopathic cases of anterior uveitis tend to resolve in 6 weeks and do not necessarily require an extensive diagnostic workup as the process tends not to recur [19].

Infectious etiologies

Anterior uveitis may be caused by infectious etiologies, including syphilis, herpes simplex virus (HSV), and herpes zoster virus. Infectious causes should be suspected when symptoms do not resolve with anti-inflammatory therapy. Iritis associated with syphilis is usually acute and unilateral [18]. HSV-associated iritis usually occurs in the setting of stromal keratitis [21]. Zoster iritis may be due to viral infection of the iris itself, and often occurs when skin lesions are observed on the tip of the nose [21].

Treatment of anterior uveitis

There is a paucity of randomized controlled trials to support the current treatment of anterior uveitis [19]. Treatment may require a multidisciplinary approach, including consultation with a rheumatologist and an ophthalmologist. Topical corticosteroids are used for anterior uveitis and the dosing depends on the severity of disease [18]. Topical prednisolone acetate 1% achieves a high concentration within the anterior chamber and initially may be administered hourly in severe cases. Dosing can be slowly reduced as a therapeutic result is achieved [7]. Cataracts and glaucoma are not only complications of uveitis, but of treatment with long-term topical steroids as well. Systemic corticosteroids and other immunosuppressive medications may be used in refractory cases or to treat a specific underlying systemic disease. Mydriatics relieve the pain associated with ciliary spasm and may prevent the development of adhesions between the pupil and lens.

Uveitis due to syphilis should be treated as neurosyphilis [18]. HSV-associated iritis is treated with topical antivirals. Topical corticosteroids may also be indicated for HSV-associated iritis, but should be used only after consultation with an ophthalmologist, given the potential risk of exacerbating HSV keratitis with this therapy [21]. Zoster iritis usually requires long-term therapy with topical corticosteroids, and there does not seem to be the same risk of worsening the infection as with HSV. Zoster iritis can last for months to years and often causes significant visual impairment, cataracts, and glaucoma [21].

Optic neuritis

Optic neuritis is characterized by inflammatory demyelination of the optic nerve. Although optic neuritis can be associated with many systemic or infectious diseases, including sarcoidosis, systemic lupus erythematosus, syphilis, postviral syndromes, lymphoma, and leukemia, it classically occurs in the setting of multiple sclerosis [7]. In the Optic Neuritis Treatment Trial, a landmark study of the effects of corticosteroids on optic neuritis, 38% of patients with optic neuritis ultimately developed multiple sclerosis [22]. Optic neuritis affects women more commonly than men, and the median age of onset is at approximately 30 years [23].

Patients with optic neuritis complain of unilateral visual loss in most cases, and there may be associated change in color perception or visual field defects. Symptoms develop over the course of hours to days. Up to 92% of cases will be associated with pain [24], which is often worse with eye movement. Pain often begins to resolve after the first few days, as visual loss commences [25]. A small number of cases involve both eyes simultaneously, and the disease may recur in the same or opposite eye. Examination reveals visual loss, with a median acuity of 20/60 in the affected eye [24]. A visual field defect and afferent pupillary defect are also common findings. The optic disk may appear edematous in some patients, but up to two thirds will have a normal-appearing optic disk [24]. Although the diagnosis of optic neuritis is made on a clinical basis, MRI should be routinely performed primarily for prognostic reasons: patients with one or more demyelinating lesions on MRI at the time of optic neuritis have a significantly increased risk of being diagnosed with multiple sclerosis over 10 years [22]. MRI of the orbits, which reveals characteristic enhancement of the optic nerve, may also be indicated in cases where the diagnosis is in question or when there is a lack of recovery of visual acuity [25].

The acute management of patients with optic neuritis should involve admission to the hospital for intravenous methylprednisolone (250 mg every 6 hours for 3 days, followed by an oral prednisone taper), which has been shown to improve short-term recovery from optic neuritis but has not been demonstrated to improve long-term visual impairment [26]. Visual loss begins to improve rapidly with intravenous corticosteroids, but will also improve over the course of weeks without treatment [7]. Most patients eventually regain their baseline visual acuity [24], but many are left with subtle visual changes that affect their quality of life [7]. Patients who develop multiple sclerosis after initial optic neuritis generally have relatively mild neurologic disability [22]. (See the article on optic neuritis elsewhere in this issue.)

Keratitis

Keratitis is defined as inflammation of the cornea. This condition may be infectious or noninfectious in etiology. Patients with keratitis complain of photophobia, foreign body sensation, tearing, and exquisite pain due to the rich sensory innervation from the ophthalmic division of the trigeminal nerve. Herpes simplex and varicella zoster viruses, which may cause decreased corneal sensation, are often less painful than other causes of keratitis [27]. The cornea is an important refractory surface of the eye and inflammation may affect visual acuity. In both infectious and noninfectious causes, the corneal inflammation may be superficial and involve only the epithelium or deep with ulceration through the epithelium [27]. In other cases, the epithelium may remain intact while the stroma becomes inflamed. With stromal keratitis, an infiltrate is observed as a focal area of corneal opacity, which does not stain with fluorescein. Infectious and noninfectious etiologies can often be determined from a careful history and examination. Infectious keratitis may be caused by bacteria, fungi, amoeba, and viruses. Complications of keratitis include corneal ulcer and perforation, scarring with partial or complete visual loss, glaucoma, and uveitis. Examination reveals conjunctival injection, which is more pronounced at the limbus. Cells and flare in the anterior chamber may be noted on slit lamp examination, and a hypopyon may form in more severe cases. Corneal defects are seen as green-stained areas when fluorescein is applied to the affected eye. In superficial keratitis, scarring does not typically occur and vision is not permanently affected [7].

Noninfectious keratitis

Superficial punctate keratitis

Superficial punctate keratitis (SPK) is a condition characterized by pain, redness, and tiny, pinpoint areas of fluorescein uptake on examination. Noninfectious causes of SPK include Thygeson's SPK, blepharoconjunctivitis, and UV light exposure.

Thygeson's SPK is a bilateral keratitis of unknown etiology. It is typically insidious in onset, lasts for months to years, and affects both men and women in the second and third decades of life. Patients experience repeated exacerbations and remissions [7]. Thygeson's SPK is unique form of keratitis in that there is no conjunctival injection. Most patients improve with topical corticosteroids without scarring or significant change in vision [7].

Chronic blepharoconjunctivitis can result in keratitis due to a hypersensitivity reaction to a *Staphylococcal* antigen associated with this condition. There are often infiltrates seen on the periphery of the cornea, and in severe cases the cornea may ulcerate. Treatment of the underlying blepharoconjunctivitis involves warm compresses and topical or systemic antibiotics [27]. Topical steroids are indicated for associated keratitis after infectious etiologies have been excluded.

Most cases of keratitis caused by UV light exposure occur in welders with inadequate eye protection [28]. UV keratitis has also been described with tanning booths, other UV lamp exposure, and sunlight reflecting off snow. The onset of pain and photophobia occurs several hours after the UV exposure [28]. Treatment of UV keratitis includes avoidance of further light exposure and topical lubricants. In most cases, the cornea heals without consequence, but permanent corneal damage has been reported [28].

Other causes of SPK include dry eye syndrome, mechanical trauma from chronic eye rubbing, topical drug toxicity (tobramycin, neomycin, eye drop preservatives, and topical antivirals), mild chemical injury, and contact lens use [7,27]. Treatment of SPK in these cases should be directed toward the underlying cause, as well as appropriate oral analgesics, artificial tears, or other lubricants, such as erythromycin ointment. In contact lens wearers with SPK, contact use should be discontinued and a topical antibiotic with activity against *Pseudomonas* should be prescribed. Patients should be reexamined daily until the cornea has healed.

Ulcerative keratitis

Extensive inflammation of the corneal epithelium may result in ulceration. Although corneal ulcers often result from infectious causes, many non-infectious etiologies can cause this condition, such as neurotrophic keratitis, atopic keratoconjunctivitis, vitamin A deficiency, rosacea, and collagen vascular diseases [27]. When ulceration does occur, the cornea is at increased risk of infection and scarring.

Neurotrophic keratitis results from recurrent injury to the cornea in patients with decreased corneal sensation. Neurotrophic keratitis can be caused by HSV and VZV infection, diabetes mellitus, chemical burns, stroke, and trigeminal nerve palsy [7]. Corneal perforation may result if the condition goes unrecognized. Treatment is primarily focused on maintaining eye lubrication and addressing the underlying disease process.

Atopic keratconjunctivitis is associated with allergic conjunctivitis and is often seen in patients with a history of other allergic disease, such as atopic dermatitis. The inflamed tarsal conjunctiva initially results in SPK, but these areas often coalesce to form a corneal ulcer. Treatment depends on the severity of disease, but may include oral antihistamines, topical steroids, topical mast cell stabilizers, and topical NSAIDs [7].

Ulcerative keratitis may be seen in a wide range of collagen vascular diseases, including RA, sarcoidosis, and many of the vasculitides. Ulcerative keratitis may be the initial presentation of the underlying disease in some cases. Approximately 20% to 30% of patients with RA have keratoconjunctivitis sicca [27,29], which increases the risk of ulcerative keratitis. Corneal involvement in RA may also present as peripheral corneal ulceration from vasculitis [29]. Corneal involvement is common in systemic lupus erythematosus (SLE) and may be a result of autoimmunity or keratoconjunctivitis sicca. Ocular involvement in sarcoidosis may occur at any time during the disease. Single or multiple round opacities may be observed on the cornea, and the condition is often bilateral. The diagnosis may be difficult in the absence of systemic evidence of sarcoidosis [27]. The vasculitides, including Wegener's granulomatosis and polyarteritis nodosa, and Churg-Strauss, typically cause a peripheral ulcerative keratitis, sparing the avascular central cornea [29]. Such corneal ulcers are susceptible to infection and this complication must be excluded before starting corticosteroid therapy. Treatment of keratitis related to collagen vascular disease is typically directed toward the underlying disease process and is best undertaken after consultation with a rheumatologist and ophthalmologist.

Infectious keratitis

Bacterial

Bacterial keratitis is one of the leading causes of blindness in the developing world [7]. The relatively avascular cornea predisposes to infection, particularly when the epithelium is compromised. The incidence of bacterial keratitis is increasing in developed countries, and contact lens use is the most common risk factor [30], followed by ocular surface disease. In the United States, the incidence of bacterial keratitis is 10 to 30 per 100,000 in contact lens wearers [7]. A change in the pathogens implicated in bacterial keratitis can also be attributed to increased contact lens use: *Streptococcus pneumoniae* has traditionally been the most common bacterium isolated from corneal ulcers, but *Pseudomonas*, *Staphylococcus aureus*, and *Serratia* are now the most commonly isolated organisms in contact lens wearers [7]. Although *Neisseria gonorrhea*, *Corynebacterium diphtheriae*, *Shigella*, and *Listeria* can invade an intact cornea [31], disruption of the cornea from underlying corneal disease, corneal trauma and foreign bodies, poor tear production, contact lens use, or corneal surgery allows for adherence and invasion of more commonly isolated bacteria. Diabetes, allergy, and topical steroid use may also increase the risk of bacterial keratitis [30]. Advanced HIV does not seem to increase the risk of bacterial keratitis, but patients may have a more aggressive course once infection occurs.

Examination often reveals a corneal infiltrate, and there may be associated conjunctival injection and chemosis. Cells and flare are found in the anterior chamber in up to 25% of cases [30], which may be severe enough to develop a sterile hypopyon. Familiarity with *Pseudomonas* keratitis has become important not only because of its increasing incidence related to contact lens use, but also owing to its virulence: if improperly treated, this infection can spread rapidly, invading the entire cornea in a matter of hours. A yellow-green discharge may be seen over the affected areas of the cornea and ulceration may progress to perforation of the cornea. Anterior chamber inflammation and hypopyon are commonly seen in *Pseudomonas* keratitis.

The vast majority of bacterial infections will respond to broad-spectrum empiric antibiotics, but culture of corneal scrapings may be prudent when less-common organisms are suspected, when the etiology is not clear from the history, or in more severe cases. Although combination therapy with a cephalosporin, such as cefazolin and an aminoglycoside or floroquinolone is typically recommended, antibiotic choice should be tailored based on clinical features, suspected pathogens, and local resistance patterns. Topical antibiotics, which achieve high concentrations in infected tissue without systemic side effects, are generally preferred over systemic antibiotics. Frequent, repetitive dosing, (every 2 minutes for the first five doses) is usually used as a loading dose. Antibiotics are then instilled approximately every 30 minutes for the first 24 to 36 hours depending on the severity of the infection [31]. Antibiotic therapy should not be delayed for any reason, as site-threatening complications can occur rapidly. Many patients require admission, particularly if treatment noncompliance is a concern or if there is site-threatening infection. Large, central ulcers or extensive infiltrates can result in scarring and varying degrees of visual loss.

Viral

Common causes of viral keratitis include HSV, VZV, Epstein-Barr virus, and adenovirus. HSV is one of the most common causes of corneal blindness in the world. Initial infection with HSV, which often occurs in childhood, is asymptomatic in most cases. In symptomatic cases of primary ocular infection, periorbital cutaneous vesicles are noted and there may be associated blepharitis, conjunctivitis, malaise, fevers, and local lymphadenopathy [21]. Keratitis occurs in 33% to 50% of primary infections, and usually appears 1 to 2 weeks after the appearance of skin lesions. Recurrent disease accounts for most cases of ocular HSV, and classically presents with unilateral dendritic corneal defects (Fig. 4), but the lid and conjunctiva may be involved as well. Within 1 to 2 years, 25% of patients will have a recurrence after an initial infection [21]. Stress, trauma, surgery, and menstrual period often trigger

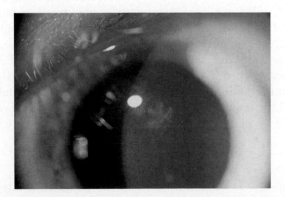

Fig. 4. Dendritic lesion of herpes simplex keratitis. (*Reprinted from* Auerback PS. Wilderness medicine, 5th edition. Philadelphia: Mosby; 2007. Fig. 25–8; with permission.)

recurrent attacks, which lead to corneal scarring and visual loss. Examination with fluorescein reveals superficial punctate lesions or characteristic dendrites, which can coalesce and enlarge. Recurrent disease may also be isolated to the stroma, appearing as a white infiltrate, which tends to be a more severe and difficult to treat form of HSV keratitis [21]. Interestingly, there is decreased corneal sensation associated with HSV keratitis. The diagnosis is often made clinically, but viral culture can be performed if there is uncertainty.

Trifluridine is the drug of choice for topical treatment owing to its high degree of ocular penetration. Trifluridine is administered six to eight times per day for the first several days and then the frequency is reduced as healing occurs [21]. Up to 97% of patients with dendritic lesions will heal within 2 weeks of trifluridine therapy [21]. Oral acyclovir 400 mg five times per day is used as alternative or adjunctive treatment to topical therapy. Topical steroids are contraindicated in the epithelial stage, but may be used in stromal stages after consultation with ophthalmologist. HSV keratitis can resolve spontaneously or with treatment over 1 to 2 weeks. Most patients will have minimal change in visual acuity, but others will be left with significant visual impairment.

VZV keratitis, similar to HSV, may result in a painful, red eye with fever and malaise. The skin findings of VZV are painful vesicular lesions over the ophthalmic division of the trigeminal nerve (forehead and upper eyelid), and typically do not cross the midline. Less commonly, patients will present with isolated corneal involvement [32]. The dendritic lesions of VZV keratitis do not have well-stained terminal bulbs and ulceration is uncommon, in contradistinction to HSV keratitis [21]. Corneal sensation is often markedly impaired, even in mild cases [27].

VZV keratits is treated with oral acyclovir 800 mg five times per day or oral valacyclovir 1000 mg three times per day for 7 to 10 days [32]. Therapy is most effective when started in the first 3 days, but may have some efficacy within 5 days of the onset of symptoms [21]. There is no clear evidence for the efficacy of topical antiviral medications for VZV keratitis [21].

There are at least 50 types of adenovirus, and not surprisingly the spectrum of symptoms is broad, ranging from isolated ocular involvement to ocular disease associated with pharyngitis or gastroenteritis [21]. Adenovirus is quite contagious, and ocular disease appropriately has been termed epidemic keratoconjunctivitis. In corneal involvement with adenovirus, patients complain of severe pain and often have bilateral conjunctivitis with a palpable preauricular lymph node. Diffuse punctate keratitis, which typically resolves without treatment in 7 to 10 days, is followed by subepithelial infiltrates. Topical steroids may provide pain relief and improve vision at this later stage [21].

Fungal

Fungal keratitis is commonly seen in the southern United States and tropical regions of the world. Infection with *Fusarium* and *Aspergillus* is often caused by traumatic injury from vegetable matter, and *Candida albicans* is seen in patients with underlying eye disease [33]. Signs and symptoms are similar to that of bacterial keratitis, and fungal infections are often treated as bacterial until culture results are available. Topical therapy is used for mild keratitis and systemic antifungal therapy is added in more severe cases. Patients are usually admitted to the hospital for hourly dosing of topical antifungal therapy, which may be required for several days [33]. Topical steroids are contraindicated. Anterior uveitis is a common finding and cycloplegics are often used in these cases. Improvement usually occurs over weeks; corneal transplant is reserved for refractory cases.

Amoebic

The first case of *Acanthamoeba* keratitis was described in 1973 [34]. Infection with this amoeba, which is abundant in the environment, usually occurs in young, healthy adults and the majority of cases are contact lens related. Symptoms are similar to bacterial keratitis, although the pain seems to be more severe and the infection progresses more slowly in the case of *Ancanthamoeba* keratitis [34]. Slit lamp examination may reveal dendritiform lesions that can be confused with HSV keratitis. *Ancanthamoeba* keratitis should be suspected in any contact lens wearer with dendriform keratitis, and cultures of the corneal epithelium and contact lenses should be sent in such cases. Treatment typically involves combination therapy with topical amoebicidal agents after consultation with an ophthalmologist.

Corneal abrasion

Patients with corneal abrasions are commonly seen in the emergency department. A corneal abrasion is a traumatic defect in the corneal epithelium, which may result from direct mechanical trauma, contact lens related injury, foreign bodies, or motor vehicle accidents with airbag deployment [35]. Patients complain of pain, sensitivity to light, and excessive tearing following trauma to the eye. The patient may recollect injury from a fingernail, makeup applicator, or excessive rubbing of the eyes. In other cases the trauma may be so minor that it is not remembered by the patient at all. Trauma to the eye of a machine worker or as a result of metal striking metal should raise suspicion for penetrating globe injury. In contact lens wearers, specific history about poorly fitting lenses and prolonged wearing should be elicited.

Application of a short-acting topical anesthetic, such as proparacaine, will facilitate examination of the painful eye. Visual acuity is typically normal unless the abrasion involves the visual axis or there is significant corneal edema. There may be blepharospasm of the affected eye as a result of photophobia. Ciliary spasm may cause miosis. The cornea can appear hazy if there is edema. Conjunctival injection is classically present and is most pronounced at the limbus. The diagnosis is confirmed by green fluorescence in damaged areas of the cornea seen under Wood's lamp or cobalt blue light on slit lamp examination after the application of fluorescein (Fig. 5). Contact lens-related abrasions may be punctate or coalesce to form a larger, round central abrasion. Multiple vertical abrasions suggest a foreign body and should prompt the examiner to flip the upper eye lid for careful examination. Siedel's sign or the presence of a hyphema on slit lamp examination suggests penetrating trauma to the globe.

Current treatment for corneal abrasions is largely based on theoretical benefit and general consensus rather than on rigorous study. Primary goals of therapy are pain control, prevention of infection, and rapid healing of the corneal epithelium. In a systematic review of five randomized controlled trials, topical NSAIDs, such as ketorolac, diclofenac, and indomethacin, resulted in a modest decrease in pain without a delay in wound healing or an increased risk of infection [36]. Patients who use topical NSAIDs may also return to work earlier and require fewer oral analgesics, including narcotics. Topical NSAIDs are, however, relatively expensive. Cycloplegics should theoretically relieve pain and photophobia related to ciliary spasm, but a systematic review showed no clear evidence to support their use in corneal abrasion [37]. Patching of the eye following a corneal abrasion has been shown to be of no benefit in pain relief or rate of healing, and is no longer recommended [38]. Concerns over the safety of patching have also been raised, as this treatment leaves the patient effectively monocular, thus impairing ambulation and driving. Contact lens-related abrasions in particular are at increased risk of infection when patched, and the eye should not be covered in these cases. Patients with contact lens-related abrasions should be instructed to discontinue contact lens use until the defect heals and symptoms resolve. Oral analgesics, such as acetaminophen, ibuprofen, or opoids,

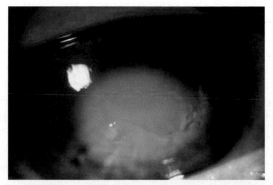

Fig. 5. Large corneal abrasion confirmed by fluorescein illumination under cobalt blue light. (*Reprinted from* Goldman L, Ausiello D. Cecil text book of medicine, 22nd edition. Philadelphia: WB Saunders; 2004. Fig. 465–8; with permission.)

are typically prescribed for pain control. The decision to use oral NSAIDs or opioids should be made on an individual patient basis. In cases where oral analgesics are contraindicated, topical NSAIDs may be of benefit. A topical antibiotic, such as erythromycin, is commonly prescribed four times per day for 3 to 5 days to prevent infection, although there is no strong evidence to support this practice. Because of their lubricating effect, antibiotic ointments are generally preferred over drops. Patients with contact lens abrasions should be treated with prophylactic topical antibiotics to cover *Pseudomonas*, such as gentamycin or ciprofloxacin. There is no convincing evidence in the literature to support tetanus prophylaxis in patients with nonpenetrating corneal abrasions [39].

Most abrasions heal within 1 to 3 days, although defects involving greater than half of the surface of cornea may require 4 to 5 days to fully heal [40]. Patients with small corneal abrasions will heal quickly and generally require only a single 24-hour follow-up examination to ensure healing. Patients with contact lens-related corneal abrasions should be reexamined daily to ensure prompt healing and to exclude infection. Referral to an ophthalmologist is indicated for large abrasions, defects over the visual axis, abrasions that become larger or more symptomatic the next day, or for patients who develop a corneal infiltrate or ulcer.

References

[1] Chang BM, Ritch R, Liebmann JM. Angle closure in younger patients. Ophthalmology 2003;110(10):1880–9.
[2] Khaw PT, Shah P, Elkington AR. Glaucoma-1: diagnosis. BMJ 2004;328:97–9.
[3] Gordon-Bennett P, Ung T, Stephenson C, et al. Misdiagnosis of angle closure glaucoma. BMJ 2006;333(7579):1157–8.
[4] Zenzen CT, Eliott D, Balok EM, et al. Acute angle-closure glaucoma associated with intranasal phenylephrine to treat epistaxis. Arch Ophthalmol 2004;122(4):655–6.
[5] Fraunfelder FW, Fraunfelder FT, Keates EU. Topiramate-associated acute, bilateral, secondary angle-closure glaucoma. Ophthalmology 2004;111(1):109–11.
[6] Rho D. Acute angle-closure glaucoma after albuterol nebulizer treatment. Am J Ophthalmol 2000;130(1):123–4.
[7] Yanoff M, Duker JS, Augsburger JJ, et al. Ophthalmology. 2nd edition. St. Louis (MO): Mosby; 2004. p. 512–8, 1117–20, 1177–80, 11263–7, 1491–8, 465–91.
[8] Dayan M, Turner B, McGhee C. Acute angle closure glaucoma masquerading as systemic illness. BMJ 1996;313(7054):413–5.
[9] Leibowitz HM. The red eye. N Engl J Med 2000;343:345–51.
[10] Berkoff DJ, Sanchez LD. An uncommon presentation of acute angle closure glaucoma. J Emerg Med 2005;29(1):43–4.
[11] Rosenberg CA, Adams SL. Narrow-angle glaucoma presenting as acute, painless visual impairment. Ann Emerg Med 1991;20(9):1020–2.
[12] Coleman AL. Glaucoma. Lancet 1999;354(9192):1803–10.
[13] Khaw PT, Shaw P, Elkington AR. Glaucoma-2: treatment. BMJ 2004;328:156–8.
[14] Okhravi N, Odufuwa B, McCluskey P, et al. Scleritis. Surv Ophthalmol 2005;50:351–63.
[15] Jabs DA, Mudun A, Dunn JP, et al. Episcleritis and scleritis: clinical features and treatment results. Am J Ophthalmol 2000;130:469–76.

[16] Hamideh F, Prete PE. Ophthalmologic manifestations of rheumatic diseases. Semin Arthritis Rheum 2001;30(4):217–41.

[17] Chang J, McCluskey PJ, Wakefield D. Acute anterior uveitis and HLA-B27. Surv Ophthalmol 2005;50(4):364–88.

[18] Hajj-Ali RA, Lowder C, Mandell BF. Uveitis in the internist's office: are a patient's eye symptoms serious? Cleve Clin J Med 2005;72(4):329–39.

[19] Pras E, Neumann R, Zandman-Goddard G, et al. Intraocular inflammation in autoimmune diseases. Semin Arthritis Rheum 2004;34(3):602–9.

[20] Klippel JH. Primer on the Rheumatic Diseases. 12th edition. Atlanta (Georgia): Arthritis Foundation; 2001. p. 245–9, 415–8, 455–8, 534–40, 233–8, 250–4.

[21] Kaufman HE. Treatment of viral diseases of the cornea and external eye. Prog Retin Eye Res 2000;19(1):69–85.

[22] Kupersmith MJ, Miller NR, Moke PS, et al. (Optic Neuritis Study Group): neurologic impairment 10 years after optic neuritis. Arch Neurol 2004;61(9):1386–9.

[23] Pirko I, Blauwet LK, Lesnick TG, et al. The natural history of recurrent optic neuritis. Arch Neurol 2004;61(9):1401–5.

[24] Balcer LJ. Optic Neuritis. N Engl J Med 2006;354(12):1273–80.

[25] Arnold AC. Evolving management of optic neuritis and multiple sclerosis. Am J Ophthalmol 2005;139(6):1101–8.

[26] Beck RW, Cleary PA, Anderson MM Jr, et al. A randomized, controlled trial of corticosteroids in the treatment of acute optic neuritis. N Engl J Med 1992;326:581–8.

[27] Sharma S. Keratitis. Biosci Rep 2001;21(4):419–44.

[28] Yen YL, Lin HL, Lin HJ, et al. Photokeratoconjunctivitis caused by different light sources. Am J Emerg Med 2004;22:511–21.

[29] Messemer EM, Foster S. Vasculitic peripheral ulcerative keratitis. Surv Ophthalmol 1999; 43(5):379–96.

[30] Bourcier T, Thomas F, Borderie V, et al. Bacterial keratitis: predisposing factors, clinical and microbiological review of 300 cases. Br J Ophthalmol 2003;87(7):834–8.

[31] O'Brien TP. Management of bacterial keratitis: beyond exorcism towards consideration of organism and host factors. Eye 2003;17(8):957–74.

[32] Shaikh S, Ta CN. Evaluation and management of herpes zoster ophthalmicus. Am Fam Physician 2002;66(9):1723–30.

[33] Thomas PA. Fungal infections of the cornea. Eye 2003;17(8):852–62.

[34] Illingworth CD, Cook SD. Acanthamoeba keratitis. Surv Ophthalmol 1998;42(6):493–508.

[35] Duma SM, Jernigan MV, Stitzel JD, et al. The effect of frontal air bags on eye injury patterns in automobile crashes. Arch Ophthalmol 2002;120(11):1517–22.

[36] Weaver CS, Terrell KM. Evidence-based emergency medicine. Update: do ophthalmic non-steroidal anti-inflammatory drugs reduce the pain associated with simple corneal abrasion without delaying healing? Ann Emerg Med 2003;41:134–40.

[37] Carley F, Carley S. Towards evidence based emergency medicine: best BETs from the Manchester Royal Infirmary. Mydriatics in corneal abrasion. Emerg Med J 2001;18(4):273.

[38] Turner A, Rabiu M. Patching for corneal abrasion. Cochrane Database Syst Rev 2006: CD004764.

[39] Mukherjee P, Sivakumar A, Mackway-Jones K. Tetanus prophylaxis in superficial corneal abrasions. Emerg Med J 2003;20(1):62–4.

[40] Wilson SA, Last A. Management of corneal abrasions. Am Fam Physician 2004;70(1):123–8.

ELSEVIER
SAUNDERS

Emerg Med Clin N Am
26 (2008) 217–231

EMERGENCY
MEDICINE
CLINICS OF
NORTH AMERICA

Ophthalmologic Complications of Systemic Disease

Jean E. Klig, MD, FAAP

*Division of Pediatric Emergency Medicine, Boston University School of Medicine,
Boston Medical Center, 1 Boston Medical Center Place, Boston, MA 02118, USA*

The human eye, as an organ, can offer critical clues to the presence of systemic illness. Ocular changes are common in the early course of many systemic infections and inflammatory diseases that may be diagnosed in the emergency department. A careful and thorough eye examination is paramount during routine evaluation in the emergency department because it can provide primary information on otherwise undetected systemic illness and corroborative data for known problems. This article reviews various ophthalmologic complications of systemic disease that can be detected by an emergency department provider, as well as key findings that can be discerned with specialty consultation.

Acquired syphilis

Infection with *Treponema pallidum* affects most organ systems if untreated. In fact, acquired syphilis was a common cause of ocular inflammation before the introduction of effective antimicrobial treatment. Although the prevalence of acquired syphilis has diminished overall in the post-antibiotic era, it still remains an important clinical entity [1]. Current worldwide estimates suggest the occurrence of approximately 12 million new cases of syphilis each year, 90% of which are in developing countries [1]. Rates of primary and secondary syphilis infection in the United States have risen markedly since 2000, primarily among male homosexuals. Although ocular syphilis is now rare overall, prolonged untreated syphilis-related ocular disease can produce destructive changes in the eye; therefore, clinical suspicion is vital to early intervention. If present, ocular syphilis will manifest during the second or third stages of clinical illness. A key triad that should prompt

E-mail address: jean.klig@bmc.org

0733-8627/08/$ - see front matter © 2008 Elsevier Inc. All rights reserved.
doi:10.1016/j.emc.2007.10.003   *emed.theclinics.com*

clinical suspicion of syphilis infection is persistent headache, red eyes or eye pain, and an unexplained elevated erythrocyte sedimentation rate (ESR) [2].

There are no signs that are pathognomonic of ocular syphilis, and it can readily mimic other ocular disorders. Madarosis, or loss of the eyelashes or eyebrows, can occur. Uveitis is the most common eye finding [3], accounting for the red eyes or eye pain in the triad detailed previously. Eye involvement usually is evident beyond the primary stage of syphilis, but a primary chancre of the conjunctiva is possible [4]. Anterior segment eye findings that may be evident to the emergency department physician on direct and slit lamp examination include keratitis (interstitial or stromal) and iridocyclitis or anterior uveitis [1,4]. Prolonged syphilitic interstitial keratitis can result in closed angle glaucoma, which can be a presenting sign of the disease [5]. Acute iridocyclitis occurs in approximately 4% of patients with secondary syphilis, with bilateral involvement in approximately 50% of cases [4]. A red eye–type finding that the emergency department provider may note is dilated iris capillaries, or roseolae, often in early iridocyclitis. Roseolae may progress to discrete papules and then to larger yellow nodules [4].

Posterior segment ocular changes in syphilis include chorioretinitis (unifocal, multifocal, or neuroretinitis), posterior uveitis, vaso-occlusive retinal changes, and retinal detachment [1,4]. The emergency department provider is most likely to detect associated visual changes and eye redness or ocular pain on examination, although it may be possible to discern inflammatory changes to the fundus. Neuro-ophthalmologic changes that may be appreciated are an Argyll Robertson pupil (unilateral or bilateral small pupils that accommodate to near vision but do not react to light), third and sixth cranial nerve palsies, and visual field defects from brain involvement. Ophthalmologic consultation is important in cases of suspected ocular syphilis, because many of the changes that occur are reversible if detected and monitored during treatment. In addition to a more extensive examination of the fundus that is performed by an ophthalmologist, additional testing via MRI, angiography, and other modalities may be performed. Ophthalmologic consultation is critical in HIV patients with evidence of ocular syphilis because more severe eye disease and greater rates of complication are common [4]. In turn, HIV testing should be considered in patients with suspected ocular syphilis given the common risk factors for both diseases [3].

Varicella-zoster virus infection

Varicella and herpes zoster infections are due to the same human herpes virus 3, also known as varicella-zoster virus (VZV). Immunization against varicella has diminished the incidence and severity of the disease overall; however, primary infections and reactivation as herpes zoster continue to occur in persons who are un-immunized or immunocompromised, or as "break-through disease" in vaccinated patients [6]. Ocular manifestations of primary varicella infection are generally uncommon. Nonetheless, the following have been reported as isolated or combined findings during primary varicella illness: lid, conjunctival, and corneal vesicles; iridocyclitis; glaucoma; cataracts; chorioretinitis; optic neuritis or atrophy; and internal ophthalmoplegia [7]. The common viral prodrome and typical skin lesions of varicella infection will precede or accompany any ocular involvement. Ocular changes can also be seen as a late complication of primary varicella illness [7].

Herpes zoster infection (shingles) results from reactivation of latent VZV in sensory nerve ganglia, with migration down the nerves to the related dermatome where severe pain and characteristic skin lesions result [8]. Risk factors for herpes zoster include advanced age, poor nutrition, immune compromise, fatigue, and physical or emotional stress [9]. The lifetime risk of herpes zoster is about 10% to 20% overall; approximately 10% to 25% of cases involve the ophthalmic division of the trigeminal nerve, which is known as herpes zoster ophthalmicus (Fig. 1). Ocular lesions develop in approximately half of patients with herpes zoster ophthalmicus [8]. Damage to the eye and surrounding structures occurs owing to inflammation of sensory nerves, with the potentially serious sequelae of chronic ocular inflammation, vision loss, or severe pain [9]. Although acute herpes zoster ophthalmicus typically entails the classic VZV rash in the specific dermatome, ocular changes can occur with minimal or no rash [8,9]. Up to one third of patients with herpes zoster ophthalmicus also have involvement of the nasociliary nerve that innervates the tip of the nose. This involvement is known as Hutchinson's sign and is a strong predictor of ocular inflammation and corneal denervation [8,10]. Patients with Hutchinson's sign are reported to have twice the incidence of ocular changes overall. Patients

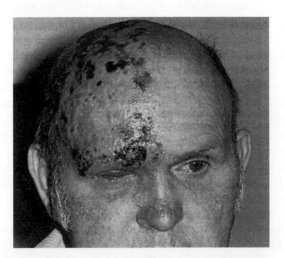

Fig. 1. Herpes zoster ophthalmicus. (*From* Wipf JE, Paauw DS. Ophthalmologic emergencies in the patient with diabetes. Endocrinol Metab Clin North Am 2000;29(4):825; with permission.)

without Hutchinson's sign may have eye involvement in up to one third of cases [8,9].

External ocular manifestations of acute herpes zoster ophthalmicus that may be observed by the emergency department provider include blepharitis, conjunctivitis, episcleritis, and scleritis. Blepharitis can entail vesicular lesions on the eyelids or lid edema and inflammation. The latter may cause ptosis on the affected side [9]. Conjunctivitis is a common early complication of herpes zoster ophthalmicus that is associated with vesicles on the lid margin; the conjunctivae will appear red and swollen and may have petechial hemorrhages [8]. Episcleritis may be seen in as many as one third of herpes zoster ophthalmicus cases and includes erythema, pain, and swelling of the episclera that can be masked by overlying conjunctivitis. Scleritis is a less common but more serious late finding of herpes zoster ophthalmicus following a week of illness, and the cornea is usually also involved (sclerokeratitis).

Corneal involvement occurs in 65% of patients with acute herpes zoster ophthalmicus, and a high level of suspicion for this entity is warranted if vision loss is reported by the patient or detected on visual acuity testing in the emergency department [9]. Symptoms of eye pain or light sensitivity may also occur. The spectrum of corneal changes in herpes zoster ophthalmicus correlates with the progression of disease and includes epithelial keratitis, anterior stromal keratitis, and disciform keratitis. Epithelial keratitis is usually a transient early finding of herpes zoster ophthalmicus that is initially seen on slit lamp examination as multiple swollen lesions which stain with fluorescein or rose bengal dye. VZV dendrites may appear later in a branching or "medusa-like" pattern with similar staining and examination via Wood's lamp or slit lamp [9]. Anterior stromal keratitis, or nummular keratitis, occurs in as many as 30% of patients with herpes zoster ophthalmicus during the second week of disease and likely reflects an antigen–antibody response to viral proliferation in the overlying epithelium [11]. On slit lamp examination, multiple patchy fine granular infiltrates with a halo can be seen in the anterior stroma below areas of previous epithelial keratitis [8,9]. Disciform keratitis is a late event in herpes zoster ophthalmicus that occurs in about 5% of cases, usually about 3 weeks after the onset of disease. It reflects an extension of anterior stromal keratitis that can herald chronic changes of scarring, lipid deposition, and vascularization, all of which can compromise vision.

Anterior uveitis, or inflammation of the iris and ciliary body, occurs in approximately 40% of patients with herpes zoster ophthalmicus. Patients with the Hutchinson's sign (involvement of the nasociliary nerve) are at a higher risk for anterior uveitis. Herpes zoster ophthalmicus iritis is generally mild, with small keratic precipitates and a faint flare in the anterior chamber that can be seen on slit lamp examination. A mild elevation in intraocular pressure frequently occurs. Complications of iris atrophy (20%), secondary glaucoma (10%), secondary cataracts (rare), and ischemia of the ciliary body (phthisis bulbi, very rare) can occur [8]. Timely ophthalmologic referral and treatment is essential. See the article by Mueller and McStay elsewhere in this issue for a discussion of treatment options.

Herpes zoster ophthalmicus is commonly associated with many cases of acute retinal necrosis. Presenting symptoms include blurred vision or pain in the affected eye. Peripheral patches of retinal necrosis may be evident on fundoscopic examination. Emergent ophthalmologic consultation is warranted because retinal detachment can occur.

Lyme disease

Lyme disease is endemic to many areas of the United States and Europe but is an uncommon cause of significant ocular disease [12]. The rare ocular manifestations of Lyme disease are largely known through case reports and small case series; epidemiologic studies of patients with Lyme disease have reported only a few cases of ocular involvement [13]. Ocular complications of Lyme disease can be similar to those of syphilis, presenting with both early and late findings [14]. Patients with severe ocular manifestations of Lyme disease likely have a more chronic form of the disease [15].

Clinical findings in stage 1 Lyme disease include the erythema chronicum migrans rash and flulike symptoms. Eye changes that may be noted in as many as 11% of patients are conjunctivitis, periorbital edema, and mild photophobia [14,15]. Stage 2 Lyme disease develops days to months later and reflects clinical progression of the illness that may include a relapsing migratory monoarthritis, neurologic disease (cranial neuropathy, meningitis, or radiculopathy), and cardiac atrioventricular block. Ocular manifestations that may occur in stage 2 Lyme disease result from intraocular inflammation that leads to granulomatous iridocyclitis with or without uveitis that may be seen on slit lamp examination. Further involvement of the retina may occur as retinal vasculitis, disk edema, or choroiditis. Neuroophthalmic symptoms of blurred vision, headache, Bell's palsy, cranial neuropathy, and diplopia may also be present [15]. Decreased color vision and visual field changes can occur. Other more rare ocular complications in late stage 2 Lyme disease are paralytic mydriasis, Horner's syndrome, the Argyll Robertson pupil, orbital myositis, and temporal arteritis [15].

Stage 3 Lyme disease occurs months to years afterwards and reflects persistent infection that manifests as prolonged chronic or recurrent arthritis or chronic neurologic syndromes. The severe ocular complications of Lyme disease seen during stage 3 are episcleritis, stromal keratitis, orbital myositis, vitreitis, or pars planitis. Episcleritis entails redness, pain, and swelling of the episclera that can be seen on direct examination. Complaints of photophobia or blurred vision can occur with stromal keratitis; scattered nummular opacities can be seen on slit lamp examination. Findings in orbital myositis can range from pain on movement of the affected ocular muscle to an inability to move the eye in the direction of the affected muscle.

Vitreitis is evidenced as multiple inflammatory nodules that may be seen on fundoscopic examination ("snowbank exudates"). It is referred to as pars planitis when stromal keratitis is also present. Ophthalmologic consultation is appropriate to confirm these findings and screen for additional rare complications of Lyme disease [15].

Acquired immunodeficiency syndrome

It is estimated that since the early 1980s over 50 million people have been infected with HIV worldwide, and more than 22 million deaths have resulted from AIDS [16]. The advent of highly active antiretroviral therapy has produced a remarkable decline in all manifestations of HIV infection, including ocular complications [16]. Nonetheless, ocular findings may provide important clues to HIV-related disease.

Conjunctival microvascular disease affects as many as 75% of HIV-infected patients. Changes of the conjunctiva can appear similar to sickle cell disease and are best observed on the inferior perilimbal bulbar conjunctiva [17]. Slit lamp examination may reveal capillary dilations, microaneurysms, variable short vessel segments or isolated vessel fragments, or a granular appearance of blood within dilated vessels [18]. Other common findings in HIV disease include dry eye, keratoconjunctivitis sicca, and chronic allergic conjunctivitis [17].

External ocular disease in AIDS patients manifests as opportunistic infections and tumors. The range of opportunistic infections includes viral (herpes zoster ophthalmicus, herpes simplex keratitis, molluscum contagiosum, human papillomavirus), protozoal (microsporidium), and fungal (candida and cryptococcus) sources [16–18]. Secondary bacterial infections (*Staphylococcus aureus*, *Staphylococcus epidermidis*, and *Pseudomonas aeruginosa*) may occur with opportunistic eye infections and can result in corneal ulcers. A higher incidence of preseptal cellulitis is also reported in AIDS patients. Kaposi's sarcoma is an AIDS-defining opportunistic tumor caused by human herpesvirus 8. As many as 20% of patients with Kaposi's sarcoma may have ocular involvement [19]. Kaposi's sarcoma lesions may appear on the eyelids or conjunctivae as an irregular mass that is red to purple in color, but they also appear similar to a hordeolum (stye) [17]. Conjunctival Kaposi's sarcoma lesions are possible and can be mistaken for subconjunctival hemorrhages which do not resolve [16]. Squamous cell carcinomas (associated with human papillomavirus infection) may also be seen as external ocular manifestations of AIDS disease.

Anterior ocular segment complications of AIDS include infectious keratitis (due to the organisms detailed previously) and anterior uveitis. The latter affects more than half of AIDS patients [20]. Mild iridocyclitis often results from VZV or herpes simplex virus infections, with inflammatory changes of the iris and anterior ciliary body seen on slit lamp examination [16]. More severe anterior uveitis occurs in association with posterior segment infections. Symptoms may include photophobia, pain, redness, decreased vision, or lacrimation.

Posterior segment eye complications occur in as many as 75% of AIDS patients and often can lead to vision impairment or blindness [19]. Retinal microangiopathy and cytomegalovirus (CMV) retinitis are most common, affecting 30% to 40% of AIDS patients overall [16]. The former is of non-infectious origin and is characterized by cotton-wool spots on fundoscopic examination that may be asymptomatic and transient. Retinal hemorrhages and microaneurysms may also be reported on examination by an ophthalmologist. CMV retinitis is usually associated with low CD4 T-lymphocyte levels and severe systemic disease, although it may be a rare presenting manifestation of AIDS [19]. Symptoms of CMV retinitis include floaters, blurred vision, and visual field loss [16]. Ophthalmologic consultation is needed given that retinal detachment (30%) and optic nerve involvement (5%) are possible. The range of optic findings includes granular retinitis, hemorrhagic retinitis, and perivascular retinitis. Other posterior eye segment AIDS-related infections are retinitis due to other viruses (VZV, herpes simplex) or bacteria (ocular syphilis), choroiditis (*Pneumocystis carinii*, *Cryptococcus neoformans*, *Mycobacterium tuberculosis*), and retinochoroiditis (*Toxoplasma gondii*) [16,19]. Neuro-ophthalmic complications of AIDS-related intracranial infections or tumors may also occur. Cerebral toxoplasmosis is most common and can present with cranial nerve palsies, visual field loss, or papilledema [16].

Reiter's syndrome

Reiter's syndrome is a multisystem disease that entails a symptom triad of urethritis, conjunctivitis, and arthritis with negative serology [21,22]. It is an uncommon disease overall that is diagnosed more frequently in men (typically those aged more than 30 years) but can also occur in women [23]. The onset of Reiter's syndrome is often preceded by genitourinary infection or bacterial enteric infection [22]. As many as 75% of patients with Reiter's syndrome test positive for HLA-B27 histocompatibility antigens.

The most consistent ocular manifestation of Reiter's syndrome is a mild bilateral mucopurulent conjunctivitis that is part of the diagnostic triad and that occurs in up to 58% of patients [24]. Mucopurulent eye discharge will be noted, and a papillary or follicular reaction is also common [24]. The conjunctivitis may occur up to 2 weeks after the onset of symptoms of urethritis but often precedes the onset of arthritis. Acute iritis that is detectable on slit lamp examination develops in as many as 20% of patients with Reiter's syndrome [25]. Keratitis may also be evident as subepithelial opacities (keratic precipitates) with overlying punctate lesions [24–26]. These findings of anterior uveitis are more common in patients who test positive for HLA-B27 antigens [26,27]. Other eye complications of Reiter's syndrome that have been reported include scleritis, episcleritis, disk edema, retinal edema, and retinal vasculitis [24]. Chronic recurrent ocular inflammation may occur following the acute eye changes and can result in posterior synechiae, glaucoma, cystoid macular edema, and cataracts [24].

Infectious endocarditis

Ocular complications of infectious endocarditis typically result from some type of septic embolic event to the retina. Emergency department providers may be familiar with the finding of a Roth's spot, which is commonly seen in endocarditis and other diseases. A Roth's spot is a cluster of superficial retinal hemorrhages that can be seen on fundoscopic examination as oval hemorrhages with pale centers, often located near the optic disk [28]. In endocarditis, this cluster represents red blood cells which surround inflammatory cells that have collected in the area in response to a septic embolus [29].

A full spectrum of retinal complications may occur in patients with infectious endocarditis. Most are described in case reports and include focal retinitis, embolic retinopathy, subretinal abscesses, choroidal septic metastasis, choroiditis, endophthalmitis (Fig. 2), papillitis, and optic neuritis [30–36]. Clinical vigilance for symptoms of ocular pain, injection, and vision loss is critical in patients with known or suspected endocarditis. Any of these symptoms should prompt an immediate complete examination of the eyes and consultation with an ophthalmologist.

Kawasaki's disease

Mucocutaneous lymph node syndrome, or Kawasaki's disease, is an acute multi-organ vasculitis that primarily affects children aged 1 to 8 years.

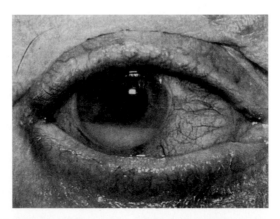

Fig. 2. Enophthalmitis. (*From* Wipf JE, Paauw DS. Ophthalmologic emergencies in the patient with diabetes. Endocrinol Metab Clin North Am 2000;29(4):821; with permission.)

It presents with fever and the following symptoms: (1) bilateral bulbar conjunctivitis without exudates; (2) dryness of the lips and oral cavity, with reddening of the mucosa; (3) polymorphous truncal rash without vesicles or crusts; (4) erythema and edema of the palms and soles, or periungual desquamation; and (5) acute nonpurulent cervical lymphadenopathy [37,38]. Incomplete or atypical presentations of Kawasaki's disease are also possible [38]. The primary ocular manifestation of Kawasaki's disease is bilateral bulbar conjunctivitis (often with limbal sparing); any additional inflammatory eye changes are similarly bilateral [39]. A recent study of conjunctival swabs from patients with Kaposi's sarcoma bulbar conjunctivitis reported a predominance of neutrophils, or "neutrophilic conjunctivitis," as a cytopathologic change that can be followed as Kawasaki's disease progresses [40].

Anterior uveitis can occur in 25% to 50% of patients with Kawasaki's disease [38]. The initial bulbar conjunctivitis can readily progress to bilateral iridocyclitis. Symptoms of photophobia, pain, redness, decreased vision, or lacrimation may occur. Subconjunctival hemorrhages or circumcorneal injection with a violaceous hue may be noted on examination of the eyes. Slit lamp examination may reveal superficial punctate keratitis, keratitic precipitates, vitreous opacities, or aqueous cells and a flare response [39,41].

Posterior segment changes have also been reported in Kawasaki's disease. Papilledema may occur, for which fluorescein angiography is needed to detect vasculitis-related changes [39,42]. Retinal ischemia may also occur as the Kawasaki's disease vasculitis progresses [43]; therefore, prompt ophthalmologic consultation is necessary, particularly if more advanced Kawasaki's disease ocular complications are suspected. Dacrocystitis has been reported as an eye complication following resolution of acute Kawasaki's disease [37].

Temporal arteritis

Giant cell arteritis, or temporal arteritis, is the most common vasculitis in patients over 50 years of age. The disease involves T cell–mediated inflammation of medium-to-large caliber arteries which produces tissue destruction, vascular occlusion, and end organ ischemia [44,45]. Although giant cell arteritis may affect the vascular supply of any organ, cranial ischemic complications are common and often include the eyes. Patients with giant cell arteritis have a significant risk of irreversible blindness [45]. As many as 90% of patients with giant cell arteritis initially complain of headache, but a wide array of symptoms is possible, including a classic symptom of jaw pain or claudication [44]. An elevated ESR is also commonly noted, but a normal ESR does not exclude the disease. Key symptoms of eye involvement in giant cell arteritis include variable loss of vision, amaurosis fugax, diplopia, and eye pain [46,47]. Amaurosis fugax has been reported to be a significant predictor of subsequent irreversible blindness in patients with giant cell arteritis [45].

Anterior ischemic optic neuropathy is the most common cause of visual loss in giant cell arteritis. Changes may be seen on fundoscopic examination as a pale or chalky white swelling of the optic nerve, and splinter hemorrhages may also be present [44]. Diminished intraocular pressure and hypotony of the ciliary body with decreased pupillary response may also be evident [48–50]. These findings can occur in both eyes [51]. Other ocular ischemic lesions that can result from giant cell arteritis but may elude detection on routine examination are central retinal artery occlusion, cilioretinal artery occlusion, posterior optic neuropathy, and choroidal ischemia [50,51]. Overall, emergency ophthalmologic consultation is essential to ensure detection of potential ocular complications of giant cell arteritis.

Giant cell arteritis–related eye changes can progress to irreversible blindness within weeks without immediate treatment. Early diagnosis and a high level of clinical suspicion for eye complications are vital to achieve the best possible outcomes. The treatment of temporal arteritis is discussed in more detail by Vortmann and Schneider elsewhere in this issue.

Hypertension

Hypertension, especially when longstanding or inadequately controlled, causes a broad array of end organ damage. Ocular complications of hypertension result from direct effects on the eye, as well as secondary effects of other ophthalmologic conditions [52]. Although hypertensive eye changes are a major risk factor in patients with diabetes, 2% to 14% of non-diabetic patients aged more than 40 years are also at risk [53,54]. The primary effects of hypertension on the eye cause pathologic changes to the retina through a range that begins with vasoconstriction and progresses to leakage at the blood–retinal barrier and arteriosclerotic changes.

Hypertensive retinopathy is classically described by four grades of retinal change based on advanced ophthalmologic examination [55]; however, clinicians may observe an array of eye findings on simple fundoscopy that correspond to mild, moderate, and severe hypertensive changes [52]. Mild retinopathy entails arteriolar narrowing, often seen as arteriovenous "nicking" or "nipping." Moderate hypertensive retinopathy can entail findings of "flame" or "blot" hemorrhages, cotton-wool spots, microaneurysms, and hard exudates [52]. All of these findings may occur with severe retinopathy, as well as swelling of the optic disk. When blood pressure is extremely high, increased intracranial pressure with resultant optic ischemia (hypertensive optic neuropathy) will be evident as papilledema on fundoscopic examination [52]. Overall, hypertensive retinopathy is a well-established sign of systemic vascular disease and is associated with subsequent stroke [52].

Other retinopathies that are known complications of hypertension are as follows: retinal vein occlusion, retinal emboli, retinal artery occlusion, retinal macroaneurysm, ischemic optic neuropathy, and diabetic retinopathy. Many of these conditions have common findings, and urgent ophthalmologic consultation is essential for a correct diagnosis and prompt treatment. Retinal vein occlusion is a common disorder from which vision loss can occur. Patients typically present with poor visual acuity; fundoscopic findings may include retinal hemorrhages, cotton-wool spots, and edema of the macular and optic disk. Retinal emboli may be single or multiple and are often asymptomatic with transient changes, although frank retinal artery occlusion can occur [52]. These emboli may be seen as punctate pale defects on fundoscopy. Retinal emboli signal a high risk of thromboembolic stroke and cardiovascular disease [52]. Retinal artery occlusion is most common in hypertensive patients over 60 years old and presents with symptoms of a painless and sudden unilateral vision loss. A "cherry red spot" may be seen on fundoscopic examination. A retinal arterial macroaneurysm is a more rare disorder that is somewhat unique to patients with hypertension. It can present with acute vision loss but is more likely discovered incidentally on advanced ophthalmologic examination of an asymptomatic patient. Ischemic optic neuropathy is the most common acute optic neuropathy of patients aged more than 50 years and is more common in patients with diabetes. Up to 90% of cases are anterior and present with abrupt vision loss and edema of the optic disk. Diabetic retinopathy is detailed in the following section.

Diabetes

Emergency department providers are likely to encounter many of the complications of type 1 and type 2 diabetes mellitus, especially as the overall incidences of diabetes and obesity continue to rise. Ocular complications of diabetes are no exception. Indeed, diabetic retinopathy remains the most common cause of legal blindness in patients between 18 and 74 years of age. Early recognition with prompt treatment can dramatically affect outcome [56]. Other ocular complications of diabetes include vascular events and severe eye infections.

The prevalence of diabetic retinopathy is markedly higher in patients who have type 1 diabetes (estimated at 40% to 80%), but it also affects 20% to 30% of patients who have type 2 diabetes [56,57]. Hypertension is also a significant risk factor for diabetic retinopathy. Intensive medical control of blood glucose levels has been shown to significantly reduce both the incidence of new retinopathy and the progression of pre-existing retinopathy. Moreover, control of hypertension with angiotensin-converting enzyme inhibitors can reduce the progression of diabetic retinopathy. Despite the routine monitoring for diabetic retinopathy as a standard, diabetic patients may still present to the emergency department with complaints of vision change. In these cases, prompt ophthalmologic consultation is required for an optimal outcome.

Three main types of diabetic retinopathy form the spectrum of progression of ocular changes: non-proliferative (background), pre-proliferative, and proliferative retinopathy [57]. Non-proliferative diabetic retinopathy may be evident on simple fundoscopic examination as dilated veins, microaneurysms temporal to the macula, and small hemorrhages in either a "dot and blot" pattern (deeper) or flame shape (more superficial) [56]. More extensive ophthalmologic examination and imaging may reveal additional findings of hard exudates, retinal edema, and arteriovenous shunting. Preproliferative diabetic retinopathy entails lesions resulting from retinal ischemia. The lesions may be evident on simple fundoscopic examination as multiple cotton-wool spots, vascular changes (narrowed arterioles; dilated veins in bead, loop, or sausage-like patterns), or dark blot hemorrhages [56]. The last change is more likely seen on further retinal examination or fluorescein angiography, along with capillary non-perfusion filling defects, macular edema, and intraretinal microvascular abnormalities. Proliferative diabetic retinopathy is best detected by an ophthalmologist. Findings include retinal scars (retinitis proliferans), new vessel formation, vitreous hemorrhage, and retinal detachment [56].

Diabetic patients are at risk for ocular vasocclusive events, presumably due to a hypercoaguable state [56]. Complications include central retinal artery occlusion (Fig. 3), central retinal vein occlusion, and ocular motor nerve palsies. Central retinal artery occlusion presents with sudden near complete or complete vision loss. Fundoscopic examination may reveal retinal edema and pallor and a darkened macula; further findings are possible on fluorescein angiography [56]. Central retinal vein occlusion presents with a slower onset of blurred vision and variable loss of vision. Fundoscopic examination may show retinal edema, dilated and twisted retinal veins, and retinal hemorrhages with cotton-wool spots ("blood and thunder") [56]. Ocular motor nerve palsies can result from ischemic cranial nerve injuries, which in diabetic patients most commonly involve the oculomotor (third)

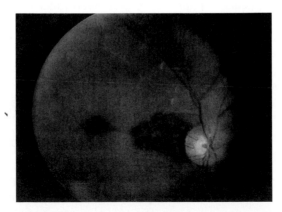

Fig. 3. Central retinal artery occlusion. (*From* Wipf JE, Paauw DS. Ophthalmologic emergencies in the patient with diabetes. Endocrinol Metab Clin North Am 2000;29(4):819; with permission.)

nerve. The sixth and fourth nerves can also be affected but in decreasing order of frequency. Symptoms of third nerve palsy can include diplopia, ptosis, and sometimes headache and eye pain; a slight anisocoria may be noted, although the pupil is usually spared. Interestingly, ocular motor nerve palsies usually occur in diabetic persons who do not have diabetic retinopathy.

Severe eye infections are rare in diabetes but are uniformly destructive when present. Two ocular infections that occur primarily in diabetic patients are bacterial endophthalmitis (see Fig. 2) and rhinocerebral mucormycosis. The former is a severe ocular complication that often results in blindness. A wide array of bacterial causes is possible and includes *Staphylococcus aureus*, *Escherichia coli*, and *Klebsiella pneumoniae*. Presenting symptoms include pain, photophobia, floaters, and reduced vision. Hypopyon (pus) can be seen in the anterior chamber on examination. Rhinocerebral mucormycosis is a rare but serious fungal complication of type 1 diabetes that presents in combination with diabetic ketoacidosis. Initial clinical symptoms include eye pain, headache, and nasal stuffiness. Periorbital swelling and proptosis may be noted, along with necrotic lesions on the palate and nasal mucosa [56]. Further complications include cavernous sinus thrombosis, internal carotid artery thrombosis, and death.

Summary

A wide array of ocular changes is possible in many systemic diseases. Emergency department providers may encounter ophthalmologic signs or symptoms during the evaluation of a patient with known systemic disease, or in a patient with as yet undiagnosed illness. Careful screening of visual acuity, a complete external eye and fundoscopic examination, as well as slit lamp examination are needed in any patient with eye complaints and especially when progression of known systemic disease is suspected. Emergent ophthalmology consultation is critical if any degree of vision loss is reported or detected on screening. Many ocular complications of systemic disease also require urgent ophthalmologic evaluation to ensure the best possible treatment outcomes are achieved.

References

[1] Gaudio PA. Update on ocular syphilis. Curr Opin Ophthalmol 2006;17:562–6.
[2] Mikita C, Truesdell A, Katial RK. A 48-year-old woman with red eyes and a rash. Ann Allergy Asthma Immunol 2004;93:526–31.
[3] Aldave AJ, King JA, Cunningham ET. Ocular syphilis. Curr Opin Ophthalmol 2001;12: 433–41.
[4] Kanski JJ. Acquired syphilis. In: Clinical ophthalmology. London: Butterworth; 1994. p. 173–4.
[5] Matsuo T, Taira Y, Nagayama M, et al. Angle-closure glaucoma as a presumed presenting sign in patients with syphilis. Jpn J Ophthalmol 2000;44:305–8.

[6] Committee on Infectious Diseases, American Academy of Pediatrics. Varicella-zoster infections. In: The red book. Illinois: The American Academy of Pediatrics; 2006. p. 711–24.
[7] Fernandez de Castro LE, Al Sarraf O, Hawthorne KM, et al. Ocular manifestations after primary varicella infection. Cornea 2006;25(7):866–7.
[8] Kanski JJ. Herpes zoster ophthalmicus. In: Clinical ophthalmology. London: Butterworth; 1994. p. 112–5.
[9] Shaikh S, Ta CN. Evaluation and management of herpes zoster ophthalmicus. Am Fam Physician 2002;66:1723–30.
[10] Liesegang TJ. Herpes zoster virus infection. Curr Opin Ophthalmol 2004;15:531–6.
[11] Marsh RJ. Herpes zoster keratitis. Trans Ophthalmol Soc U K 1973;93:181–92.
[12] Lesser RL. Ocular manifestations of Lyme disease. Am J Med 1995;8(Suppl 4A):60–2.
[13] Karma A, Mikkila H. Ocular manifestations and treatment of Lyme disease. Curr Opin Ophthalmol 1996;7(1):7–12.
[14] Kanski JJ. Lyme disease. In: Clinical ophthalmology. London: Butterworth; 1994. p. 175.
[15] Zaidman GW. The ocular manifestations of Lyme disease. Int Ophthalmol Clin 1997;37(2):13–28.
[16] Moraes HV. Ocular manifestations of HIV/AIDS. Curr Opin Ophthalmol 2002;13:397–403.
[17] Chronister CL. Review of external ocular diseases associated with AIDS and HIV infection. Optom Vis Sci 1996;73(4):225–30.
[18] Shuler JD, Engstrom RE, Holland GN. External ocular disease and anterior segment disorders associated with AIDS. Int Ophthalmol Clin 1989;29:98–104.
[19] Kanski JJ. Acquired immune deficiency syndrome. In: Clinical ophthalmology. London: Butterworth; 1994. p. 168–71.
[20] Cunningham ET Jr. Uveitis in HIV positive patients. Br J Ophthalmol 2000;84:233–5.
[21] Mahoney BP. Rheumatologic disease and associated ocular manifestations. J Am Optom Assoc 1993;64(6):403–15.
[22] Schneider JM, Matthews JH, Graham BS. Reiter's syndrome. Cutis 2003;71(3):198–200.
[23] Neuwelt CM, Borenstein DG, Jacobs RP. Reiter's syndrome: a male and female disease. J Rheumatol 1982;9(2):268–72.
[24] Kiss S, Letko E, Qamruddin S, et al. Long-term progression, prognosis, and treatment of patients with recurrent ocular manifestations of Reiter's syndrome. Ophthalmology 2003;110(9):1764–9.
[25] Kanski JJ. Reiter's syndrome. In: Clinical ophthalmology. London: Butterworth; 1994. p. 157–8.
[26] Lowder CY, Char DH. Uveitis, a review. West J Med 1984;140(3):421–32.
[27] Ostler CR, Dawson J, Schachter J, et al. Reiter's syndrome. Am J Ophthalmol 1971;71:986–91.
[28] Horton JC. Roth's spots. In: Knoop KJ, Stack LB, Storrow AB, editors. Atlas of emergency medicine. 2nd edition. New York: McGraw-Hill; 2002. p. 80.
[29] Kanski JJ. Anaemias. In: Clinical ophthalmology. London: Butterworth; 1994. p. 373.
[30] Disorders of the eye. In: Kasper DL, Braunwald E, Hauser S, et al, editors. Harrison's principles of internal medicine. 16th edition. Iowa: McGraw-Hill; Part 2, Section 4, Chapter 25.
[31] Zayit-Soudry S, Neudorfer M, Barak A, et al. Endogenous phialemonium curvatum endophthalmitis. Am J Ophthalmol 2005;140(4):755–7.
[32] Arcieri ES, Jorge EF, de Abrea Ferreira L, et al. Bilateral endogenous endophthalmitis associated with infective endocarditis: case report. Braz J Infect Dis 2001;5(6):356–9.
[33] Shmuely H, Kremer I, Sagie A, et al. Candida tropicalis multifocal endophthalmitis as the only initial manifestation of pacemaker endocarditis. Am J Ophthalmol 1997;123(4):559–60.
[34] Verweij PE, Rademakers AJ, Koopmans PP, et al. Endophthalmitis as presenting symptoms of group G streptococcal endocarditis. Infection 1994;22(1):56–7.
[35] Munier F, Othenin-Girard P. Subretinal neovascularization secondary to choroidal septic metastasis from acute bacterial endocarditis. Retina 1992;12:108–12.

[36] Herschorn BJ, Brucker AJ. Embolic retinopathy due to *Corynebacterium minutissimum* endocarditis. Br J Ophthalmol 1985;69:29–31.
[37] Mauriello JA, Stabile C, Wagner RS. Dacrocystitis following Kawasaki's disease. Ophthal Plast Reconstr Surg 1986;2(4):209–11.
[38] Committee on Infectious Diseases, American Academy of Pediatrics. Kawasaki's disease. In: The red book. Illinois: The American Academy of Pediatrics; 2006. p. 412–5.
[39] Ohno S, Miyajima T, Higuchi M, et al. Ocular manifestations of Kawasaki's disease. Am J Ophthalmol 1982;93(6):713–7.
[40] Al-abbadi MA, Abuhammour W, Harasheh A, et al. Conjunctival changes in children with Kawasaki disease: cytopathologic characterization. Acta Cytol 2007;51(3):370–4.
[41] Jacob JK, Polomeno RC, Chad Z, et al. Ocular manifestations of Kawasaki disease. Can J Ophthalmol 1982;17(5):199–202.
[42] Anand S, Yang YC. Optic disc changes in Kawasaki disease. J Pediatr Ophthalmol Strabismus 2004;41(3):177–9.
[43] Font RL, Mehta RS, Streusand SB, et al. Bilateral retinal ischemia in Kawasaki disease. Ophthalmology 1983;90(5):569–77.
[44] Bhatti MT, Tabandeh H. Giant cell arteritis: diagnosis and management. Curr Opin Ophthalmol 2001;12:393–9.
[45] Gonzalez-Gay MA, Garcia-Porrua C, Llorca J, et al. Visual manifestations of giant cell arteritis: trends and clinical spectrum in 161 patients. Medicine 2000;79(5):283–92.
[46] Paraskevas KI, Boumpas DT, Vrentzos GE, et al. Oral and ocular/orbital manifestations of temporal arteritis: a disease with deceptive clinical symptoms and devastating consequences. Clin Rheumatol 2007;26(7):1044–8.
[47] Hayreh SS, Podhajsky PA, Zimmerman B. Ocular manifestations of giant cell arteritis. Am J Ophthalmol 1998;125(4):509–20.
[48] Huna-Baron R, Mizrachi IB, Glovinsky Y. Intraocular pressure is low in eyes with giant cell arteritis. J Neuroophthalmol 2006;26(4):273–5.
[49] Radda TM, Bardach H, Riss B. Acute ocular hypotony. Ophthalmologica 1981;182(3):148–52.
[50] Calcagni CA, Claes CA, Maheshwari M, et al. Hypotony as a presentation of giant cell arteritis. Eye 2007;21:123–4.
[51] Casson RJ, Fleming FK, Shaikh A, et al. Bilateral ocular ischemic syndrome secondary to giant cell arteritis. Arch Ophthalmol 2001;119:306–7.
[52] Wong T, Mitchell P. The eye in hypertension. Lancet 2007;369:425–35.
[53] Yu T, Mitchell P, Berry G, et al. Retinopathy in older persons without diabetes and its relationship to hypertension. Arch Ophthalmol 1998;116:83–9.
[54] Wong TY, Mitchell P. Hypertensive retinopathy. N Engl J Med 2004;351:2310–7.
[55] Kanski JJ. Hypertensive retinopathy. In: Clinical ophthalmology. London: Butterworth; 1994. p. 367–70.
[56] Wipf JE, Paauw DS. Ophthalmologic emergencies in the patient with diabetes. Endocrinol Metab Clin North Am 2000;29(4):813–29.
[57] Kanski JJ. Diabetic retinopathy. In: Clinical ophthalmology. London: Butterworth; 1994. p. 344–57.

ELSEVIER
SAUNDERS

Emerg Med Clin N Am
26 (2008) 233–238

EMERGENCY
MEDICINE
CLINICS OF
NORTH AMERICA

Conditions Requiring Emergency Ophthalmologic Consultation

Brendan Magauran, MD, MBA

*Department of Emergency Medicine, Boston University School of Medicine,
Boston Medical Center, 1 Boston Medical Center Place, Boston, MA 02118, USA*

Ophthalmologic complaints in the Emergency Department (ED) are estimated to represent 3% of all visits [1]. Emergency physicians are well prepared to diagnose and manage the majority of these visits. Corneal abrasions, conjunctivitis, and conjunctival or corneal foreign bodies comprise 75% of ED visits [2]. The challenge for the emergency physician is to decide which cases require the expertise of an ophthalmologist and in what time frame. Optimally, the decision should be evidence based and in accordance with clinical guidelines developed collaboratively between emergency physicians and ophthalmologists. Hopefully, in the not too distant future, this will be the case. This article reviews the instances where emergency consultation with an ophthalmologist is warranted, with specific reference to each article contained in this issue of *Clinics*.

Emergency ophthalmology consultation caveats

The availability of on-call specialists to the ED on a 24-hour a day basis is not uniform across EDs in the United States. Specialty eye hospitals and tertiary care centers, which also function as Level 1 Trauma Centers, for the most part, do have around-the-clock ophthalmology coverage. Many other hospitals, however, do not have this level of coverage or lack subspecialty services in ophthalmology. Ophthalmology has subspecialties, including oculo-plastics, neuro-ophthalmology, and retina. A general ophthalmologist may feel uncomfortable with a particular request for consultation and ask that the patient be referred to a facility with a higher level of care and ophthalmologic subspecialization. This is particularly true for cases involving possible postoperative complications from eye surgeries. It is therefore

E-mail address: brendan.magauran@bmc.org

0733-8627/08/$ - see front matter © 2008 Elsevier Inc. All rights reserved.
doi:10.1016/j.emc.2007.11.008   *emed.theclinics.com*

important for emergency medicine practitioners who find themselves in such a situation to have referral hospitals that can be contacted to accept patients in transfer.

Emergency diagnoses requiring emergency ophthalmology consultation

The following box contains a list of diagnoses or conditions that generally warrant an emergency ophthalmologic consultation (Box 1).

There are also cases where emergency ophthalmologic consultation is reasonable, and these include patients with one good eye experiencing vision changes, patients with a complicated ocular history, as well as cases where the ED practitioner is unsure of a diagnosis and is concerned about vision loss. A telephone discussion to determine the timing of the consultation with the ophthalmologist will usually answer such questions.

Trauma

Emergency physicians are well versed in the management of trauma. The basic ABC principle (Airway, Breathing, Circulation) in ED trauma management takes precedence over eye injuries. Evaluation for life and limb-threatening injuries is the first priority. Most patients with multiple trauma and an eye injury will require ophthalmologic consultation, but the timing of this consultation is dependent on the severity of other injuries. Most often, this consultation occurs at some point during the in-patient stay after life threatening conditions have been addressed. This article reviews the conditions that usually require ophthalmologic consultation from the ED.

Box 1. Conditions that generally warrant an emergency ophthalmologic consultation

Trauma
   Ruptured globe
   Lid laceration through margin, nasolacrimal system,
      or cannaliculus
Endophthalmitis
Angle closure glaucoma
Severe uveitis
Corneal ulceration
Acute vision loss
   Central retinal artery occlusion
   Temporal arteritis
   Retinal detachment
   Optic Neuritis
Orbital cellulitis

CT scan is the imaging modality of choice in defining the extent of blunt and penetrating trauma to the eye and orbit. Orbital fractures are not an emergency unless there is vision loss or globe injury. Retrobulbar hemorrhage may occur with nondisplaced orbital fractures and may result in acute vision loss. Penetrating injuries with globe rupture also require CT scanning for retained foreign bodies, but sensitivity is only 75% [3]. These entities are discussed in detail in the article by Linden and Bord elsewhere in this issue.

Direct trauma to the eyelid involving the nasolacrimal system, lid margin, or tarsal plate requires specialized repair by either a plastic surgeon or an ophthalmologist, depending on institutional preference and availability. The timing of this repair should occur after any life or limb-threatening injuries are addressed.

Endophthalmitis

Endophthalmitis represents inflammation of the aqueous or vitreous humor. It may result from infection, trauma, or as a postoperative complication. This is generally a difficult diagnosis to make in the ED. Suspicion of the diagnosis requires emergent ophthamologic consultation for diagnostic evaluation, hospital admission, and surgery as necessary.

Acute angle closure glaucoma

Acute angle closure glaucoma (AACG) is generally painful and occasionally associated with headache, nausea, vomiting, and abdominal pain. The diagnosis may be difficult to establish when abdominal complaints are prominent [4]. Intraocular pressure generally rises beyond 50 mm Hg and may induce optic nerve atrophy if untreated. The emergency physician can certainly initiate therapy and consult an ophthalmologist. The issue is then response to treatment and monitoring of the intraocular pressure. Generally, patients with a new diagnosis of AACG are admitted to the hospital and an ophthalmologist oversees medical therapy. Cases refractory to medical therapy may require surgical intervention. AACG is discussed in detail in the article by Lowenstein and Dargin elsewhere in this issue.

Severe uveitis

Anterior uveitis (iridocyclitis) is inflammation of the iris (iritis) and ciliary body (cyclitis) and accounts for the majority of uveitis in Western countries [5]. It typically occurs in patients between the ages of 20 and 50 [5]. Inflammatory cells and flare in the anterior chamber associated with conjunctival injection primarily involving the limbus help confirm the diagnosis. The etiology of anterior uveitis is broad and may include infection, rheumatologic disease (HLA-B27 particularly), idiopathic, or even a malignancy which may mimic anterior uveitis. Given the broad differential diagnosis associated with this condition, consultations with specialists in rheumatology, infectious diseases, oncology, and ophthalmology may be warranted. A complete discussion of uveitis is found elsewhere in this issue in the article by Klig, entitled "Ophthalmologic Complications of Systemic Disease"; the article by Mahmood and Narang, entitled "Diagnosis and Management of the Red Eye"; and the article by Mueler and McStay, entitled "Ocular Infection and Inflammation".

Corneal ulceration

Degradation of the corneal stroma leads to ulceration of the cornea and is associated with numerous types of infection, systemic diseases, and glucocorticoid usage, and may lead to permanent vision loss. The depth of the ulceration may lead to corneal perforation with extension of the infection into the anterior chamber. Corneal ulcerations tend to heal with scarring, resulting in corneal opacification and decreased visual acuity. Ophthalmologic consultation and diagnosis of the etiology of the ulceration may decrease permanent damage to the cornea and resultant vision loss. The article by Klig, entitled "Ophthalmologic Complications of Systemic Disease"; the article by Mahmood and Narang, entitled "Diagnosis and Management of the Red Eye"; and the article by Mueler and McStay, entitled "Ocular Infection and Inflammation" found elsewhere in this issue discuss this topic in greater detail with reference to the etiology of the corneal ulceration.

Acute visual loss

Acute visual loss is a concerning complaint and can be difficult to diagnose. Presenting symptoms can be numerous and seemingly unrelated to the eye. It can be a painful or painless condition. The four major diagnoses addressed in this article include temporal arteritis, optic neuritis, central retinal artery occlusion, and retinal detachment.

Temporal arteritis

Temporal arteritis is a diagnosis that is in the differential diagnosis for acute vision loss. The gold standard for diagnosis is a temporal artery biopsy positive for giant cell arteritis. The end result of this condition is retinal ischemia and vision loss. Fundoscopic abnormalities or optic atrophy are not helpful in establishing or eliminating the diagnosis [6]. Suspicion of the diagnosis with prompt referral to an ophthalmologist is important, as the administration of high dose steroids may help prevent further vision loss [7]. Improvement in vision loss was present in only 4% of patients in one retrospective study [8].

Optic neuritis

Patients with optic neuritis generally present with pain on eye movement associated with unilateral vision loss, visual field defects, and change in color perception. Pain resolves as visual loss commences [9]. MRI reveals demyelinating lesions and may be helpful in establishing the diagnosis of multiple sclerosis. The vision loss is progressive and may occur rapidly over several hours or more slowly over days. Treatment with steroids generally leads to improved vision over several weeks [10]. Consultation with neurology as well as ophthalmology is generally warranted, given the likelihood of other conditions, such as multiple sclerosis, as well as other etiologies of acute vision loss.

Central retinal artery occlusion

Central retinal artery occlusion (CRAO) results in a sudden painless loss of vision. The primary cause of CRAO is embolic disease, but there are numerous other conditions that may cause CRAO as well. Immediate ophthalmologic consultation is warranted as vision may be preserved with treatment. Irreversible vision loss generally occurs after 4 hours of ischemia [11]. Visual acuity at presentation is predictive of final visual acuity. However, in a 1980 experimental study of ischemic time after retinal artery occlusion, restoration of blood flow at 100 minutes was associated with preservation of vision [12]. That being said, the medical and surgical treatments for CRAO have marginal benefit overall in preserving vision. Unfortunately, spontaneous resolution of an embolus is quite rare [13].

Retinal detachment

Retinal detachment is characterized by the separation of the retina from the underlying retinal epithelium. The incidence of retinal detachment is roughly one to two cases per ten thousand people [14,15]. Patients complain of new floaters, squiggly lines, or cobwebs that appear abruptly, associated with visual field loss. Examination with an ophthalmoscope is generally insufficient as the detachment may be at the periphery of the retina where the retina is the thinnest. The classic finding of a white billowing retinal separation is helpful if present, but the presence of a new visual field deficit with new "floaters" requires a dilated examination by an ophthalmologist [16].

The above causes of acute visual loss are all covered in more detail in the article by Vortmann and Schneider elsewhere in this issue.

Orbital cellulitis

Cellulitis involving the orbital tissues is usually an extension of an infection involving the sinuses. Patients may present with significant pain, swelling, and even proptosis, with increased risk of permanent ocular damage and vision loss. Potentially fatal complications of orbital cellulitis include meningitis and cavernous sinus thrombosis. CT scan can define the limits of infection and the presence of an abscess. Admission and emergent ophthalmologic consultation are warranted. This is discussed in detail elsewhere in this issue by Mueller and McStay.

In summary, this article has attempted to provide guidelines to the emergency physician regarding when to call for emergency ophthalmology consultation. It is not intended to provide an exhaustive list of every possible problem that may be encountered in the ED requiring the expertise of an ophthalmologist.

References

[1] Nawar EW, Niska RW, Xu J. National hospital ambulatory medical care survey: 2005 emergency department summary. Advance Data from Vital and Health Statistics 2007;386:1–32.

[2] Nash EA, Margo CE. Patterns of emergency department visits for disorders of the eye and ocular adnexa. Arch Ophthalmol 1998;116:1222–6.

[3] Joseph D, Pieramici D, Beauchamp N. Computed tomography in the diagnosis and prognosis of open-globe injuries. Ophthalmology 2000;107:1899–906.

[4] Leibowitz HM. The red eye. N Engl J Med 2000;343:345–51.

[5] Chang J, McCluskey PJ, Wakefield D. Acute anterior uveitis and HLA-B27. Surv Ophthalmol 2005;50(4):364–88.

[6] Smetana GW, Shmerling RH. Does this patient have temporal arteritis? JAMA 2002;287(1):92–101.

[7] Aiello PD, Trautmann JC, McPhee TG, et al. Visual prognosis in giant cell arteritis. Ophthalmology 1993;100(4):550–5.

[8] Hayreh SS, Zimmerman B, Kardon R. Visual improvement with corticosteroid therapy in giant cell arteritis. Report of a large study and review of literature. Acta Ophthalmol Scand 2002;80(4):355–67.

[9] Beck RW, Cleary PA, Anderson MM Jr, et al. A randomized, controlled trial of corticosteroids in the treatment of acute optic neuritis. N Engl J Med 1992;326:581–8.

[10] Beck RW, Gal RL, Bhatti MT, et al. Visual function more than 10 years after optic neuritis: experience of the Optic Neuritis Treatment Trial. Am J Ophthalmol 2004;137(1):77–83 [Erratum in: Am J Ophthalmol 2004].

[11] Hayreh SS, Zimmerman MB, Kimura A, et al. Central retinal artery occlusion. Retinal survival time. Exp Eye Res 2004;78(3):723–36.

[12] Hayreh SS, Weingeist TA. Experimental occlusion of the central artery of the retina. Retinal tolerance time to acute ischaemia. Br J Ophthalmol 1980;64(11):818–25.

[13] Rumelt S, Dorenboim Y, Rehany U. Aggressive systematic treatment for central retinal artery occlusion. Am J Ophthalmol 1999;128:733–8.

[14] Algvere PV, Jahnberg P, Textorius O. The Swedish retinal detachment register. I. A database for epidemiological and clinical studies. Graefes Arch Clin Exp Ophthalmol 1999;237:137–44.

[15] Rowe JA, Erie JC, Baratz KH, et al. Retinal detachment in Olmsted County, Minnesota, 1976 through 1995. Ophthalmology 1999;106:154–9.

[16] Shingleton BJ, O'Donoghue MW. Blurred vision. N Engl J Med 2000;343(8):556–62.

ELSEVIER
SAUNDERS

Emerg Med Clin N Am
26 (2008) 239–243

EMERGENCY
MEDICINE
CLINICS OF
NORTH AMERICA

Index

Note: Page numbers of article titles are in **boldface** type.

Moving?

Make sure your subscription moves with you!

To notify us of your new address, find your **Clinics Account Number** (located on your mailing label above your name), and contact customer service at:

E-mail: elspcs@elsevier.com

800-654-2452 (subscribers in the U.S. & Canada)
407-345-4000 (subscribers outside of the U.S. & Canada)

Fax number: 407-363-9661

Elsevier Periodicals Customer Service
6277 Sea Harbor Drive
Orlando, FL 32887-4800

*To ensure uninterrupted delivery of your subscription, please notify us at least 4 weeks in advance of move.

ELSEVIER